Respiratory Care

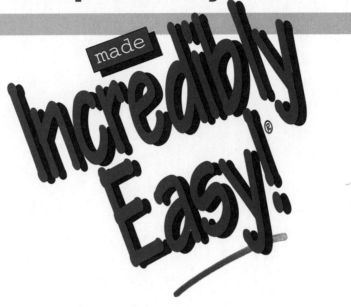

Respiratory Care

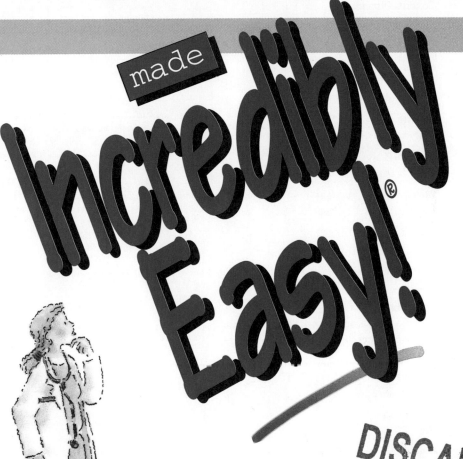

made **Incredibly Easy!**®

LIPPINCOTT WILLIAMS & WILKINS
A **Wolters Kluwer** Company

Philadelphia • Baltimore • New York • London
Buenos Aires • Hong Kong • Sydney • Tokyo

Staff

Executive Publisher
Judith A. Schilling McCann, RN, MSN

Editorial Director
David Moreau

Clinical Director
Joan M. Robinson, RN, MSN

Senior Art Director
Arlene Putterman

Art Director
Mary Ludwicki

Editorial Project Manager
Tracy S. Diehl

Clinical Project Manager
Beverly Ann Tscheschlog, RN, BS

Editors
Laura Bruck, Brenna H. Mayer

Clinical Editors
Maryann Foley, RN, BSN; Tamara Kear, RN, MSN, CNN

Copy Editors
Kimberly Bilotta (supervisor), Heather Ditch,
Lisa Stockslager, Kelly Taylor, Dorothy P. Terry,
Pamela Wingrod

Designer
Lynn Foulk

Illustrator
Bot Roda

Digital Composition Services
Diane Paluba (manager), Joyce Rossi Biletz

Manufacturing
Patricia K. Dorshaw (director), Beth Janae Orr

Editorial Assistants
Megan L. Aldinger, Tara L. Carter-Bell, Linda K. Ruhf

Librarian
Wani Z. Larsen

Indexer
Karen C. Comerford

RCIE010504—030706

Library of Congress Cataloging-in-Publication Data
Respiratory care made incredibly easy.
    p. ; cm.
    Includes bibliographical references and index.
    1. Respiratory organs — Diseases — Nursing. I. Lippincott Williams & Wilkins.
    [DNLM: 1. Respiratory Therapy — nursing. 2. Respiratory Tract Diseases — nursing. WY 163 R4333 2005]
RC735.5.R4645 2005
616.2'004231 — dc22
ISBN 1-58255-335-1 (alk. paper)   2003027704

Contents

Contributors and consultants

W. Chad Barefoot, RN, MSN, CRNP, ACNP
Acute Care Nurse Practitioner
Abington (Pa.) Memorial Hospital

Cheryl A. Bean, RN, DSN, APRN,BC, ANP, AOCN
Associate Professor
Indiana University School of Nursing
Indianapolis

Nancy P. Blumenthal, RN, MSN, CS, CRNP
Senior Nurse Practitioner, Lung Transplant
   Program
University of Pennsylvania Medical Center
Philadelphia

Arlene M. Clarke Coughlin, RN, MSN
Nursing Instructor/Nursing Supervisor
Holy Name Hospital
Teaneck, N.J.

Shelba Durston, RN, MSN, CCRN
Nursing Instructor
San Joaquin Delta College
Stockton, Calif.
Staff Nurse
San Joaquin General Hospital
French Camp, Calif.

Carrin Dvorak, RN, MSN
Assistant Professor of Nursing
Cuyahoga Community College
Cleveland

Henry B. Geiter, Jr., RN, ADN, CCRN, TNCC
Adjunct Instructor
St. Petersburg (Fla.) College
Critical Care Nurse
Bayfront Hospital
St. Petersburg, Fla.
Critical Care Transport Nurse
Sunstar AMR
Largo, Fla.

Timothy B. Mahan, RN, MS, ANP, CCPT, CS, RRT
Nurse Practitioner
Smithtown (N.Y.) Medical Specialists

Robin Walsh, RN, BSN, CCRN, CEN
Triage/Observation Nurse
University Health Services
University of Massachusetts at Amherst

Foreword

During my 20 years as a pulmonary clinical nurse specialist, I've always been on a search to find relevant, clinically accurate respiratory care information. There's such a vast shortage of books pertaining to respiratory care that it's often difficult to find quality resources.

Now—finally—we have a new respiratory nursing care book: *Respiratory Care Made Incredibly Easy!*

With a fresh approach, this book provides coverage across the continuum of respiratory nursing care. Its chapters include anatomy and physiology, assessment, diagnostic procedures, treatment, infection and inflammation, obstructive disorders, restrictive disorders, vascular lung disorders, neoplastic disorders, traumatic injuries, and respiratory emergencies.

Respiratory Care Made Incredibly Easy! is loaded with helpful features. Color illustrations in the anatomy and physiology chapter allow you to visualize parts of the body. A *Quick quiz* at the end of each chapter provides rationales that will help you remember key topics.

The book also offers easy-to-understand logos that make learning simple:

Kids' korner identifies assessment techniques, treatments, procedures, and diseases specific to the pediatric population.

No place like home provides key information about adaptations in treatment and care when the patient goes home.

Now I get it explains important aspects of a disorder, procedure, test, or treatment.

Advice from the experts offers tips and tricks for nurses and key troubleshooting techniques.

With all of these features, plus the wide range of respiratory care topics, *Respiratory Care Made Incredibly Easy!* is a "must have" reference for all acute care nurses who have respiratory care patients—whether they're in medical-surgical nursing units, critical care nursing units, emergency departments, or pediatric nursing units. Home care and hospice nurses can also use this book to supplement their knowledge of respiratory care modalities.

Nurses obtain certification in specialized areas of nursing when they demonstrate their expertise by passing examinations. *Respiratory Care Made Incredibly Easy!* will be an asset for nurses who require respiratory nursing knowledge to be able to pass certification exams in medical-surgical, critical care, or pediatric nursing. When respiratory nursing certification is offered in the future, this book will be an excellent reference.

Although challenging, respiratory nursing care is also very rewarding. Do yourself and your patients a favor by learning all that you can about respiratory nursing care. And enjoy doing it with this incredible new book!

Debra Siela, RN, DNSc, CCNS, APRN,BC, CCRN, RRT
Assistant Professor of Nursing
Ball State University
Intensive Care Unit Clinical Nurse Specialist
Ball Memorial Hospital
Muncie, Ind.
Past President Respiratory Nursing Society
Latham, N.Y.

Anatomy and physiology

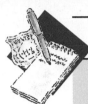

Just the facts

In this chapter, you'll learn:

♦ structures of the respiratory system and their functions

♦ how inspiration and expiration occur

♦ how gas exchange takes place in the alveoli

♦ how problems with the nervous, musculoskeletal, and pulmonary systems can affect breathing

♦ role of the lungs in acid-base balance.

Understanding respiratory anatomy and physiology

The respiratory system consists of the:
• upper respiratory tract
• lower respiratory tract
• lungs
• thoracic cavity.

The respiratory system maintains the exchange of oxygen and carbon dioxide in the lungs and tissues. This system also helps to regulate the body's acid-base balance.

Upper respiratory tract

The upper respiratory tract consists primarily of the nose, mouth, nasopharynx, oropharynx, laryngopharynx, and larynx. These structures warm, humidify, and filter inspired air and protect the lower airway from foreign matter. They're also responsible for tasting, smelling, and chewing and swallowing food. (See *Structures of the respiratory system*, page 2.)

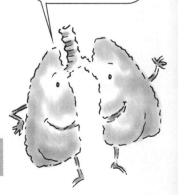

The respiratory system maintains the exchange of oxygen and carbon dioxide in the lungs and tissues.

Structures of the respiratory system

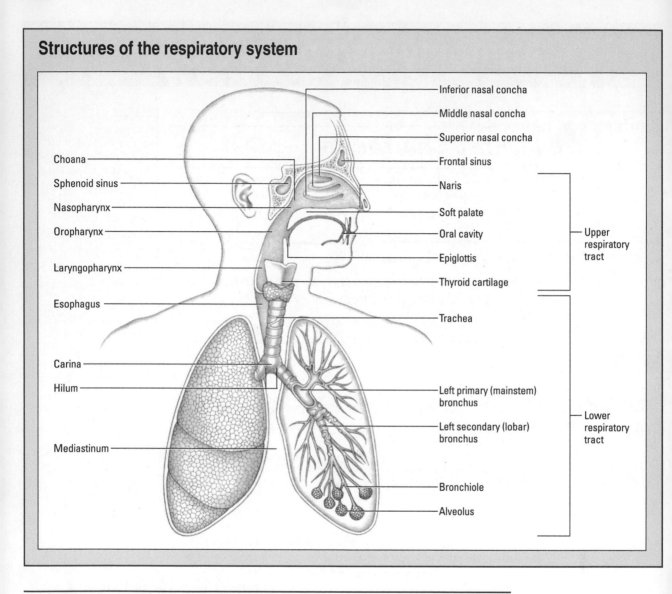

Nostrils and nasal passages

Air enters the body through the nostrils (nares). In the nostrils, small hairs, known as *vibrissae*, filter out dust and large foreign particles. Air then passes into the two nasal passages, which are separated by the nasal septum. Cartilage forms the anterior walls of the nasal passages; bony structures (called *conchae* or *turbinates*) form the posterior walls.

Just passing through

The conchae warm and humidify air before it passes into the nasopharynx. Their mucus layers also trap finer foreign particles, which the cilia carry to the pharynx to be swallowed.

Sinuses and nasopharynx

The four paranasal sinuses are located in the frontal, sphenoid, and maxillary bone and provide speech resonance. Air passes from the nasal cavity into the muscular nasopharynx through the choanae, a pair of openings in the posterior nasal cavity that are constantly open.

Oropharynx and laryngopharynx

The oropharynx is the posterior wall of the mouth. It connects the nasopharynx and the laryngopharynx. The laryngopharynx extends to the esophagus and larynx.

Larynx

The larynx contains the vocal cords and connects the pharynx with the trachea. Muscles and cartilage form the walls of the larynx, including the large, shield-shaped thyroid cartilage situated just under the jaw line. (See *Two things at once.*)

Lower respiratory tract

The lower respiratory tract consists of the trachea, lungs, right and left mainstream bronchi, five secondary bronchi, and bronchioles. Functionally, the lower tract is subdivided into the conducting airways and the acinus. A mucous membrane that contains hairlike cilia lines the lower tract. Cilia constantly clean the tract and carry foreign matter upward for swallowing or expectoration.

Conducting airways

The conducting airways, which contain the trachea and bronchi, help facilitate gas exchange in the acinus.

Kids' korner

Two things at once

During swallowing, the infant's nasopharynx is in a direct path to the larynx. This positioning allows two separate pathways: one for breathing and one for swallowing, enabling the infant to suckle and breathe at the same time.

Trachea

The trachea extends from the cricoid cartilage (at the top) to the carina (at the bottom). Also called the *tracheal bifurcation*, the carina is a ridge-shaped structure at the level of the sixth or seventh thoracic vertebra. C-shaped cartilage rings reinforce and protect the trachea to prevent it from collapsing.

> The conducting airways help conduct gas exchange. And a-one, and a-two, and a-one, two, three...

Bronchi

The primary bronchi begin at the carina. The right mainstem bronchus — shorter, wider, and more vertical than the left — supplies air to the right lung. The left mainstem bronchus delivers air to the left lung.

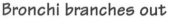

Secondary bronchi and the hilum

The mainstem bronchi divide into the five lobar (secondary) bronchi. Along with blood vessels, nerves, and lymphatics, the lobar bronchi enter the pleural cavities and lungs at the *hilum*. Located behind the heart, the hilum is a slit on the lung's medial surface where the lungs are anchored.

Bronchi branches out

Each lobar bronchus enters a lobe in each lung. Within its lobe, each of the lobar bronchi branches into segmental bronchi (tertiary bronchi). The segments continue to branch into smaller and smaller bronchi, finally branching into bronchioles.

The larger bronchi consist of cartilage, smooth muscle, and epithelium. As the bronchi become smaller, they first lose cartilage and then smooth muscle; as a result, the smallest bronchioles consist of just a single layer of epithelial cells.

> These involuntary defense mechanisms help protect the respiratory system from infection and prevent foreign-body inhalation.

Defending the lungs

In addition to warming, humidifying, and filtering inspired air, the lower airway provides the lungs with defense mechanisms, including:

- irritant reflex
- mucociliary system
- secretory immunity.

The irritant reflex is triggered when inhaled particles, cold air, or toxins stimulate irritant receptors. Reflex bronchospasm then occurs to limit exposure, followed by coughing, which expels the irritant.

Look out! It's a trap!

The mucociliary system produces mucus, which traps foreign particles. Foreign matter is then swept to the upper airway for expec-

Involuntary defense mechanisms

- Sneezing
- Coughing
- Gagging
- Spasms

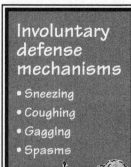

toration. A breakdown in the epithelium of the lungs or the mucociliary system can cause defense mechanisms to malfunction and allow atmospheric pollutants and irritants to enter and inflame the lungs.

Secrete weapon

Secretory immunity protects the lungs by releasing an antibody in the respiratory mucosal secretions that initiates an immune response against antigens contacting the mucosa.

Acinus

Each bronchiole includes terminal bronchioles and the acinus—the chief respiratory unit for gas exchange. Each bronchiole descends from a lobule and contains terminal bronchioles. (See *A close look at a lobule.*)

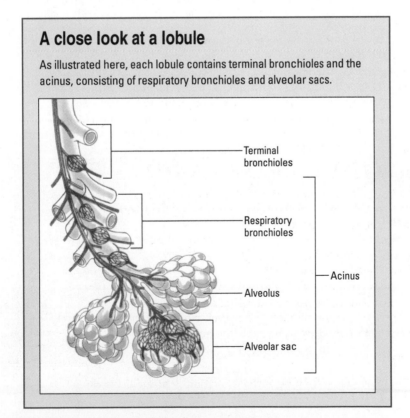

A close look at a lobule

As illustrated here, each lobule contains terminal bronchioles and the acinus, consisting of respiratory bronchioles and alveolar sacs.

Terminal bronchioles

Respiratory bronchioles

Acinus

Alveolus

Alveolar sac

Respiratory bronchioles

Within the acinus, terminal bronchioles branch into yet smaller respiratory bronchioles. Terminal bronchioles are considered anatomic "dead spaces" because they don't participate in gas exchange. The respiratory bronchioles feed directly into alveoli at sites along their walls.

Alveoli

The lungs contain about 300 million pulmonary alveoli, which are grapelike clusters of air-filled sacs at the ends of the respiratory passages. Here, gas exchange takes place by diffusion (the passage of gas molecules through respiratory membranes).

Alveolar walls contain two basic epithelial cell types:

Type I cells are the most abundant. These cells are thin, flat, squamous cells across which gas exchange occurs.

Type II cells produce a lipid-like substance, called *surfactant*, that coats the alveolus. During inspiration, alveolar surfactant allows the alveoli to expand uniformly. During expiration, surfactant prevents alveolar collapse.

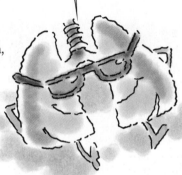

Yeah, I'm just movin' and diffusin'—it's all good.

No more diffusion confusion

In diffusion, oxygen is passed to the blood for circulation through the body. At the same time, carbon dioxide—a cellular waste product that's gathered by the blood as it circulates—is collected from the blood for disposal out of the body through the lungs.

Lungs and accessory structures

The cone-shaped lungs hang suspended in the right and left pleural cavities, straddling the heart, and anchored by root and pulmonary ligaments. The right lung is shorter, broader, and larger than the left. It has three lobes and handles 55% of gas exchange. The left lung has two lobes. Each lung's concave base rests on the diaphragm; the apex extends about 1¼" (3 cm) above the first rib.

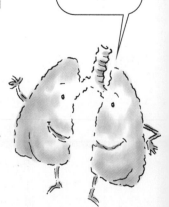

I hang in the right and left pleural cavities, Daddio.

Pleura and pleural cavities

The pleura—the membrane that totally encloses the lung—is composed of a visceral layer and a parietal layer. The visceral pleura lines the entire lung surface, including the areas between the lobes. The parietal pleura lines the inner surface of the chest wall and upper surface of the diaphragm.

Serious serous fluid

The pleural cavity — the tiny area between the visceral and parietal pleura — contains a thin film of serous fluid. This fluid has two functions:

☝ It lubricates the pleural surfaces so that they slide smoothly against each other as the lungs expand and contract.

✌ It creates a bond between the layers that causes the lungs to move with the chest wall during breathing.

Thoracic cavity

The thoracic cavity is an area that's surrounded by the diaphragm (below), the scalene muscles and fasciae of the neck (above), and the ribs, intercostal muscles, vertebrae, sternum, and ligaments (around the circumference).

Mediastinum

The space between the lungs is called the *mediastinum*. It contains the:
- heart and pericardium
- thoracic aorta
- pulmonary artery and veins
- venae cavae and azygos vein
- thymus, lymph nodes, and vessels
- trachea, esophagus, and thoracic duct
- vagus, cardiac, and phrenic nerves.

Thoracic cage

The thoracic cage is composed of bone and cartilage. It supports and protects the lungs, allowing them to expand and contract. The ribs form the major portion of the thoracic cage. (See *Lung structures in the thoracic cage*, page 8.)

Posterior thoracic cage

The vertebral column and 12 pairs of ribs form the posterior portion of the thoracic cage. The ribs extend from the posterior thoracic vertebrae toward the anterior thorax.

Lung structures in the thoracic cage

The ribs, vertebrae, and other structures of the thoracic cage act as landmarks that you can use to identify underlying structures.

From an anterior view
• The base of each lung rests at the level of the sixth rib at the midclavicular line and the eighth rib at the midaxillary line.
• The apex of each lung extends about ¾" to 1½" (2 to 4 cm) above the inner aspects of the clavicles.
• The upper lobe of the right lung ends level with the fourth rib at the midclavicular line and with the fifth rib at the midaxillary line.
• The middle lobe of the right lung extends triangularly from the fourth to the sixth rib at the midclavicular line and to the fifth rib at the midaxillary line.
• Because the left lung doesn't have a middle lobe, the upper lobe of the left lung ends level with the fourth rib at the midclavicular line and with the fifth rib at the midaxillary line.

From a posterior view
• The lungs extend from the cervical area to the level of the tenth thoracic vertebra (T10). On deep inspiration, the lungs may descend to T12.
• An imaginary line, stretching from the T3 level along the inferior border of

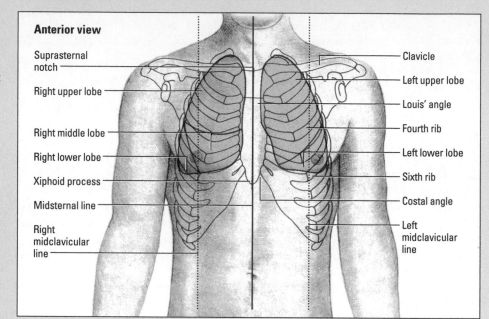

Anterior view

Suprasternal notch
Right upper lobe
Right middle lobe
Right lower lobe
Xiphoid process
Midsternal line
Right midclavicular line

Clavicle
Left upper lobe
Louis' angle
Fourth rib
Left lower lobe
Sixth rib
Costal angle
Left midclavicular line

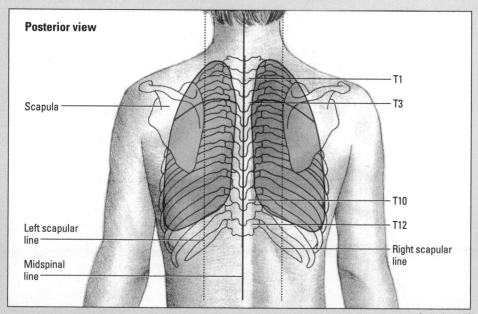

Posterior view

Scapula
Left scapular line
Midspinal line

T1
T3
T10
T12
Right scapular line

(continued)

Lung structures in the thoracic cage *(continued)*

the scapulae to the fifth rib at the midaxillary line, separates the upper lobes of both lungs.

• The upper lobes are above T3; the lower lobes are below T3 and extend to T10.

• The diaphragm originates around the ninth or tenth rib.

From a lateral view

• The right and left lateral rib cages cover the lobes of the right and left lungs, respectively.

• Beneath the rib cages, the lungs extend from just above the clavicles to the level of the eighth rib.

• The left lateral thorax allows access to two lobes; the right lateral thorax, to three lobes.

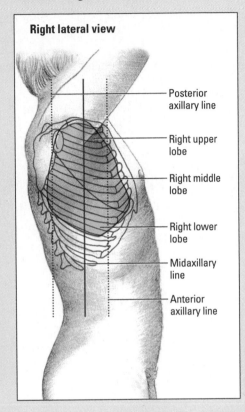

Right lateral view

- Posterior axillary line
- Right upper lobe
- Right middle lobe
- Right lower lobe
- Midaxillary line
- Anterior axillary line

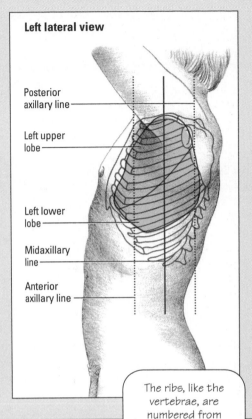

Left lateral view

- Posterior axillary line
- Left upper lobe
- Left lower lobe
- Midaxillary line
- Anterior axillary line

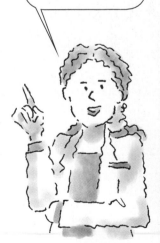

The ribs, like the vertebrae, are numbered from top to bottom.

Anterior thoracic cage

The anterior thoracic cage consists of the manubrium, sternum, xiphoid process, and ribs. It protects the mediastinal organs that lie between the right and left pleural cavities.

Rib numbers

Ribs 1 through 7 attach directly to the sternum; ribs 8 through 10 attach to the cartilage of the preceding rib. The other 2 pairs of ribs are "free-floating"—they don't attach to any part of the anterior thoracic cage. Rib 11 ends anterolaterally, and rib 12 ends laterally.

Bordering on the costal angle

The lower parts of the rib cage (costal margins) near the xiphoid process form the borders of the costal angle — an angle of about 90 degrees in a normal person.

It's suprasternal

Above the anterior thorax is a depression called the *suprasternal notch*. Because the suprasternal notch isn't covered by the rib cage like the rest of the thorax, the trachea and aortic pulsation can be palpated here.

Inspiration and expiration

Breathing involves two actions: inspiration (an active process) and expiration (a relatively passive process). Both actions rely on respiratory muscle function and the effects of pressure differences in the lungs. (See *Tracing pulmonary circulation.*)

It's perfectly normal!

During normal respiration, the external intercostal muscles aid the diaphragm, the major muscle of respiration. The diaphragm descends to lengthen the chest cavity, while the external intercostal muscles (located between and along the lower borders of the ribs) contract to expand the anteroposterior diameter. This co-ordinated action causes inspiration. Rising of the diaphragm and relaxation of the intercostal muscles causes expiration. (See *Mechanics of respiration*, page 12.)

Accessory muscles

During exercise, when the body needs increased oxygenation, or in certain disease states that require forced inspiration and active expiration, the accessory muscles of respiration also participate.

Forced inspiration

During forced inspiration:
• the pectoral muscles (upper chest) raise the chest to increase the anteroposterior diameter
• the sternocleidomastoid muscles (side of the neck) raise the sternum

Tracing pulmonary circulation

The right and left pulmonary arteries carry de-oxygenated blood from the right side of the heart to the lungs. These arteries divide into distal branches, called *arterioles,* which eventually terminate as a concentrated capillary network in the alveoli and alveolar sac, where gas exchange occurs.

Venules—the end branches of the pulmonary veins—collect oxygenated blood from the capillaries and transport it to larger vessels, which in turn lead to the pulmonary veins. The pulmonary veins enter the left side of the heart and distribute oxygenated blood throughout the body.

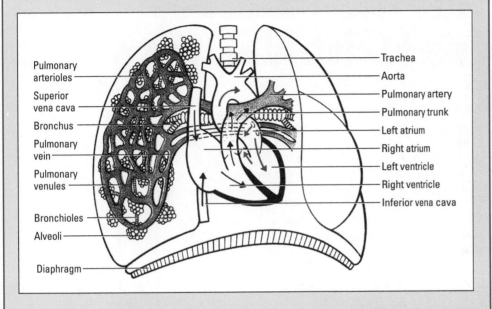

- Pulmonary arterioles
- Superior vena cava
- Bronchus
- Pulmonary vein
- Pulmonary venules
- Bronchioles
- Alveoli
- Diaphragm
- Trachea
- Aorta
- Pulmonary artery
- Pulmonary trunk
- Left atrium
- Right atrium
- Left ventricle
- Right ventricle
- Inferior vena cava

• the scalene muscles (in the neck) elevate, fix, and expand the upper chest
• the posterior trapezius muscles (upper back) raise the thoracic cage.

Active expiration

During active expiration, the internal intercostal muscles contract to shorten the chest's transverse diameter and the abdominal rectus muscles pull down the lower chest, thus depressing the lower ribs.

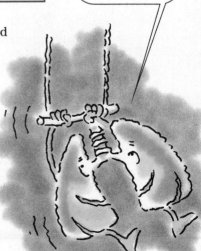

The posterior trapezius muscles raise the thoracic cage so I can fill with air during forced inspiration.

Mechanics of respiration

The muscles of respiration help the chest cavity expand and contract. Pressure differences between atmospheric air and the lungs help produce air movement. These illustrations show the muscles that work together to allow inspiration and expiration.

Anterior view

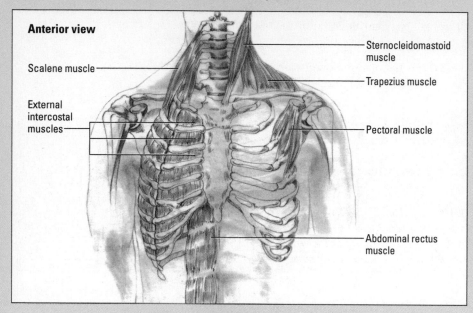

Scalene muscle

External intercostal muscles

Sternocleidomastoid muscle

Trapezius muscle

Pectoral muscle

Abdominal rectus muscle

Posterior view

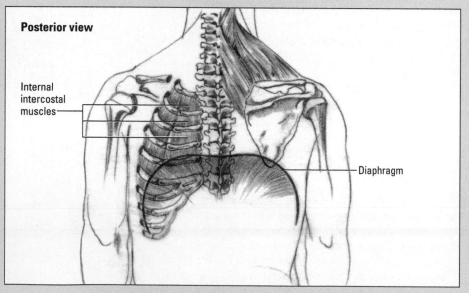

Internal intercostal muscles

Diaphragm

External and internal respiration

Effective respiration consists of gas exchange in the lungs, called *external respiration*, and gas exchange in the tissues, called *internal respiration*.

External respiration occurs through three processes:

☝ *ventilation* — gas distribution into and out of the pulmonary airways

✌ *pulmonary perfusion* — blood flow from the right side of the heart, through the pulmonary circulation, and into the left side of the heart

🤟 *diffusion* — gas movement through a semipermeable membrane from an area of greater concentration to one of lesser concentration.

Internal respiration, however, occurs only through diffusion.

Ventilation

Ventilation is the distribution of gases (oxygen and carbon dioxide) into and out of the pulmonary airways. Problems within the nervous, musculoskeletal, and respiratory systems greatly compromise breathing effectiveness.

Nervous system

Involuntary breathing results from stimulation of the respiratory center in the medulla and the pons of the brain. The medulla controls the rate and depth of respiration; the pons moderates the rhythm of the switch from inspiration to expiration.

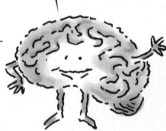

The respiratory center of the central nervous system is located in the medulla.

Musculoskeletal system

The adult thorax is flexible — its shape can be changed by contracting the chest muscles. The medulla controls ventilation primarily by stimulating contraction of the diaphragm and external intercostal muscles. These actions produce the intrapulmonary pressure changes that cause inspiration.

No room for expansion

Changes in lung or chest-wall compliance can occur. Destruction of the lung's elastic fibers, which causes the lungs to become stiff, decreases lung compliance and makes breathing difficult. This lack of elasticity occurs in acute respiratory distress syndrome (ARDS). The alveolocapillary membrane may also be affected, causing hypoxia. Chest-wall compliance is affected by thoracic deformity, muscle spasm, and abdominal distention.

Respiratory system

Airflow distribution can be affected by many factors, including:
- airflow pattern (see *Comparing airflow patterns*)
- volume and location of the functional reserve capacity (air retained in the alveoli that prevents their collapse during respiration)
- degree of intrapulmonary resistance
- presence of lung disease.

La pièce de résistance

Resistance refers to opposition to airflow. Changes in resistance may occur in the lung tissue, chest wall, or airways. Airway resistance accounts for about 80% of all respiratory system resistance. It's increased in such obstructive diseases as asthma, chronic bronchitis, and emphysema.

More work, less efficiency

With increased resistance, a person has to work harder to breathe, especially during expiration, to compensate for narrowed airways and diminished gas exchange. Other musculoskeletal and intrapulmonary factors can affect airflow and, in turn, may affect breathing. For instance, forced breathing, as in emphysema, activates accessory muscles of respiration, which require additional oxygen to work. Less efficient ventilation with an increased workload is the result.

Comparing airflow patterns

The pattern of airflow through the respiratory passages affects airway resistance.

Laminar flow
Laminar flow, a linear pattern that occurs at low flow rates, offers minimal resistance. This flow type occurs mainly in the small peripheral airways of the bronchial tree.

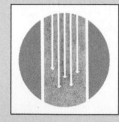

Turbulent flow
The eddying pattern of *turbulent flow* creates friction and increases resistance. Turbulent flow is normal in the trachea and large central bronchi. If the smaller airways become constricted or clogged with secretions, however, turbulent flow may also occur there.

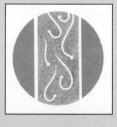

Transitional flow
A mixed pattern, known as *transitional flow,* is common at lower flow rates in the larger airways, especially where the airways narrow from obstruction, meet, or branch.

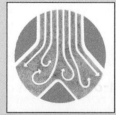

Running interference

Other airflow alterations can also increase oxygen and energy demand and cause respiratory muscle fatigue. These conditions include interference with expansion of the lungs or thorax (changes in compliance) and interference with airflow in the tracheobronchial tree (changes in resistance).

Pulmonary perfusion

Pulmonary perfusion refers to blood flow from the right side of the heart, through the pulmonary circulation, and into the left side of the heart. Perfusion aids external respiration. Normal pulmonary blood flow allows alveolar gas exchange; however, many factors may interfere with gas transport to the alveoli. Examples include:
• Cardiac output less than the average of 5 L/minute decreases gas exchange by reducing blood flow.
• Elevations in pulmonary and systemic resistance reduce blood flow.
• Abnormal or insufficient hemoglobin picks up less oxygen for exchange.

Trading places: O_2 and CO_2

How much oxygen and carbon dioxide trade places in the alveoli? That depends largely on the amount of air in the alveoli (ventilation) and the amount of blood in the pulmonary capillaries (perfusion). The ratio of ventilation to perfusion is called the $\dot{V}/\dot{Q}$ ratio. The $\dot{V}/\dot{Q}$ ratio expresses the effectiveness of gas exchange.

Make me a match

For effective gas exchange, ventilation and perfusion must match as closely as possible. In normal lung function, the alveoli receive air at a rate of about 4 L/minute while the capillaries supply blood to the alveoli at a rate of about 5 L/minute, creating a $\dot{V}/\dot{Q}$ ratio of 4:5, or 0.8. (See *Understanding ventilation and perfusion*, page 16.)

Uh-oh, mismatch!

A $\dot{V}/\dot{Q}$ mismatch, resulting from ventilation-perfusion dysfunction or altered lung mechanics, accounts for most of the impaired gas exchange in respiratory disorders. Ineffective gas exchange between the alveoli and the pulmonary capillaries can affect all body systems by altering the amount of oxygen delivered to living cells.

Ineffective gas exchange from an abnormality causes three outcomes:

 shunting (reduced ventilation to a lung unit)

Now I get it!

Understanding ventilation and perfusion

Effective gas exchange depends on the relationship between ventilation and perfusion, or the $\dot{V}/\dot{Q}$ ratio. These diagrams show what happens when the $\dot{V}/\dot{Q}$ ratio is normal and abnormal.

Normal ventilation and perfusion

When ventilation and perfusion are matched, unoxygenated blood from the venous system returns to the right side of the heart through the pulmonary artery to the lungs, carrying carbon dioxide (CO_2). The arteries branch into the alveolar capillaries. Gas exchange takes place in the alveolar capillaries.

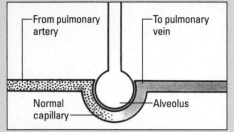

From pulmonary artery — To pulmonary vein — Normal capillary — Alveolus

Inadequate perfusion (dead-space ventilation)

When the $\dot{V}/\dot{Q}$ ratio is high, as shown here, ventilation is normal, but alveolar perfusion is reduced or absent. Note the narrowed capillary, indicating poor perfusion. This commonly results from a perfusion defect, such as pulmonary embolism or a disorder that decreases cardiac output.

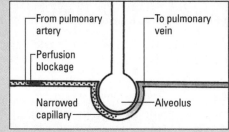

From pulmonary artery — Perfusion blockage — To pulmonary vein — Narrowed capillary — Alveolus

Inadequate ventilation (shunt)

When the $\dot{V}/\dot{Q}$ ratio is low, pulmonary circulation is adequate but not enough oxygen (O_2) is available to the alveoli for normal diffusion. A portion of the blood flowing through the pulmonary vessels doesn't become oxygenated.

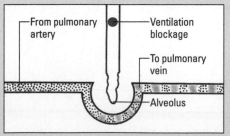

From pulmonary artery — Ventilation blockage — To pulmonary vein — Alveolus

Inadequate ventilation and perfusion (silent unit)

The silent unit indicates an absence of ventilation and perfusion to the lung area. The silent unit may help compensate for a $\dot{V}/\dot{Q}$ imbalance by delivering blood flow to better-ventilated lung areas.

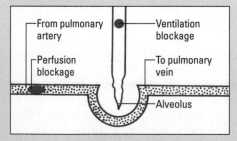

From pulmonary artery — Ventilation blockage — Perfusion blockage — To pulmonary vein — Alveolus

▓▓▓ Blood with CO_2 ▭ Blood with O_2 ▦ Blood with CO_2 and O_2

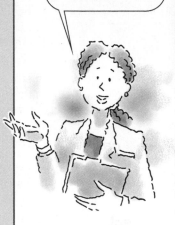

A high $\dot{V}/\dot{Q}$ ratio results from reduced or absent alveolar perfusion.

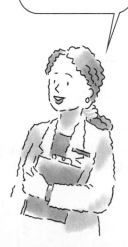

A silent unit can stem from various causes, including pulmonary embolism and chronic alveolar collapse.

dead-space ventilation (reduced perfusion to a lung unit)

 silent unit (combination of the above).

Don't shunt me out

Shunting causes the movement of unoxygenated blood from the right side of the heart to the left side of the heart. A shunt may occur from a physical defect that allows unoxygenated blood to bypass fully functioning alveoli. It may also result when airway obstruction prevents oxygen from reaching an adequately perfused area of the lung.

Respiratory disorders are commonly classified as shunt producing if the $\dot{V}/\dot{Q}$ ratio falls below 0.8 and dead-space producing if the $\dot{V}/\dot{Q}$ ratio exceeds 0.8.

Dead calm

Dead-space ventilation occurs when alveoli don't have adequate blood supply for gas exchange to occur. This occurs with pulmonary emboli, pulmonary infarction, and cardiogenic shock.

The science of silence

A silent unit occurs when little or no ventilation and perfusion are present, such as in cases of pneumothorax and ARDS.

Diffusion

In diffusion, oxygen and carbon dioxide molecules move between the alveoli and capillaries. The direction of movement is always from an area of greater concentration to one of lesser concentration. In the process, oxygen moves across the alveolar and capillary membranes, dissolves in the plasma, and then passes through the red blood cell (RBC) membrane. Carbon dioxide moves in the opposite direction. (See *Exchanging gases*, page 18.)

Spaces in between

The epithelial membranes lining the alveoli and capillaries must be intact. Both the alveolar epithelium and the capillary endothelium are composed of a single layer of cells. Between these layers are tiny spaces (interstices) filled with elastin and collagen.

From the RBCs to the alveoli

Normally, oxygen and carbon dioxide move easily through all of these layers. Oxygen moves from the alveoli into the bloodstream, where it's taken up by

> Between the epithelium and endothelium are tiny spaces filled with elastin and collagen.

Now I get it!

Exchanging gases

Gas exchange occurs very rapidly in the millions of tiny, thin-membraned alveoli within the respiratory units. Inside these air sacs, oxygen from inhaled air diffuses into the blood while carbon dioxide diffuses from the blood into the air and is exhaled. Blood then circulates throughout the body, delivering oxygen and picking up carbon dioxide. Finally, the blood returns to the lungs to be oxygenated again.

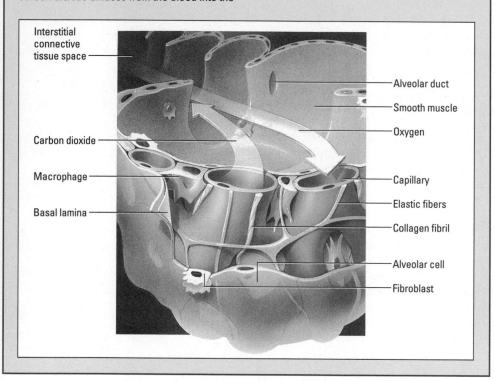

- Interstitial connective tissue space
- Carbon dioxide
- Macrophage
- Basal lamina
- Alveolar duct
- Smooth muscle
- Oxygen
- Capillary
- Elastic fibers
- Collagen fibril
- Alveolar cell
- Fibroblast

hemoglobin in the RBCs. When it arrives in the bloodstream, it displaces carbon dioxide (the byproduct of metabolism), which diffuses from RBCs into the blood and then to the alveoli.

To bind or not to bind

Most transported oxygen binds with hemoglobin to form oxyhemoglobin; however, a small portion dissolves in the plasma. The portion of oxygen that dissolves in plasma can be measured as the partial pressure of oxygen in arterial blood (PaO_2).

After oxygen binds to hemoglobin, RBCs travel to the tissues. Through cellular diffusion, internal respiration occurs when the RBCs release oxygen and absorb carbon dioxide. The RBCs then transport the carbon dioxide back to the lungs for removal during expiration.

Acid-base balance

Oxygen taken up in the lungs is transported to the tissues by the circulatory system, which exchanges it for carbon dioxide produced by metabolism in body cells. Because carbon dioxide is more soluble than oxygen, it dissolves in the blood. Most of the oxygen in the blood forms bicarbonate (base) and smaller amounts form carbonic acid (acid).

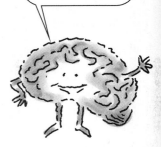

Respiration takes cooperation! I send the messages...

Respiratory responses

The lungs control bicarbonate levels by converting bicarbonate to carbon dioxide and water for excretion. In response to signals from the medulla, the lungs can change the rate and depth of breathing. This change allows for adjustments in the amount of carbon dioxide lost while helping maintain acid-base balance.

Metabolic alkalosis

For example, in *metabolic alkalosis* (a condition resulting from excess bicarbonate retention), the rate and depth of ventilation decrease so that carbon dioxide can be retained, which increases carbonic acid levels.

Metabolic acidosis

In *metabolic acidosis* (a condition resulting from excess acid retention or excess bicarbonate loss), the lungs increase the rate and depth of ventilation to eliminate excess carbon dioxide, thus reducing carbonic acid levels.

Broken balance beam

When the lungs don't function properly, an acid-base imbalance results. For example, they can cause respiratory acidosis through *hypoventilation* (reduced rate and depth of ventilation), which leads to carbon dioxide retention.

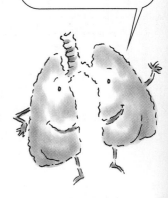

...and I change the rate and depth of breathing. Together we adjust levels of carbon dioxide and maintain acid-base balance.

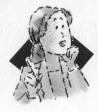

Quick quiz

1. The chief respiratory unit for gas exchange is the:
A. acinus.
B. alveoli.
C. terminal bronchiole.
D. hilum.

Answer: A. The acinus is the chief respiratory unit for gas exchange.

2. The number of lobes in the right lung is:
A. two.
B. three.
C. four.
D. six.

Answer: B. The right lung has three lobes.

3. During gas exchange, oxygen and carbon dioxide diffusion occurs in the:
A. venules.
B. alveoli.
C. RBCs.
D. bronchioles.

Answer: B. Oxygen and carbon dioxide diffusion occurs in the alveoli.

4. Oxygen passes through the alveoli into the bloodstream and binds with hemoglobin to form:
A. RBCs.
B. carbon dioxide.
C. oxyhemoglobin.
D. myoglobin.

Answer: C. When oxygen passes through the alveoli into the bloodstream, it binds with hemoglobin to form oxyhemoglobin.

Thanks for studying hard. I feel much safer now!

Scoring

☆☆☆ If you answered all four items correctly, extraordinary! Take a deep breath! You've responded extremely well to the respiratory system.

☆☆ If you answered three items correctly, fascinating! You're breezing through these systems like a whirlwind.

☆ If you answered fewer than three items correctly, get inspired! There are 10 more quick quizzes to go!

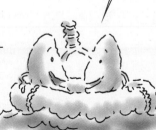

Assessment

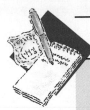

Just the facts

In this chapter, you'll learn:

♦ how to obtain a health history for respiratory disorders

♦ how to assess the respiratory system using the four components of a physical examination

♦ normal breath sounds

♦ abnormal respiratory system findings.

Understanding respiratory assessment

Performing a respiratory system assessment includes obtaining a careful history and performing a complete physical examination of the patient, which will provide you with essential information about the thorax and lungs. Knowing the basic structures and functions of the respiratory system will help you perform a comprehensive respiratory assessment and recognize any abnormalities.

> Explore the patient's chief complaint during your assessment.

Obtaining a health history

Any assessment begins with a health history, including exploration of the patient's chief complaints. (See *Hidden agendas*, page 22.) A patient with a respiratory disorder may complain of shortness of breath, cough, sputum production, wheezing, and chest pain. (See *Breathtaking facts*, page 22.)

Some questions are helpful in gaining information about certain signs and symptoms. (See *Listen and learn, then teach*, page 23.)

Breathtaking facts

Here are some facts about the roles of coughing, pain, and shortness of breath in abnormal respiratory function.

Cough it up
• Coughing clears unwanted material from the tracheobronchial tree.
• Sputum from the bronchial tubes traps foreign matter and protects the lungs from damage.

Pain sites
The lungs themselves don't contain pain receptors; however, chest pain may be caused by inflammation of the pleura or the costochondral joints at the midclavicular line or edge of the sternum.

How much oxygen?
Patients with chronically high partial pressure of arterial carbon dioxide ($Paco_2$), such as those with chronic obstructive pulmonary disease or a neuromuscular disease, may be stimulated to breathe by a low oxygen level (the hypoxic drive) rather than by a slightly high $Paco_2$ level, as is normal. For such patients, supplemental oxygen therapy should be provided cautiously because it may depress the stimulus to breathe, further increasing $Paco_2$.

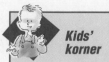

Kids' korner

Hidden agendas

Most information that you obtain about a child will come from the family. In some instances, the chief complaint that the parent expresses may not be the actual reason she's seeking medical attention.

Always ask the parent if there are other concerns about the child. Asking such questions as "Was there anything else you wanted to ask me today?" or "Do you have other concerns?" may invite the parent to share her concerns for the visit.

If the child is an adolescent, she'll usually respond to those who pay attention to her. Showing interest in the adolescent (and not her problems) early in the interview will help build trust and begin a rapport with her. Start the interview by first informally asking about her friends, school, or hobbies. When rapport has been established, you can return to more open-ended questioning.

Asking about shortness of breath

You can gain a history of the patient's shortness of breath by using several scales. Ask the patient to rate his usual level of dyspnea on a scale of 1 to 10, in which 1 means no dyspnea and 10 means the worst he has experienced. Then ask him to rate the level that day.

Other scales grade dyspnea as it relates to activity. In addition to using one of the severity scales, you might also ask these questions: What do you do to relieve the dyspnea? How well does it work? (See *Grading dyspnea*.)

Asking about orthopnea

A patient with orthopnea (shortness of breath when lying down) tends to sleep with his upper body elevated. Ask the patient how many pillows he uses. His answer describes the severity of orthopnea. For instance, a patient who uses three pillows can be said to have "three-pillow orthopnea."

Asking about cough

Ask the patient with a cough these questions:
• Is the cough productive?
• If the cough is a chronic problem, has it changed recently? If so, how?
• What makes the cough better? What makes it worse?

Advice from the experts

Listen and learn, then teach

Listening to what your patient says about his respiratory problems will help you know where he needs education. These typical responses indicate that the patient needs to know more about self-care techniques:

• "Whenever I feel breathless, I just take a shot of my inhaler." This patient needs to know more about proper use of an inhaler and when to call the doctor.

• "If I feel all congested, I just smoke a cigarette, and then I can cough up that phlegm!" This patient needs to know about the dangers of cigarette smoking.

• "None of the other guys wear a mask when we're working." This patient needs to know the importance of wearing an appropriate safety mask when working around heavy dust and particles in the air, such as sawdust or powders.

Asking about sputum

When a patient produces sputum, ask him to estimate the amount in teaspoons or some other common measurement. Also ask him these questions:

• At what time of day do you cough most often?
• What's the color and consistency of the sputum?
• If sputum is a chronic problem, has it changed recently? If so, how?
• Do you cough up blood? If so, how much and how often?

Asking about wheezing

If a patient wheezes, ask him these questions:
• When does wheezing occur?
• What makes you wheeze?
• Do you wheeze loudly enough for others to hear it?
• What helps stop your wheezing?

Asking about chest pain

If the patient has chest pain, ask him these questions:
• Where is the pain?
• What does it feel like? Is it sharp, stabbing, burning, or aching?
• Does it move to another area?
• How long does it last?
• What causes it to occur? What makes it better?

Chest pain that occurs from a respiratory problem is usually the result of pleural inflammation, inflammation of the costochondral junctions, soreness of chest muscles because of coughing, or

Grading dyspnea

To assess dyspnea as objectively as possible, ask your patient to briefly describe how various activities affect his breathing. Then document his response using this grading system:

• *Grade 0*—not troubled by breathlessness except with strenuous exercise
• *Grade 1*—troubled by shortness of breath when hurrying on a level path or walking up a slight hill
• *Grade 2*—walks more slowly on a level path because of breathlessness than do people of the same age or has to stop to breathe when walking on a level path at his own pace
• *Grade 3*—stops to breathe after walking about 100 yards (91 m) on a level path
• *Grade 4*—too breathless to leave the house or breathless when dressing or undressing.

indigestion. Less common causes of pain include rib or vertebral fractures caused by coughing or osteoporosis.

Check the broader health history

Remember to look at the patient's medical and family history, being particularly watchful for a smoking habit, allergies, previous operations, and respiratory diseases, such as pneumonia and tuberculosis.

Also, ask about environmental exposure to irritants such as asbestos. People who work in mining, construction, or chemical manufacturing are commonly exposed to environmental irritants.

Using a systematic approach

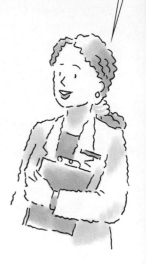

Don't overlook the patient's medical and family history.

Any patient can develop a respiratory disorder. By using a systematic assessment, you can detect subtle or obvious respiratory changes. The depth of your assessment will depend on several factors, including the patient's primary health problem and his risk of developing respiratory complications.

A physical examination of the respiratory system follows four steps: inspection, palpation, percussion, and auscultation. Before you begin, make sure the room is well-lit and warm.

Make a few observations about the patient as soon as you enter the room. Note how the patient is seated, which will most likely be the position most comfortable for him. Take note of his level of awareness and general appearance. Does he appear relaxed? Anxious? Uncomfortable? Is he having trouble breathing? You'll include these observations in your final assessment.

Inspecting the chest

Introduce yourself and explain why you're there. Help the patient into an upright position. The patient should be undressed from the waist up or clothed in an examination gown that allows you access to his chest.

Back, then front

Examine the back of the chest first, using inspection, palpation, percussion, and auscultation. Always compare one side with the other. Then examine the front of the chest using the same sequence. The patient can lie back when you examine the front of the chest if that's more comfortable for him.

Beauty in symmetry

Note masses or scars that indicate trauma or surgery. Look for chest wall symmetry. Both sides of the chest should be equal at rest and expand equally as the patient inhales. The diameter of the chest, from front to back, should be about half the width of the chest.

A new angle

Look at the angle between the ribs and the sternum at the point immediately above the xiphoid process. This angle—the costal angle—should be less than 90 degrees in an adult. The angle will be larger if the chest wall is chronically expanded because of an enlargement of the intercostal muscles, as can happen with chronic obstructive pulmonary disease (COPD).

Breathing rate and pattern

To find the patient's respiratory rate, count for a full minute—longer if you note abnormalities. Don't tell him what you're doing or he might alter his natural breathing pattern.

Adults normally breathe at a rate between 12 and 20 breaths/minute. (See *Look at the tummy.*) The respiratory pattern should be even, coordinated, and regular, with occasional sighs. The ratio of inspiration to expiration is about 1:2.

Men, children, and infants usually use abdominal, or diaphragmatic, breathing. Athletes and singers do as well. Most women, however, usually use chest, or intercostal, breathing.

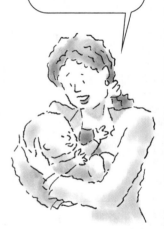

Infants usually use abdominal, or diaphragmatic, breathing but most women usually use chest, or intercostal, breathing.

Kids' korner

Look at the tummy

In infancy and early childhood, diaphragmatic breathing is predominant and thoracic excusing is minimal. Therefore, observe the respiratory rate by looking at the abdominal excursion—not the chest excursion. You can also place your hand directly on the thorax to determine the respiratory rate.

An infant's or child's breathing rate is very susceptible to illness, exercise, and emotion, so observe the respiratory rate when the child is asleep or quiet. The respiratory rate can range between 30 and 60 breaths/minute in the neonate, 20 and 40 breaths/minute in early childhood, and 15 and 25 breaths/minute in late childhood.

Raising a red flag

Watch for paradoxical (uneven) movement of the chest wall. Paradoxical movement may appear as an abnormal collapse of part of the chest wall when the patient inhales or an abnormal expansion when the patient exhales. In either case, this uneven movement indicates a loss of normal chest wall function.

Muscles in motion

When the patient inhales, his diaphragm should descend and the intercostal muscles should contract. This dual motion causes the abdomen to push out and the lower ribs to expand laterally.

When the patient exhales, his abdomen and ribs return to their resting position. The upper chest shouldn't move much. Accessory muscles may hypertrophy, indicating frequent use. Frequent use of accessory muscles may be normal in some athletes, but for other patients it indicates a respiratory problem, particularly when the patient purses his lips and flares his nostrils when breathing.

Inspecting related structures

Inspection of the skin, tongue, mouth, fingers, and nail beds may also provide information about respiratory status.

Skin color and nail beds

Skin color varies considerably among patients; however, typically, a patient with a bluish tint to his skin and mucous membranes is considered cyanotic. Cyanosis, which occurs when oxygenation to the tissues is poor, is a late sign of hypoxemia.

The most reliable place to check for cyanosis is the tongue and mucous membranes of the mouth. A chilled patient may have cyanotic nail beds, nose, or ears, indicating low blood flow to those areas but not necessarily to major organs.

Clubbing clues

When you check the fingers, look for clubbing, a possible sign of long-term hypoxia. (See *Assessing for clubbing*.)

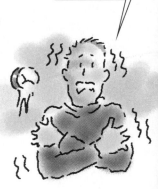

Brrrr! It's cold in here. I may have cyanotic nail beds, nose, or ears.

Palpating the chest

Palpation of the chest provides some important information about the respiratory system and the processes involved in breathing. (See *Palpating the chest*, page 28.) Here's what to look for when palpating the chest.

Assessing for clubbing

To assess for chronic tissue hypoxia, check the patient's fingers for clubbing. Normally, the angle between the fingernail and the point where the nail enters the skin is about 160 degrees. Clubbing occurs when that angle increases to 180 degrees or more, as shown below.

Normal finger

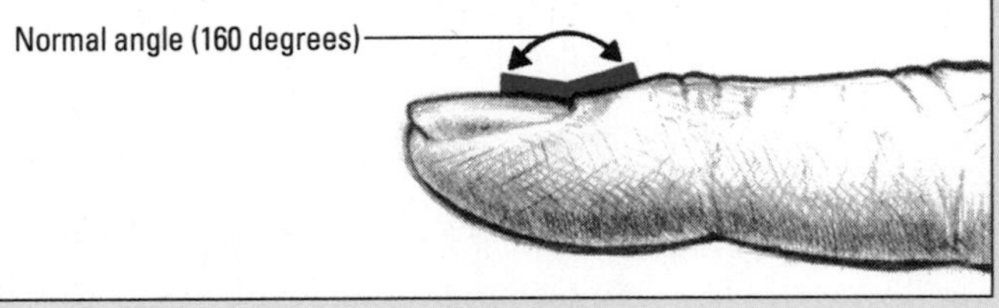

Normal angle (160 degrees)

Clubbed finger

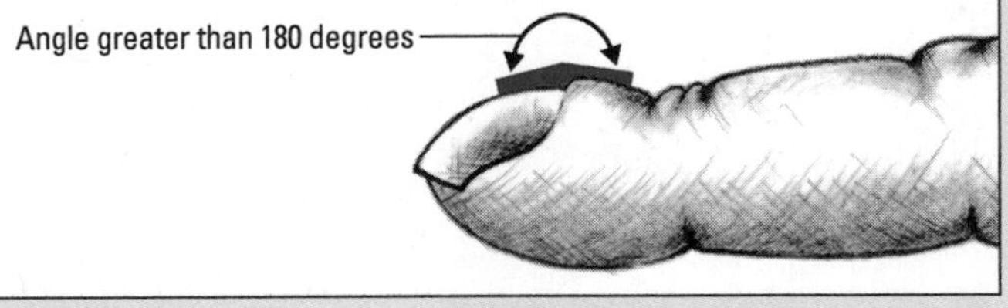

Angle greater than 180 degrees

No extra air

The chest wall should feel smooth, warm, and dry. Crepitus indicates subcutaneous air in the chest, an abnormal condition. Crepitus feels like puffed-rice cereal crackling under the skin and indicates that air is leaking from the airways or lungs.

If a patient has a chest tube, you may find a small amount of subcutaneous air around the insertion site. If the patient has no chest tube or the area of crepitus is getting larger, alert the doctor immediately.

No pain

Gentle palpation shouldn't cause the patient pain. If the patient complains of chest pain, try to find a painful area on the chest wall. Painful costochondral joints are typically located at the midclavicular line or next to the sternum. Rib or vertebral fractures will be quite painful over the fracture, though pain may radiate around the chest as well. Pain may also result from sore muscles as a result of protracted coughing. A collapsed lung may cause pain.

Advice from the experts

Palpating the chest

To palpate the chest, place the palm of your hand (or hands) lightly over the thorax, as shown below left. Palpate for tenderness, alignment, bulging, and retractions of the chest and intercostal spaces. Assess the patient for crepitus, especially around drainage sites. Repeat this procedure on the patient's back.

Next, use the pads of your fingers, as shown below right, to palpate the front and back of the thorax. Pass your fingers over the ribs and any scars, lumps, lesions, or ulcerations. Note the skin temperature, turgor, and moisture. Also note tenderness and bony or subcutaneous crepitus. The muscles should feel firm and smooth.

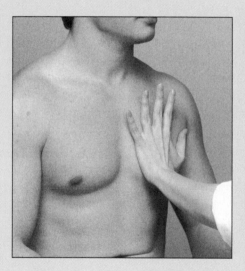

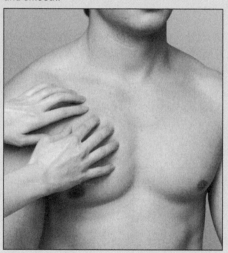

Vibratin' fremitus

Palpate for tactile fremitus, palpable vibrations caused by the transmission of air through the bronchopulmonary system. Fremitus is decreased over areas where pleural fluid collects, at times when the patient speaks softly and in pneumothorax, atelectasis, and emphysema. Fremitus is increased normally over the large bronchial tubes and abnormally over areas in which alveoli are filled with fluid or exudate, as happens in pneumonia. (See *Checking for tactile fremitus.*)

Measuring the symmetry

To evaluate the patient's chest wall symmetry and expansion, place your hands on the front of the chest wall with your thumbs touching each other at the second intercostal space. As the patient

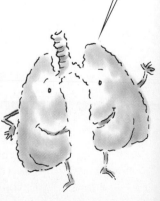

Symmetry is beautiful when it comes to the chest wall!

Advice from the experts

Checking for tactile fremitus

When you check the back of the thorax for tactile fremitus, ask the patient to fold his arms across his chest. This movement shifts the scapulae out of the way.

What to do
Check for tactile fremitus by lightly placing your open palms on both sides of the patient's back, as shown, without touching his back with your fingers. Ask the patient to repeat the phrase "ninety-nine" loudly enough to produce palpable vibrations. Then palpate the front of the chest using the same hand positions.

What the results mean
Vibrations that feel more intense on one side than the other indicate tissue consolidation on that side. Less intense vibrations may indicate emphysema, pneumothorax, or pleural effu-

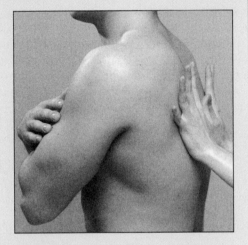

sion. Faint or no vibrations in the upper posterior thorax may indicate bronchial obstruction or a fluid-filled pleural space.

inhales deeply, watch your thumbs. They should separate simultaneously and equally to a distance several centimeters away from the sternum.

Repeat the measurement at the fifth intercostal space. The same measurement may be made on the back of the chest near the tenth rib.

Warning signs

The patient's chest may expand asymmetrically if he has pleural effusion, atelectasis, pneumonia, or pneumothorax. Chest expansion may be decreased at the level of the diaphragm if the patient has emphysema, respiratory depression, diaphragm paralysis, atelectasis, obesity, or ascites.

Percussing the chest

You'll percuss the chest to find the boundaries of the lungs; to determine whether the lungs are filled with air, fluid, or solid material; and to evaluate the distance the diaphragm travels between the patient's inhalation and exhalation. (See *Percussing the chest.*)

Different sites, different sounds

Percussion allows you to assess structures as deep as 3″ (7.6 cm). You'll hear different percussion sounds in different areas of the chest. (See *Percussion sounds.*)

You also may hear different sounds after certain treatments. For instance, if your patient has atelectasis and you percuss his chest before chest physiotherapy, you'll hear a high-pitched, dull, soft sound. After physiotherapy, you should hear a low-pitched, hollow sound. In all cases, make sure you use other assessment techniques to confirm percussion findings. (See *Double-check percussion findings.*)

Ringing with resonance

You'll hear resonant sounds over normal lung tissue, which you should find over most of the chest. In the left front chest from the third or fourth intercostal space at the sternum to the third or fourth intercostal space at the midclavicular line, you should hear a dull sound. Percussion is dull there because the heart occupies that space. Resonance resumes at the sixth intercostal space. The

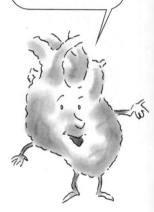

Percussion over me is dull. Of course, that doesn't mean I'm dull. I'm a pretty dynamic guy — handsome, muscular, always moving...

Advice from the experts

Percussing the chest

To percuss the chest, hyperextend the middle finger of your left hand if you're right-handed or the middle finger of your right hand if you're left-handed. Place your hand firmly on the patient's chest. Use the tip of the middle finger of your dominant hand — your right hand if you're right-handed, left hand if you're left-handed — to tap on the middle finger of your other hand just below the distal joint (as shown).

The movement should come from the wrist of your dominant hand, not your elbow or upper arm. Keep the fingernail you use for tapping short so you won't hurt yourself. Follow the standard percussion sequence over the front and back chest walls.

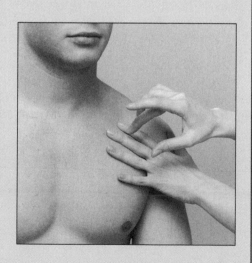

Percussion sounds

Use this chart to help you become more comfortable with percussion and to interpret percussion sounds quickly. Learn the different percussion sounds by practicing on yourself, your patients, and any other person willing to help.

Sound	Description	Clinical significance
Flat	Short, soft, high-pitched, extremely dull, found over the thigh	Consolidation, as in atelectasis and extensive pleural effusion
Dull	Medium in intensity and pitch, moderate length, thudlike, found over the liver	Solid area, as in pleural effusion
Resonant	Long, loud, low-pitched, hollow, found over the left front chest at sixth intercostal space	Normal lung tissue
Hyperresonant	Very loud, lower-pitched, found over the stomach	Hyperinflated lung, as in emphysema or pneumothorax
Tympanic	Loud, high-pitched, moderate length, musical, drumlike, found over a puffed-out cheek	Air collection, as in a gastric air bubble or air in the intestines

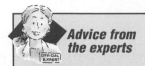

Advice from the experts

Double-check percussion findings

Use other assessment findings to verify the results of respiratory percussion. For example, if an X-ray report on a patient with chronic obstructive pulmonary disease indicates findings consistent with emphysema, you should hear low-pitched, loud booming sounds when you percuss the chest.

sequence of sounds in the back is slightly different. (See *Percussion sequences*, page 32.)

Problem sounds

When you hear hyperresonance during percussion, it means you've found an area of increased air in the lung or pleural space. Expect hyperresonance with pneumothorax, acute asthma, bullous emphysema (large holes in the lungs from alveolar destruction), or gastric distention that pushes up on the diaphragm.

When you hear abnormal dullness, it means you've found areas of decreased air in the lungs. Expect abnormal dullness in the presence of pleural fluid, consolidation, atelectasis, or a tumor.

Movement of the diaphragm

Percussion also allows you to assess how much the diaphragm moves during inspiration and expiration. The normal diaphragm descends 1¼" to 2" (3 to 5 cm) when the patient inhales. The diaphragm doesn't move as far in patients with emphysema, respiratory depression, diaphragm paralysis, atelectasis, obesity, or ascites. (See *Measuring diaphragm movement*, page 33.)

Percussion sequences

Follow these percussion sequences to distinguish between normal and abnormal sounds in the patient's lungs. Remember to compare sound variations from one side with the other as you proceed. Carefully describe abnormal sounds you hear and include their locations. You'll follow the same sequences for auscultation.

Anterior

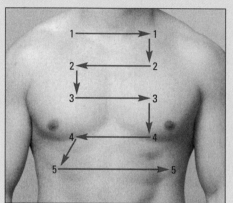

Posterior

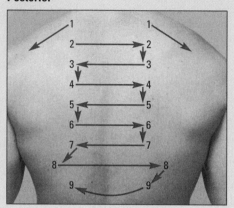

Auscultating the chest

As air moves through the bronchi, it creates sound waves that travel to the chest wall. The sounds produced by breathing change as air moves from larger airways to smaller airways. Sounds also change if they pass through fluid, mucus, or narrowed airways. Auscultation helps you to determine the condition of the alveoli and surrounding pleura.

Preparing to auscultate

Auscultation sites are the same as percussion sites. Using the diaphragm of the stethoscope, listen to a full inspiration and a full expiration at each site. Ask the patient to breathe through his mouth; nose breathing alters the pitch of breath sounds. If the patient has abundant chest hair, mat it down with a damp washcloth so the hair doesn't make sounds like crackles.

Be firm

To auscultate for breath sounds, press the stethoscope firmly against the skin. Remember, if you listen through clothing or dry chest hair, you may hear unusual and deceptive sounds.

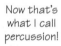

Now that's what I call percussion!

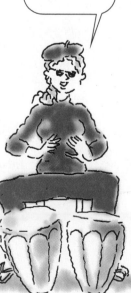

Advice from the experts

Measuring diaphragm movement

You can measure how much the diaphragm moves by asking the patient to exhale. Percuss the back on one side to locate the upper edge of the diaphragm, the point at which normal lung resonance changes to dullness. Use a pen to mark the spot indicating the position of the diaphragm at full expiration on that side of the back.

Then ask the patient to inhale as deeply as possible. Percuss the back when the patient has inhaled until you locate the diaphragm. Use the pen to mark this spot as well. Repeat on the opposite side of the back.

Measure
Use a ruler or tape measure to determine the distance between the marks. The distance, normally 1¼" to 2" (3 to 5 cm) long, should be equal on both the right and left sides.

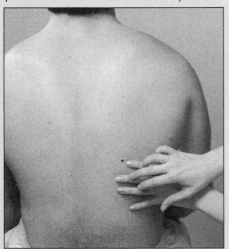

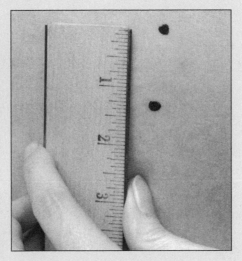

Normal breath sounds

You'll hear four types of breath sounds over normal lungs. (See *Qualities of normal breath sounds*, page 34.) The type of sound you hear depends on where you listen. (See *Locations of normal breath sounds*, page 34.) These are the four normal breath sounds:

• Tracheal breath sounds, heard over the trachea, are harsh and discontinuous. They occur when a patient inhales or exhales.

• Bronchial breath sounds, usually heard next to the trachea, are loud, high-pitched, and discontinuous. They're loudest when the patient exhales.

Qualities of normal breath sounds

This chart lists types of normal breath sounds along with their quality, ratio of inspiration (I) to expiration (E), and location.

Breath sound	Quality	Inspiration-expiration ratio	Location
Tracheal	Harsh, high-pitched	I < E	Over trachea
Bronchial	Loud, high-pitched	I > E	Next to trachea
Bronchovesicular	Medium in loudness and pitch	I = E	Next to sternum, between scapulae
Vesicular	Soft, low-pitched	I > E	Remainder of lungs

Locations of normal breath sounds

These photographs show the normal locations of different types of breath sounds.

Anterior thorax

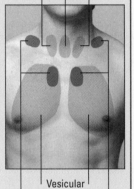

Bronchial
Tracheal
Vesicular
Bronchovesicular

Posterior thorax

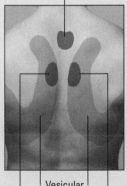

Tracheal
Vesicular
Bronchovesicular

• Bronchovesicular sounds, heard when the patient inhales or exhales, are medium-pitched and continuous. They're best heard over the upper third of the sternum and between the scapulae.
• Vesicular sounds, heard over the rest of the lungs, are soft and low-pitched. They're prolonged during inhalation and shortened during exhalation. (See *Quieter and softer.*)

What a change means

If you hear diminished but normal breath sounds in both lungs, the patient may have emphysema, atelectasis, severe bronchospasm, or shallow breathing. If you hear breath sounds in one lung only, the patient may have pleural effusion, pneumothorax, a tumor, or mucus plugs in the airways. In such cases, the doctor may order pulmonary function tests to further assess the patient's condition.

Interpreting what you hear

Classify each sound according to its intensity, location, pitch, duration, and characteristic. Note whether the sound occurs when the patient inhales, exhales, or both. If you hear a sound in an area other than that in which you would expect to hear it, consider the sound abnormal.

For instance, bronchial or bronchovesicular breath sounds found in an area where vesicular breath sounds would normally be heard indicates that the alveoli and small bronchioles in that area might be filled with fluid or exudate, as occurs in pneumonia and atelectasis. You won't hear vesicular sounds in those areas because no air is moving through the small airways.

Abnormal voice sounds

To assess for abnormal voice sounds, ask the patient to repeat the words below while you listen. Auscultate over an area where you heard abnormally located bronchial breath sounds.

Bronchophony

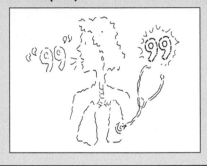

Egophony

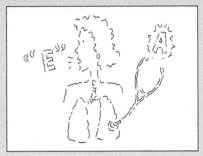

Whispered pectoriloquy

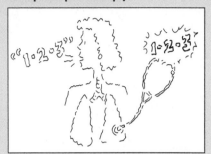

The next step

A patient with abnormal findings during a respiratory assessment may be further evaluated using such diagnostic tests as arterial blood gas analysis and pulmonary function tests.

Vocal fremitus

Vocal fremitus is the sound produced by chest vibrations as the patient speaks. Abnormal transmission of voice sounds may occur over consolidated areas. (See *Abnormal voice sounds*.) The most common abnormal voice sounds are:
- *bronchophony*. Ask the patient to say "ninety-nine" or "blue moon." Over normal lung tissue, the words sound muffled. Over consolidated areas, the words sound unusually loud.
- *egophony*. Ask the patient to say "E." Over normal lung tissue, the sound is muffled. Over consolidated lung tissue, it will sound like the letter *a*.
- *whispered pectoriloquy*. Ask the patient to whisper "1, 2, 3." Over normal lung tissue, the numbers will be almost indistinguishable. Over consolidated lung tissue, the numbers will be loud and clear.

Abnormal findings

Your assessment of the chest may reveal any of a number of abnormalities of the chest wall and lungs. Let's look first at chest abnormalities, which may be congenital or acquired. (See *Identifying chest abnormalities*, page 36.)

Kids' korner

Quieter and softer

When listening for breath sounds in a child, remember that adult breath sounds are harsher and louder because the stethoscope is closer to the source of the sound. In a neonate, breathing is intermittent, shallow, and slow, and then deep and rapid. In addition, breath sounds are commonly diminished on the opposite side to which the child's head is turned. Normal neonates and older infants may have fine crackles at the end of deep inspiration.

Identifying chest abnormalities

As you inspect the patient's chest, note deviations in size and shape. These illustrations show a normal adult chest and four common chest deformities.

Normal adult chest

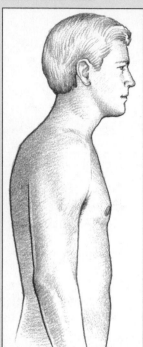

Barrel chest
Increased anteroposterior diameter

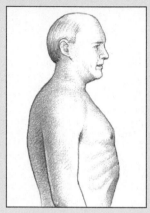

Pectus excavatum (funnel chest)
Depression on all or part of the sternum

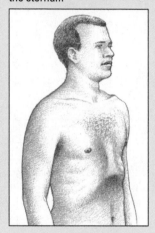

Pectus carinatum (pigeon chest)
Anteriorly displaced sternum with sternum protruding beyond front of abdomen; increased front-to-back diameter of chest

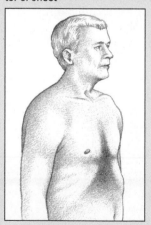

Thoracic kyphoscoliosis
Raised shoulder and scapula, thoracic convexity, flared interspaces, curvature of spine; rotation of vertebrae; distorted lung tissues

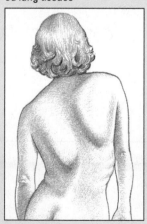

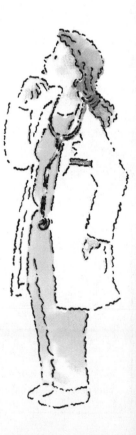

Chest abnormalities

As you examine a patient for chest abnormalities, keep in mind that a patient with a deformity of the chest wall might have completely normal lungs and that the lungs might be cramped within the chest. The patient might have a smaller-than-normal lung capacity and limited exercise tolerance, or he may more easily develop respiratory failure from a respiratory tract infection. (See *What pediatric chest abnormalities mean*.)

Barrel chest

A barrel chest looks like its name implies — the chest is abnormally round and bulging, with a greater-than-normal front-to-back diameter. Barrel chest may be normal in infants and elderly patients.

In other patients, barrel chest occurs as a result of COPD. In patients with COPD, barrel chest indicates that the lungs have lost their elasticity and that the diaphragm is flattened. You'll note that this patient typically uses accessory muscles when he inhales and easily becomes breathless. You'll also note kyphosis of the thoracic spine, ribs that run horizontally rather than tangentially, and a prominent sternal angle.

Pectus carinatum

A patient with pectus carinatum, or *pigeon chest*, has a chest with a sternum that protrudes beyond the front of the abdomen. The

---

Kids' korner

What pediatric chest abnormalities mean

When examining a child, note these structural abnormalities of the chest:

• *Barrel chest* may indicate chronic respiratory disease, such as cystic fibrosis or asthma.

• *Funnel chest* may indicate rickets or Marfan syndrome.

• *Localized bulges* may indicate underlying pressures, such as cardiac enlargement or aneurysm.

• *More than five café-au-lait spots* may indicate neurofibromatosis. Note that these spots may occur elsewhere on the body.

• *Pigeon chest* may indicate Marfan or Morquio's syndrome or a chronic upper respiratory tract condition.

• *Rachitic beads* (bumps at the costochondral junction of the ribs) may indicate rickets.

• *An unusually wide space between the nipples* may indicate Turner's syndrome (the distance between the outside areolar edges shouldn't be more than one-fourth of the patient's chest circumference).

displaced sternum increases the front-to-back diameter of the chest. Most patients are asymptomatic; however, some may develop a rigid chest wall in which the anteroposterior diameter is almost fixed in full inspiration, making respiratory efforts less effective. As the lungs lose compliance, incidence of emphysema and frequency of infection increase.

Pectus excavatum

A patient with pectus excavatum, or *funnel chest*, has a funnel-shaped depression on all or part of the sternum. The shape of the chest may interfere with respiratory and cardiac function. Compression of the heart and great vessels may cause murmurs.

Thoracic kyphoscoliosis

In thoracic kyphoscoliosis, the patient's spine curves to one side and the vertebrae are rotated. Because the rotation distorts lung tissues, it may be more difficult to assess respiratory status.

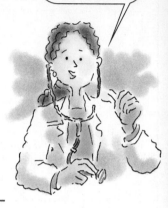

Compression of the heart and great vessels due to funnel chest may cause murmurs.

Abnormal respiratory patterns

Identifying abnormal respiratory patterns can help you make a more complete assessment of a patient's respiratory status and his overall condition. (See *Spotting abnormal respiratory patterns.*)

Tachypnea

Tachypnea is a respiratory rate greater than 20 breaths/minute with shallow breathing. It's commonly seen in patients with restrictive lung disease, pain, sepsis, obesity, and anxiety. Fever may be another cause. The respiratory rate may increase by 4 breaths/minute for every 1° F (0.6° C) rise in body temperature.

Bradypnea

Bradypnea is a respiratory rate below 10 breaths/minute and is commonly noted just before a period of apnea or full respiratory arrest. Patients with bradypnea might have central nervous system (CNS) depression as a result of excessive sedation, tissue damage, or diabetic coma, which all depress the brain's respiratory control center. (The respiratory rate normally decreases during sleep.)

Apnea

Apnea is the absence of breathing. Periods of apnea may be short and occur sporadically during Cheyne-Stokes respirations, Biot's

Spotting abnormal respiratory patterns

Here are typical characteristics of the more common abnormal respiratory patterns.

Tachypnea
Shallow breathing with increased respiratory rate

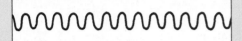

Bradypnea
Decreased rate but regular breathing

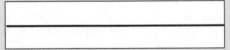

Apnea
Absence of breathing; may be periodic

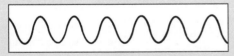

Hyperpnea
Deep breathing at a normal rate

Kussmaul's respirations
Rapid, deep breathing without pauses; in adults, more than 20 breaths/minute; breathing that usually sounds labored with deep breaths that resemble sighs

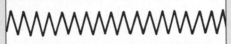

Cheyne-Stokes respirations
Breaths that gradually become faster and deeper than normal, then slower, during a 30- to 170-second period; alternates with 20- to 60-second periods of apnea

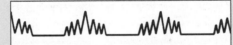

Biot's respirations
Rapid, deep breathing with abrupt pauses between each breath; equal depth to each breath

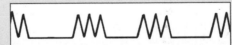

respirations, or other abnormal respiratory patterns. This condition may be life threatening if periods of apnea last long enough.

Hyperpnea

Characterized by deep breathing, hyperpnea occurs in patients who exercise or those with anxiety, pain, or metabolic acidosis. In a comatose patient, hyperpnea may indicate hypoxia or hypoglycemia.

Kussmaul's respirations

Kussmaul's respirations are rapid, deep, sighing breaths that occur in patients with metabolic acidosis, especially when associated with diabetic ketoacidosis.

Cheyne-Stokes respirations

Cheyne-Stokes respirations have a regular pattern of variations in the rate and depth of breathing. Deep breaths alternate with short periods of apnea. This respiratory pattern is seen in patients with heart failure, kidney failure, or CNS damage. Cheyne-Stokes respirations may be normal during sleep in children and elderly patients.

Biot's respirations

Biot's respirations involve rapid, deep breaths that alternate with abrupt periods of apnea. Biot's respirations are an ominous sign of severe CNS damage.

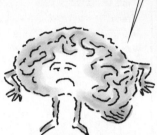

Biot's respirations are an ominous sign of severe CNS damage. Oy!

Abnormal breath sounds

Because solid tissue transmits sound better than air or fluid, breath sounds (as well as spoken or whispered words) will be louder than normal over areas of consolidation. If pus, fluid, or air fills the pleural space, breath sounds will be quieter than normal. If a foreign body or secretions obstruct a bronchus, breath sounds will be diminished or absent over lung tissue located distal to the obstruction. (See *Abnormal breath sound types*.)

Adventitious sounds are abnormal no matter where you hear them in the lungs. They include fine and coarse crackles, wheezes, rhonchi, stridor, and pleural friction rub.

Crackles

Crackles are intermittent, nonmusical, brief crackling sounds that are caused by collapsed or fluid-filled alveoli popping open. Heard primarily when the patient inhales, crackles are classified as either fine or coarse and usually don't clear with coughing. If crackles do clear with coughing, secretions most likely caused them. (See *Types of crackles*.)

Wheezes

Wheezes are high-pitched sounds heard first when a patient exhales. The sounds occur when airflow is blocked. As severity of the block increases, wheezes may also be heard when the patient inhales. The sound of a wheeze doesn't change with coughing. Patients may wheeze as a result of asthma, infection, heart failure, or airway obstruction from a tumor or foreign body. (See *Signs and symptoms of upper airway obstruction*.)

Abnormal breath sound types

These are types of abnormal breath sounds:
• *Crackles*—intermittent, nonmusical, crackling sounds heard during inspiration; classified as fine or coarse
• *Wheezes*—high-pitched sounds caused by blocked airflow, heard on exhalation
• *Rhonchi*—low-pitched snoring or rattling sound; heard primarily on exhalation
• *Stridor*—loud, high-pitched sound heard during inspiration
• *Pleural friction rub*—low-pitched, grating sound heard during inspiration and expiration; accompanied by pain.

Types of crackles

Here's how to differentiate fine crackles from coarse crackles, a critical distinction when assessing the lungs.

Fine crackles

These characteristics distinguish fine crackles:
- occur when the patient stops inhaling
- are usually heard in lung bases
- sound like a piece of hair being rubbed between the fingers or like Velcro being pulled apart
- occur in restrictive diseases, such as pulmonary fibrosis, asbestosis, silicosis, atelectasis, heart failure, and pneumonia.

Coarse crackles

These characteristics distinguish coarse crackles:
- occur when the patient starts to inhale; may be present when the patient exhales
- may be heard through the lungs and even at the mouth
- sound more like bubbling or gurgling, as air moves through secretions in larger airways
- occur in chronic obstructive pulmonary disease, bronchiectasis, pulmonary edema, and with severely ill patients who can't cough; also called the "death rattle."

Signs and symptoms of upper airway obstruction

If a patient can't maintain a patent airway, he may end up in respiratory arrest. Refer to this list of potential signs and symptoms when assessing a patient for partial or complete airway obstruction:
- anxiety
- dyspnea
- stridor
- wheezing
- decreased or absent breath sounds
- use of accessory muscles
- seesaw movement between chest and abdomen
- inability to speak (complete obstruction)
- cyanosis.

Rhonchi

Rhonchi are low-pitched, snoring, rattling sounds that occur primarily when a patient exhales, although they may also be heard when the patient inhales. Rhonchi usually change or disappear with coughing. The sounds occur when fluid partially blocks the large airways.

Stridor

Stridor is a loud, high-pitched crowing sound that is heard, usually without a stethoscope, during inspiration. Stridor, which is caused by an obstruction in the upper airway, requires immediate attention.

Pleural friction rub

Pleural friction rub is a low-pitched, grating, rubbing sound heard when the patient inhales and exhales. Pleural inflammation causes the two layers of pleura to rub together. The patient may complain of pain in areas where the rub is heard.

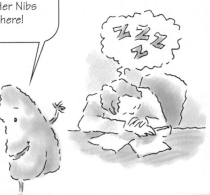

Rhonchi are low-pitched, snoring, rattling sounds. Of course, I don't snore — but get a load of Her Nibs over there!

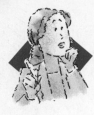

Quick quiz

1. In a patient with COPD, barrel chest indicates:
A. loss of lung elasticity.
B. rotation of the spinal column.
C. increased elasticity of the intercostal muscles.
D. displacement of the diaphragm.

Answer: A. Barrel chest in a patient with COPD is an indication of loss of elasticity in the lungs and a flattening of the diaphragm. In addition, the patient easily becomes breathless.

2. The percussion sound usually heard over most of the lungs is:
A. dullness.
B. resonance.
C. tympany.
D. hyperresonance.

Answer: B. The lungs, made up of tissue and air, make a resonant percussion sound. Solid tissue is flat or dull; air-filled spaces are hyperresonant or tympanic.

3. Fine crackles are heard in:
A. asthma.
B. pulmonary fibrosis.
C. neuromuscular disease.
D. pleurisy.

Answer: B. Crackles are heard when collapsed or stiff alveoli snap open, as in pulmonary fibrosis.

4. When you auscultate the lower lobes of a healthy patient's lungs, you would expect to hear:
A. tracheal breath sounds.
B. bronchial breath sounds.
C. vesicular breath sounds.
D. adventitious breath sounds.

Answer: C. Vesicular breath sounds, heard over the lower lobes, are soft, low-pitched, and prolonged during inspiration.

Scoring

✫✫✫ If you answered all four items correctly, excellent! You've left us breathless with your expertise!

✫✫ If you answered three items correctly, hooray! You're our resident respiratory guru!

✫ If you answered fewer than three items correctly, never fear! You're just getting started. Study on!

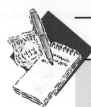

3

Diagnostic procedures

Just the facts

In this chapter, you'll learn:

♦ common diagnostic tests in respiratory care

♦ factors that can interfere with these tests

♦ what patient care is associated with these tests

♦ what test results might indicate.

Understanding respiratory diagnostic procedures

If the patient's history and physical examination reveal evidence of respiratory dysfunction, diagnostic tests will help identify and evaluate the dysfunction. These tests include blood, sputum, and pleural fluid studies; endoscopic and imaging tests; biopsies; and various other tests, including pulmonary function tests, pulse oximetry, and thoracentesis.

Blood studies

Blood studies used to diagnose respiratory disorders include arterial blood gas (ABG) analysis, white blood cell (WBC) count, and WBC differential.

Arterial blood gas analysis

ABG analysis is one of the first tests ordered to assess respiratory status because it helps evaluate gas exchange in the lungs by measuring:

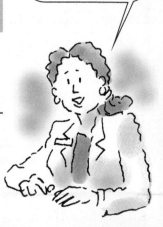

Arterial blood gas analysis is one of the first tests used to assess respiratory status because it evaluates gas exchange in the lungs.

Understanding acid-base disorders

This chart lists acid-base disorders along with their arterial blood gas (ABG) analysis results, possible causes, and signs and symptoms.

Disorder and ABG findings	Possible causes	Signs and symptoms
Respiratory acidosis (excess carbon dioxide [CO_2] retention) pH < 7.35 (SI, < 7.35) HCO_3^- > 26 mEq/L (SI, > 26 mmol/L) (if compensating) $Paco_2$ > 45 mm Hg (SI > 5.3 kPa)	• Central nervous system depression from drugs, injury, or disease • Asphyxia • Hypoventilation from pulmonary, cardiac, musculoskeletal, or neuromuscular disease	Diaphoresis, headache, tachycardia, confusion, restlessness, apprehension, flushed face
Respiratory alkalosis (excess CO_2 excretion) pH > 7.45 (SI, > 7.45) HCO_3^- < 22 mEq/L (SI, < 22 mmol/L) (if compensating) $Paco_2$ < 35 mm Hg (SI, < 4.7 kPa)	• Hyperventilation from anxiety, pain, or improper ventilator settings • Respiratory stimulation by drugs, disease, hypoxia, fever, or high room temperature • Gram-negative bacteremia	Rapid, deep respirations; paresthesias; light-headedness; twitching; anxiety; fear
Metabolic acidosis (HCO_3^- loss, acid retention) pH < 7.35 (SI, < 7.35) HCO_3^- < 22 mEq/L (SI, < 22 mmol/L) $Paco_2$ < 35 mm Hg (SI, < 4.7 kPa) (if compensating)	• HCO_3^- depletion from diarrhea • Excessive production of organic acids from hepatic disease, endocrine disorders, shock, or drug intoxication • Inadequate excretion of acids from renal disease	Rapid, deep breathing; fruity breath; fatigue; headache; lethargy; drowsiness; nausea; vomiting; coma (if severe); abdominal pain
Metabolic alkalosis (HCO_3^- retention, acid loss) pH > 7.45 (SI, > 7.45) HCO_3^- > 26 mEq/L (SI, > 26 mmol/L) $Paco_2$ > 45 mm Hg (SI, > 5.3 kPa) (if compensating)	• Loss of hydrochloric acid from prolonged vomiting or gastric suctioning • Loss of potassium from increased renal excretion (as in diuretic therapy) or steroids • Excessive alkali ingestion	Slow, shallow breathing; hypertonic muscles; restlessness; twitching; confusion; irritability; apathy; tetany; seizures; coma (if severe)

• *pH.* An indication of hydrogen ion (H^+) concentration in the blood, pH shows the blood's acidity or alkalinity.
• *partial pressure of arterial carbon dioxide* ($Paco_2$). Known as the respiratory parameter, $Paco_2$ reflects the adequacy of the lungs' ventilation and carbon dioxide elimination.
• *partial pressure of arterial oxygen* (Pao_2). Pao_2 reflects the body's ability to pick up oxygen from the lungs.
• *bicarbonate* (HCO_3^-) *level.* Known as the metabolic parameter, the HCO_3^- level reflects the kidneys' ability to retain and excrete HCO_3^-. (See *Understanding acid-base disorders.*)

Teamwork

The respiratory and metabolic systems work together to keep the body's acid-base balance within normal limits. If respiratory acidosis develops, for example, the kidneys attempt to compensate by conserving HCO_3^-. Therefore, if respiratory acidosis is present, expect to see the HCO_3^- value rise above normal. Similarly, if metabolic acidosis develops, the lungs try to compensate by increasing the respiratory rate and depth to eliminate carbon dioxide. Therefore, expect to see the $Paco_2$ level fall below normal.

Nursing considerations

• Blood for an ABG analysis should be drawn from an arterial line if the patient has one. If a percutaneous puncture must be done, the site must be chosen carefully. The brachial, radial, and femoral arteries can be used. (See *Obtaining an ABG sample*.)
• After the sample is obtained, apply pressure to the puncture site for 5 minutes and tape a gauze pad firmly in place. (Don't apply tape around the arm; it could restrict circulation.) Regularly monitor the site for bleeding and check the arm for signs of complications (such as swelling, discoloration, pain, numbness, and tingling).
• Make sure it's noted on the slip whether the patient is breathing room air or oxygen. If oxygen, document the number of liters. If the patient is receiving mechanical ventilation, the fraction of inspired oxygen should be documented.

Calling interference

• Keep in mind that certain conditions may interfere with test results — for example, failing to properly heparinize the syringe before drawing a blood sample or exposing the sample to air. Venous blood in the sample may lower Pao_2 levels and elevate $Paco_2$ levels.
• Wait at least 20 minutes before drawing blood for an ABG after initiating, changing, or discontinuing oxygen therapy; after initiating or changing settings of mechanical ventilation; after suctioning the patient; or after extubation.
• Tell the patient which site — either the radial, brachial, or femoral artery — has been selected for the puncture.
• Instruct the patient to breathe normally during the test, and warn him that he may feel brief cramping or throbbing pain at the puncture site.
• Monitor vital signs and observe for signs of circulatory impairment, such as swelling, discoloration, pain, numbness, or tingling in the bandaged arm or leg.

Obtaining an ABG sample

Follow these steps to obtain a sample for arterial blood gas (ABG) analysis:
• After Allen's test, perform a cutaneous arterial puncture (if an arterial line is in place, draw blood from the arterial line).
• Use a heparinized blood gas syringe to draw the sample.
• Eliminate all air from the sample, place it on ice immediately, and transport it for analysis.
• Apply pressure to the puncture site for 3 to 5 minutes. If the patient is receiving anticoagulants or has a coagulopathy, hold the puncture site longer than 5 minutes if necessary.
• Tape a gauze pad firmly over the puncture site. If the puncture site is on the arm, don't tape the entire circumference because this may restrict circulation.

White blood cell count

The WBC, or leukocyte count, measures the number of WBCs in a microliter of whole blood through the use of electronic devices. A WBC count can be useful in diagnosing infection and inflammation as well as in monitoring a patient's response to chemotherapy or radiation therapy. WBC counts can also help determine whether further tests are needed.

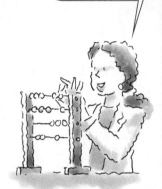

White blood cell counts help diagnose infection and inflammation as well as determine the need for further tests.

Counting high

An elevated WBC count (leukocytosis) commonly signals infection, such as an abscess, meningitis, appendicitis, or tonsillitis. A high count may also indicate leukemia or tissue necrosis caused by burns, myocardial infarction, or gangrene.

Nursing considerations

• Tell the patient that he should avoid strenuous exercise for 24 hours before the test to avoid altered readings and that he should also avoid ingesting a large meal before the test.
• Perform a venipuncture, and collect the sample in a 7-ml tube containing ethylenediaminetetraacetic acid (EDTA).
• Completely fill the sample collection tube, and invert it gently several times to adequately mix the sample and anticoagulant.

White blood cell differential

A WBC differential can provide more specific information about a patient's immune system. In a WBC differential, the laboratory classifies 100 or more WBCs in a stained film of blood according to five major types of leukocytes — neutrophils, eosinophils, basophils, lymphocytes, and monocytes — and determines the percentage of each type.

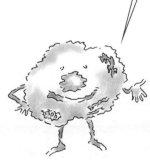

A white blood cell differential helps evaluate the body's ability to fight infection. It also helps detect allergic reactions, parasitic infections, and leukemia.

The lowdown on levels

Abnormally high levels of WBCs are associated with allergic reactions and parasitic infections. After the normal values for the patient have been determined, an assessment can be made.

Nursing considerations

• Perform a venipuncture, and collect the sample in a 7-ml tube containing EDTA.
• Completely fill the collection tube, and invert it gently several times to adequately mix the sample and anticoagulant.

Sputum and pleural fluid studies

Sputum and pleural fluid studies include sputum analysis, nasopharyngeal culture, and throat culture.

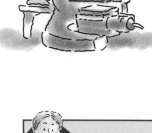

A sputum culture isolates and identifies the cause of a pulmonary infection.

Sputum analysis

Analysis of a sputum specimen (the material expectorated from a patient's lungs and bronchi during deep coughing) helps diagnose respiratory disease, determine the cause of respiratory infection (including viral and bacterial causes), identify abnormal lung cells, and manage lung disease.

A sputum specimen is stained and examined under a microscope and, depending on the patient's condition, sometimes cultured. Culture and sensitivity testing identifies a specific microorganism and its antibiotic sensitivities. A negative culture may suggest a viral infection.

Flora and fauna

Flora commonly found in the respiratory tract include alpha-hemolytic streptococci, *Neisseria* species, diphtheroids, some *Haemophilus* species, pneumococci, staphylococci, and yeasts such as *Candida*. However, the presence of normal flora doesn't rule out infection. A culture isolate must be interpreted in light of the patient's overall clinical condition.

On-site organisms

Pathogenic organisms most commonly found in sputum include *Streptococcus pneumoniae*, *Mycobacterium tuberculosis*, *Klebsiella pneumoniae* (and other Enterobacteriaceae), *H. influenzae*, *Staphylococcus aureus*, and *Pseudomonas aeruginosa*. Other pathogens, such as *Pneumocystis carinii*, *Legionella* species, *Mycoplasma pneumoniae*, and respiratory viruses, may exist in the sputum and can cause lung disease, but they usually require serologic or histologic diagnosis rather than diagnosis by sputum culture. (See *Sputum culture interference*.)

Nursing considerations

Sputum culture may be collected using one of three methods: expectoration, tracheal suctioning, or bronchoscopy:
• Include on the laboratory request the nature and origin of the specimen, the date and time of collection, the initial diagnosis, and medications the patient is currently taking.
• Send the specimen to the laboratory immediately after collection.

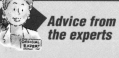

Advice from the experts

Sputum culture interference

Failure to report current or recent antimicrobial therapy may alter sputum culture results. In addition, sputum collected over an extended period may cause pathogens to deteriorate or become overgrown by commensals (one of two or more organisms that live in an intimate, nonparasitic relationship).

Expecting the expectoration

- Encourage the patient to increase his fluid intake the night before sputum collection to aid expectoration.
- Encourage the patient to obtain a sputum specimen in the morning.
- When the patient is ready to expectorate, instruct him to take three deep breaths and force a deep cough.
- To prevent foreign particles from contaminating the specimen, instruct the patient not to eat, brush his teeth, or use a mouthwash before expectorating. He may rinse his mouth with water.
- Before sending the specimen to the laboratory, make sure the specimen is sputum, not saliva. Saliva has a thinner consistency and more froth (bubbles) than sputum.
- For expectoration, put on gloves and a mask. Instruct the patient to cough deeply and expectorate into the container. If the cough is nonproductive, use chest physiotherapy or nebulization to induce sputum, as ordered. Using aseptic technique, close the container securely and place it in a leak-proof bag before sending it to the laboratory.

Lube the tube

- For tracheal suctioning, administer oxygen to the patient, before and after suctioning and as necessary. Using sterile gloves, lubricate the catheter with normal saline solution and pass the catheter through the nostril, without suction. (The patient will cough when the catheter passes through the larynx.)
- Advance the catheter into the trachea. Apply suction for no longer than 15 seconds to obtain the specimen. Stop suction and gently remove the catheter. Discard the catheter and gloves. Then detach the in-line sputum trap from the suction apparatus and cap the opening.
- If the patient becomes hypoxic or cyanotic, remove the catheter immediately and administer oxygen. (See *Using an in-line trap.*)

> If the patient becomes hypoxic or cyanotic, administer oxygen.

Brushing up

- For bronchoscopy, secretions are collected with a bronchial brush or aspirated through the inner channel of the scope using an irrigating solution such as normal saline solution, if necessary. After the specimen is obtained, the bronchoscope is removed.
- After bronchoscopy, observe the patient carefully for signs of hypoxemia, laryngospasm, bronchospasm, pneumothorax, perforation of the trachea or bronchus (subcutaneous crepitus), or trauma to respiratory structures. Check for breathing or swallowing difficulty.

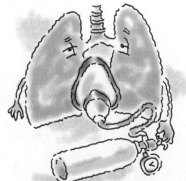

Using an in-line trap

When using an in-line trap, put on sterile gloves, push the suction tubing onto the male adapter of the trap, and follow these three steps:

Insert the suction catheter into the rubber tubing of the trap. Then suction the patient.

After suctioning, disconnect the in-line trap from the suction tubing and catheter.

To seal the container, connect the rubber tubing to the female adapter of the trap.

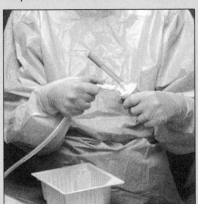
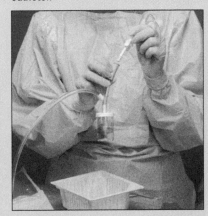
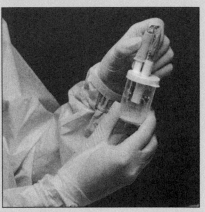

- Do *not* give liquids until the gag reflex returns. In a patient with asthma or chronic bronchitis, watch for aggravated broncho-spasms.

Nasopharyngeal culture

Direct microscopic inspection of a Gram-stained smear of a naso-pharyngeal specimen provides preliminary identification of organisms, which may guide clinical management and determine the need for additional testing. Streaking a culture plate with the swab and allowing any organisms present to grow permits isolation and identification of pathogens. Cultured pathogens may require susceptibility testing to determine the appropriate antimicrobial agent.

Found flora

Flora commonly found in the nasopharynx include nonhemolytic streptococci, alpha-hemolytic streptococci, *Neisseria* species (except *N. meningitidis* and *N. gonorrhoeae*), *Staphylococcus epidermidis* and, occasionally, *S. aureus*.

A nasopharyngeal culture can identify pathogens that can cause upper respiratory tract symptoms.

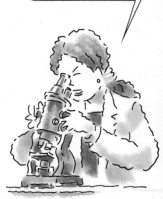

Nursing considerations

• Inform the patient how and where the specimen will be obtained and that he may experience slight discomfort and gag.
• Put on gloves and moisten a swab with sterile water or saline. Ask the patient to cough before you begin collecting the specimen, and then position the patient with his head tilted back.

Shine a light on it

• Using a penlight and tongue blade, inspect the nasopharyngeal area. Next, without touching the sides of the patient's nostril or his tongue, gently pass the swab through the nostril and into the nasopharynx, keeping the swab near the septum and floor of the nose. (See *Obtaining a nasopharyngeal specimen*.)
• If *Bordetella pertussis* is suspected, Dacron or calcium alginate mini-tipped swabs should be used for collection.

Lab notes

• If the specimen is for isolation of a virus, verify the laboratory's recommended collection and refrigeration techniques.
• Note recent antimicrobial therapy or chemotherapy on the laboratory request.
• Tell the laboratory if *Corynebacterium diphtheriae* or *B. pertussis* is suspected; these organisms need special growth media.
• Keep the container upright.

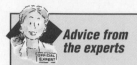

Advice from the experts

Obtaining a nasopharyngeal specimen

To collect a nasopharyngeal specimen, gently but quickly rotate the swab when it passes into the nasopharynx. Then remove the swab, taking care not to injure the nasal mucous membrane.

Throat culture

A throat culture requires swabbing the throat, streaking a culture plate, and allowing the organisms to grow for isolation and identification of pathogens. A Gram-stained smear may provide preliminary identification, which may guide clinical management and determine the need for further tests. Culture results must be interpreted in light of clinical status, recent antimicrobial therapy, and the amount of normal flora. It's preferable to obtain cultures before antimicrobial therapy has been initiated to get a more accurate count.

What it all means

Possible pathogens cultured include group A beta-hemolytic streptococci *(Streptococcus pyogenes)*, which can cause scarlet fever or pharyngitis; *Candida albicans*, which can cause thrush; *C. diphtheriae*, which can cause diphtheria; and *B. pertussis*, which can cause whooping cough. Other cultured bacteria include *Legionella* species, *Mycoplasma pneumoniae*, *Staphylococcus aureus*, *Streptococcus pneumoniae*, and *H. influenzae*.

Failure to report recent or current antimicrobial therapy may alter test results.

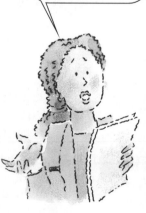

Throat culture is also used to screen for carriers of *N. meningitidis*. Fungi include *Histoplasma capsulatum*, *Coccidioides immitis*, and *Blastomyces dermatitidis*. Viruses include adenovirus, enterovirus, herpesvirus, rhinovirus, influenza virus, and parainfluenza virus.

The swab is coming! The swab is coming! Get out of town before the throat culture isolates and identifies us!

Nursing considerations

• Check for a recent history of antimicrobial therapy, and obtain the throat specimen before beginning antimicrobial therapy.
• Explain to the patient that this test helps identify microorganisms and takes about 30 seconds. Tell him he may gag during swabbing.
• Use gloves when performing the procedure and handling specimens.
• Have the patient tilt his head back and close his eyes. With the throat well-illuminated, check for inflamed areas using a tongue blade.

Swab the deck

• Swab the tonsillar areas from side to side; include inflamed or purulent sites. Do *not* touch the tongue, cheeks, or teeth with the swab.
• Immediately place the swab in the culture tube. If a commercial sterile collection and transport system is used, crush the ampule and force the swab into the medium to keep it moist.

Special delivery

• Note recent antimicrobial therapy on the laboratory request. Also indicate the suspected organism.
• Send the specimen to the laboratory immediately after collection, keeping the container upright during transport. Don't refrigerate specimens.

Endoscopic and imaging tests

Endoscopic and imaging tests include bronchoscopy, chest X-ray, fluoroscopy, mediastinoscopy, magnetic resonance imaging (MRI), pulmonary angiography, thoracic computed tomography (CT) scan, thoracoscopy, and ventilation-perfusion (V̇/Q̇) scan.

Bronchoscopy

Bronchoscopy is the direct inspection of the trachea and bronchi through a flexible fiber-optic or rigid bronchoscope. It allows the doctor to determine the location and extent of pathologic processes, assess resectability of a tumor, diagnose bleeding sites, collect tissue or sputum specimens, and remove foreign bodies, mucus plugs, or excessive secretions.

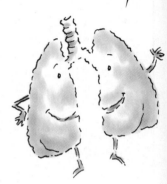

Bronchoscopy inspects the trachea and me through a bronchoscope. How do I look? Am I fabulous or what?!

Nursing considerations

• Tell the patient that he'll receive a sedative, such as diazepam (Valium), midazolam (Versed), or meperidine (Demerol).
• Tell the patient that he must fast for 4 to 6 hours before the test.
• Explain that the doctor will introduce the bronchoscope tube through the patient's nose or mouth into the airway. Then he'll flush small amounts of anesthetic through the tube to suppress coughing and gagging.
• Explain to the patient that he'll be asked to lie on his side or sit with his head elevated at least 30 degrees until his gag reflex returns. Food, fluid, and oral drugs will be withheld until this time. Hoarseness or a sore throat is temporary and, when his gag reflex returns, he can have throat lozenges or a gargle.
• Report bloody mucus, dyspnea, wheezing, or chest pain to the doctor immediately. A chest X-ray will be taken after the procedure, and the patient may receive an aerosolized bronchodilator treatment.

Creeping crepitus

• Watch for subcutaneous crepitus around the patient's face and neck, which may indicate tracheal or bronchial perforation.
• Monitor the patient for breathing problems from laryngeal edema or laryngospasm; call the doctor immediately if you note labored breathing.
• Observe the patient for signs of hypoxia, pneumothorax, bronchospasm, or bleeding.
• Keep resuscitative equipment and a tracheostomy tray available during the procedure and for 24 hours afterward.

A chest X-ray alone may not confirm a diagnosis, but it can show structural abnormalities and lesion location and size.

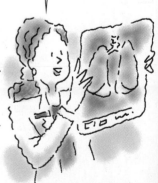

Chest X-ray

Because normal pulmonary tissue is radiolucent, foreign bodies, infiltrates, fluids, tumors, and other abnormalities appear as densities (white areas) on a chest X-ray. It's most useful when compared with the patient's previous films, which allows the radiologist to detect changes. (See *Evaluating chest X-rays.*)

Evaluating chest X-rays

To evaluate anteroposterior or postero-anterior chest X-rays, follow these guidelines:

• Examine the area around the rib cage for masses, swelling, air, or foreign objects.

• Observe the diaphragm. Normally, the right side looks higher than the left. Expect the diaphragm to curve downward, with clearly delineated margins.

• Examine the bony structures, including the proximal humeri, clavicles, scapulae, ribs, sternum, and vertebrae. Note any unusual densities.

• Count the ribs from top to bottom (including the floating ribs).

• Observe the mediastinum. Located in the middle of the chest, the mediastinum narrows at the trachea to the right of the transverse aortic arch. If the patient is intubated, the distal end of the tube appears above the carina, clearly away from the right bronchi. At the lower end of the mediastinum, look for the heart, which points to the left with the apex at the fifth intercostal space.

• Inspect the pleura, starting at the hila and moving down to the costophrenic angle. The pleura should adhere to the ribs without a distinct line inside the rib cage.

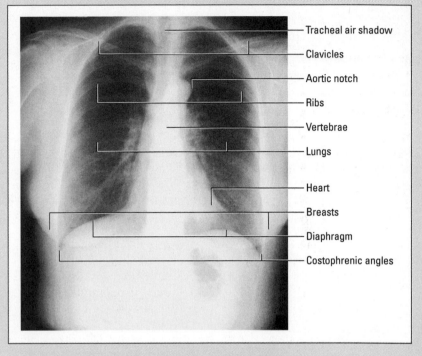

• Compare the lung fields. Look for adequate lung expansion and similar areas of density in both lungs — these areas represent blood vessels. Asymmetrical densities that look like white wisps or solid areas are abnormal.

• If the patient has an endotracheal tube or central I.V. line, check it for proper placement.

Normal chest X-ray

The photo above shows a normal chest X-ray with bony and soft landmarks in the posteroanterior view.

By itself, a chest X-ray film may not provide information for a definitive diagnosis. For example, it may not reveal mild to moderate obstructive pulmonary disease. Even so, it can show the location and size of lesions and identify structural abnormalities that influence ventilation and diffusion. Examples of abnormalities visible on X-ray include pneumothorax, fibrosis, atelectasis, and infiltrates. (See *Understanding chest X-ray findings,* pages 54 and 55.)

(Text continues on page 56.)

Advice from the experts

Understanding chest X-ray findings

This table describes how anatomic structures normally appear on chest X-ray, lists possible abnormalities, and describes the implications of these abnormalities.

Anatomic structure and normal appearance	Abnormality
Trachea Visible midline in the anterior mediastinal cavity; translucent, tubelike appearance	Deviation from midline
	Narrowing with hourglass appearance and deviation to one side
Heart Visible in the anterior left mediastinal cavity; appears solid because of blood contents; edges may be clear in contrast with surrounding air density of the lung	Shift
	Hypertrophy of right heart
	Cardiac borders obscured by stringy densities ("shaggy heart")
Mediastinum (mediastinal shadow) Visible as the space between the lungs; shadowy appearance that widens at the hilum of the lungs	Deviation to nondiseased side; deviation to diseased side by traction
	Gross widening
Ribs Visible as thoracic cavity encasement	Break or misalignment
	Widening of intercostal spaces
Mainstem bronchus Visible; part of the hila with translucent, tubelike appearance	Spherical or oval density
Bronchi Usually not visible	Visible
Lung fields Usually not visible throughout, except for the blood vessels	Visible
	Irregular, patchy densities

Implications

Tension pneumothorax, atelectasis, pleural effusion, consolidation, mediastinal nodes; in children, enlarged thymus

Substernal thyroid
Stenosis secondary to trauma

Atelectasis, pneumothorax

Cor pulmonale, heart failure

Cystic fibrosis

Pleural effusion or tumor, fibrosis or collapsed lung

Neoplasms of esophagus, bronchi, lungs, thyroid, thymus, peripheral nerves, lymphoid tissue; aortic aneurysm; mediastinitis; cor pulmonale

Fractured sternum or ribs

Emphysema

Bronchogenic cyst

Bronchial pneumonia

Atelectasis

Resolving pneumonia, infiltrates, silicosis, fibrosis, metastatic neoplasm

Nursing considerations

• Tell the patient that he must wear a gown without snaps and must remove all metal objects and jewelry from his neck and chest; however, he doesn't need to remove his pants, socks, and shoes.
• If the test is performed in the radiology department, tell the patient that he'll stand or sit in front of a machine. If it's performed at the bedside, tell him that someone will help him to a sitting position and a cold, hard film plate will be placed behind his back. He'll be asked to take a deep breath and to hold it for a few seconds while the X-ray is taken. He should remain still for those few seconds.
• Reassure the patient that the amount of radiation exposure is minimal. Facility personnel will leave the area when the technician takes the X-ray because they're potentially exposed to radiation many times each day.
• Explain that female patients of childbearing age will wear a lead apron. Males will be given a protective shield for the testes.

Fluoroscopy

In fluoroscopy, a continuous stream of X-rays passes through the patient, casting shadows of the heart, lungs, and diaphragm on a fluorescent screen. Because fluoroscopy exposes the patient to high levels of radiation and reveals less detail than standard chest radiography, it's indicated only when diagnosis depends on visualizing physiologic or pathologic motion of thoracic contents. For example, it's used to rule out paralysis in patients with diaphragmatic elevation. Normal diaphragmatic movement is synchronous and symmetrical. Normal diaphragmatic excursion ranges from ¾″ to 1⅝″ (2 to 4 cm).

Diminished excursion

Diminished diaphragmatic movement may indicate pulmonary disease. Increased lung translucency (not transparent but permitting light passage) may indicate elasticity loss or bronchiolar obstruction. In elderly people, the lowest part of the trachea may be displaced to the right by an elongated aorta. Diminished or paradoxical diaphragmatic movement may indicate diaphragmatic paralysis, which sometimes occurs after open-heart surgery. However, fluoroscopy may not detect such paralysis if the patient compensates for diminished diaphragm function by forcefully contracting abdominal muscles to aid expiration.

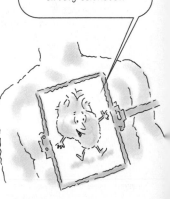

Fluoroscopy can detect bronchiolar obstructions and pulmonary disease. It also aids placement of a tube or catheter such as a pulmonary artery catheter.

Nursing considerations

• Describe the procedure to the patient, and explain that this test assesses respiratory structures and their motion. Tell the patient that the test usually takes 5 minutes.
• Instruct the patient to remove all metallic objects that might fall in the X-ray field, including jewelry.
• If necessary, assist with patient positioning. Move cardiac monitoring cables, I.V. tubing from subclavian lines, pulmonary artery catheter lines, and safety pins as far as possible from the X-ray field. During the test, cardiopulmonary motion is observed on a screen.
• If the patient is intubated, check that no tubes have been dislodged during positioning.
• To avoid exposure to radiation, leave the room or the immediate area during the test; if you must stay, wear a lead-lined apron.

Mediastinoscopy

Mediastinoscopy is performed under general anesthesia and involves insertion of a mirrored-lens instrument that's similar to a bronchoscope but is inserted through an incision at the anterior base of the neck. A biopsy of mediastinal lymph nodes is obtained. Because mediastinal lymph nodes drain lymphatic fluid from the lungs, specimens can identify carcinoma, granulomatous infection, sarcoidosis, coccidioidomycosis, or histoplasmosis. It can also be used to stage lung cancer or determine the extent of lung tumor metastasis.

Nursing considerations

• Explain to the patient that this surgical procedure requires general anesthesia.
• Tell the patient that he can't eat or drink anything for at least 8 hours before the test.
• Make sure the patient has signed a consent form.
• Inform the patient that a lighted instrument will be introduced through the anterior portion of his neck to obtain a biopsy of lymph nodes.
• Explain to the patient that this test will help identify disease, stage his lung cancer, or determine the extent of lung tumor metastasis.
• After the procedure, evaluate the patient's breathing and lung sounds and check the wound site for bleeding and hematoma.

Magnetic resonance imaging

MRI is a noninvasive test that employs a powerful magnet, radio waves, and a computer to help diagnose respiratory disorders. It provides high-resolution, cross-sectional images of lung structures and traces blood flow. MRI's greatest advantage is its ability to "see through" bone and to delineate fluid-filled soft tissue in great detail, without using ionizing radiation or contrast media.

> Tell the patient he'll lie on a table that slides into an 8' tunnel. Urge him to relax by focusing on breathing or a favorite subject.

Nursing considerations

• Tell the patient that he must remove all jewelry and take everything out of his pockets. No metal can be in the test room. The powerful magnet may demagnetize the magnetic strip on a credit card or stop a watch from ticking. If he has any metal inside his body, such as a pacemaker, orthopedic pins or disks, or bullets or shrapnel fragments, he must notify his doctor.
• Explain to the patient that he'll be asked to lie on a table that slides into an 8' (2.4 m) tunnel inside the magnet.
• Tell him to breathe normally but not to talk or move during the test to avoid distorting the results. The test usually takes 15 to 30 minutes but may take up to 45 minutes.
• Warn the patient that the machinery will be noisy with sounds ranging from a constant ping to a loud bang. He may feel claustrophobic or bored. Suggest that he try to relax and concentrate on breathing or a favorite subject or image.

Pulmonary angiography

Pulmonary angiography, also called *pulmonary arteriography*, allows radiographic examination of the pulmonary circulation. After injecting a radioactive contrast dye through a catheter inserted into the pulmonary artery or one of its branches, a series of X-rays is taken to detect blood flow abnormalities, possibly caused by emboli or pulmonary infarction. This test provides more reliable results than a V̇/Q̇ scan but carries higher risks, including cardiac arrhythmias.

Nursing considerations

• Let the patient know who will perform the test and where and when it will be done. Explain that the test takes about 1 hour and allows confirmation of pulmonary emboli.

• Tell the patient he must fast for 6 hours before the test or as ordered. He may continue his prescribed drug regimen unless the doctor orders otherwise.
• Explain that he'll be given a sedative, such as diazepam (Valium), as ordered. Diphenhydramine (Benadryl) may also be given to reduce the risk of a reaction to the dye.
• Explain the procedure to the patient. The doctor will make a percutaneous needle puncture in an antecubital, femoral, jugular, or subclavian vein. The patient may feel pressure at the site. The doctor will then insert and advance a catheter.
• After catheter insertion, check the pressure dressing for bleeding and assess for arterial occlusion by checking the patient's temperature, sensation, color, and peripheral pulse distal to the insertion site.
• After the test, monitor the patient for hypersensitivity to the contrast medium or to the local anesthetic. Keep emergency equipment nearby and watch for dyspnea.

Thoracic computed tomography scan

A thoracic CT scan provides cross-sectional views of the chest by passing an X-ray beam from a computerized scanner through the body at different angles and depths. The CT scan provides a three-dimensional image of the lung, allowing the doctor to assess abnormalities in the configuration of the trachea or major bronchi and evaluate masses or lesions, such as tumors and abscesses, and abnormal lung shadows. A contrast agent is sometimes used to highlight blood vessels and to allow greater visual discrimination.

Nursing considerations

• Tell the patient that if a contrast dye will be used, he should fast for 4 hours before the test.
• Explain that he'll lie on a large, noisy, tunnel-shaped machine. When the dye is injected into his arm vein, he may experience transient nausea, flushing, warmth, and a salty taste.
• Tell him that the equipment may make him feel claustrophobic. He shouldn't move during the test, and he should try to relax and breathe normally. Movement may invalidate the results and require repeat testing.
• Reassure the patient that radiation exposure during the test is minimal.
• Encourage fluid intake after the test if a contrast agent is used.

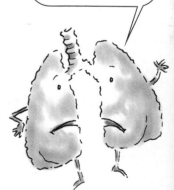

A thoracic CT scan allows assessment of tracheal and bronchial abnormalities, masses, lesions, and — gulp — abnormal shadows.

Thoracoscopy

A thoracoscopy is an invasive diagnostic procedure that uses a fiber-optic endoscope to examine the thoracic cavity. Video-assisted examination is a recent addition to the test. Thoracoscopy allows visualization of the visceral and parietal pleura, pleural spaces, mediastinum, thoracic walls, and pericardium. It can also be used to perform laser procedures, to assess pleural effusion, tumor growth, emphysema, inflammatory disease, and conditions that would predispose the patient to pneumothorax. Biopsies of the pleura, mediastinal lymph nodes, and lungs can also be confirmed through thoracoscopy.

Nursing considerations

- Obtain ordered laboratory tests as well as urinalysis and chest X-ray.
- Make sure the patient has signed a consent form.
- Explain to the patient that he must refrain from eating or drinking for at least 8 hours before the test.
- Explain to the patient that this surgical procedure requires general anesthesia.
- Obtain a postoperative chest X-ray, as ordered, to check for abnormal air or fluid in the chest cavity.
- Monitor vital signs and the amount and color of chest tube drainage.
- Encourage the patient to cough and deep breathe frequently.
- Assist the patient in splinting his incision during coughing and deep breathing to reduce discomfort.
- Check to see if the patient requires a chest tube for 24 to 48 hours after the procedure to assist with lung expansion.

Ventilation-perfusion scan

Although less reliable than pulmonary angiography, a $\dot{V}/\dot{Q}$ scan carries fewer risks. This test indicates lung perfusion and ventilation. It's used to evaluate $\dot{V}/\dot{Q}$ mismatch; detect pulmonary emboli, atelectasis, obstructing tumors, and chronic obstructive pulmonary disease; and determine pulmonary function, particularly in preoperative patients with marginal lung reserves.

The tech on technetium

In a $\dot{V}/\dot{Q}$ scan, two radionuclides are usually administered. The first, ^{99m}Tc, is used for the perfusion part of the study and is injected I.V. Decreased radioactive uptake in an area of the lung in-

Memory jogger

How can you remember the difference between hot spots and cold spots? Simple: Think about the weather. When it's **hot** outside, the temperature is **high.** So, **hot spots** have a **high** uptake of radioactive substance. Similarly, when it's **cold** outside, the temperature is **low.** So **cold spots** have **low** radioactive substance uptake.

dicates decreased blood flow to that area and, consequently, identifies that area as the site of embolization.

It's a gas, gas, gas

For the ventilation portion of the test, the other radionuclide commonly used is ^{133}Xe gas. This test, as the name implies, requires the patient to "ventilate" or breathe the radioactive particles into his lungs. Decreased areas of radioactivity correspond to some irregular lung function.

Nursing considerations

• Tell the patient that, like pulmonary angiography, a $\dot{V}/\dot{Q}$ scan requires injection of a radioactive contrast dye. Explain that he'll lie in a supine position on a table as a radioactive protein substance is injected into an arm vein.

Smile...you're on $\dot{V}/\dot{Q}$ camera

• While he remains supine, a large camera will take pictures, continuing as he lies on his side, lies prone, and sits up. When he's prone, more dye will be injected.
• Also inform the patient that during the ventilation part of the test he'll be asked to inhale a radioactive gas. He'll be asked again to remain still as a machine scans his chest after he inhales the gas and again as he exhales it. (See *Normal and abnormal ventilation scans.*)
• Reassure the patient that the amount of radioactivity in the dye is minimal. However, he may experience some discomfort from the venipuncture and from lying on a cold, hard table. He may also feel claustrophobic when surrounded by the camera equipment.

Biopsies

Biopsies include lung and pleural biopsies.

Lung biopsy

In a lung biopsy, a specimen of pulmonary tissue is excised for examination, using either the closed or the open technique. The closed technique, performed under local anesthesia, includes both needle and transbronchial biopsies. The open technique, performed under general anesthesia in the operating room, includes both limited and standard thoracotomies.

Normal and abnormal ventilation scans

The normal ventilation scan below taken 30 minutes to 1 hour after the wash-out phase, shows equal gas distribution. The abnormal scan, taken 1½ to 2 hours after the start of the wash-out phase, shows unequal gas distribution, represented by the area of poor wash-out on both the left and right sides.

Normal scan

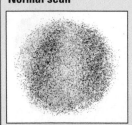

Abnormal scan

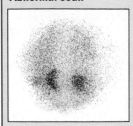

Easy access

Needle biopsy is appropriate when the lesion is readily accessible. This procedure provides a much smaller specimen than that of the open technique. Transbronchial biopsy, the removal of multiple tissue specimens through a fiber-optic bronchoscope, is appropriate for some lung abnormalities or when the patient's condition won't tolerate an open biopsy.

What it all means

Examination of lung tissue specimens can reveal squamous cell or oat cell carcinoma and adenocarcinoma.

Nursing considerations

• Describe the test to the patient and tell him that the test takes 30 to 60 minutes. Instruct him to fast after midnight before the procedure.
• Make sure the patient has signed a consent form. Check his history for hypersensitivity to the local anesthetic.

You...are...getting...very...sleepy

• Explain to the patient that a mild sedative will be administered 30 minutes before the biopsy to help the patient relax.
• Explain to the patient that after the biopsy site is selected, lead markers are placed on his skin and X-rays are ordered to verify the markers' correct placement.
• During biopsy, observe the patient for signs of respiratory distress—shortness of breath, elevated pulse rate, and cyanosis (late sign); if such signs develop, report them immediately.

Distress signals

• Check vital signs every 15 minutes for 1 hour, every hour for 4 hours, and then every 4 hours for 24 hours.
• Assess for bleeding, shortness of breath, increased pulse, diminished breath sounds on the biopsy side and, eventually, cyanosis.
• Make sure the chest X-ray is repeated immediately after the biopsy.

Pleural biopsy

Pleural biopsy is the removal of pleural tissue for examination using needle or open biopsy. Performed under local anesthesia, pleural biopsy usually follows thoracentesis (aspiration of pleural fluid), which is performed when the cause of the effusion is unknown. However, it can be performed separately. (See *Scoping out a Cope's needle*.)

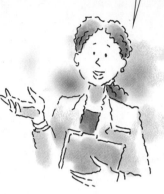

Needle biopsy provides a smaller specimen than open biopsy does.

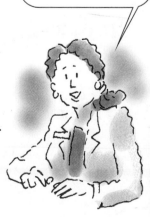

Pleural biopsy helps differentiate between nonmalignant and malignant disease. It also helps diagnose viral, fungal, parasitic, and collagen vascular disease.

Scoping out a Cope's needle

Used to obtain a pleural biopsy specimen, a Cope's needle consists of three parts: a sharp obturator (A) and a cannula (B) (that, fitted together, are called a *trocar),* and a blunt-ended, hooked stylet (C). The trocar is used to gain access to the pleural cavity. Then the obturator is re-moved, leaving the cannula in place. The stylet is passed through the cannula to excise a tissue specimen, as shown here.

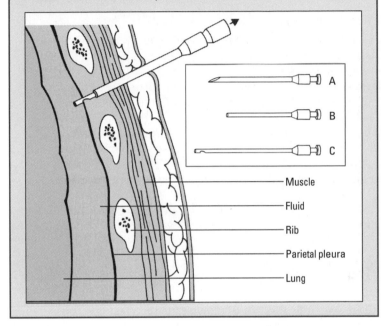

A

B

C

Muscle

Fluid

Rib

Parietal pleura

Lung

Open pleural biopsy, performed in the absence of pleural effu-sion, permits direct visualization of the pleura and the underlying lung. It's performed in the operating room. Microscopic examina-tion of the tissue specimen can reveal malignant disease, tubercu-losis, or viral, fungal, parasitic, or collagen vascular disease. Pri-mary tumors of the pleura are commonly fibrous and epithelial.

Nursing considerations

• Explain the procedure to the patient and tell him that it typically takes 30 to 45 minutes.
• Advise the patient that blood studies will be necessary before the biopsy and that chest X-rays will be taken before and after the biopsy.
• Make sure the patient has signed a consent form. Check the pa-tient's history for hypersensitivity to the local anesthetic. Just be-fore the procedure, record vital signs.

• Explain to the patient that he'll sit on the side of the bed with his feet resting on a stool and his arms supported by the overbed table or his upper body. If he can't sit up, place him in a side-lying position with the side to be biopsied facing up.

Specimen treatment

• The specimen is immediately put in a special solution in a labeled specimen bottle. Then the skin around the biopsy site is cleaned, and an adhesive bandage is applied.

Close attention

• After the biopsy, check the patient's vital signs every 15 minutes for 1 hour and then every hour for 4 hours or until his condition is stable.
• Make sure the chest X-ray is repeated immediately after the biopsy. Instruct the patient to lie on his unaffected side to promote healing of the biopsy site.
• Watch for signs of respiratory distress (shortness of breath), shoulder pain, and such other complications as pneumothorax (immediate) and pneumonia (delayed).
• Send the specimen to the laboratory immediately after collection.
• Pleural biopsy is contraindicated in patients with severe bleeding disorders.

Other diagnostic tests

Other diagnostic tests include pulmonary function tests (PFTs), pulse oximetry, and thoracentesis.

Pulmonary function tests

There are two types of PFTs: volume and capacity. These tests aid diagnosis in patients with suspected respiratory dysfunction. The doctor orders these tests to:
• evaluate ventilatory function through spirometric measurements
• determine the cause of dyspnea
• assess the effectiveness of medications, such as bronchodilators and steroids
• determine whether a respiratory abnormality stems from an obstructive or restrictive disease process
• evaluate the extent of dysfunction. (See *Interpreting PFTs*.)

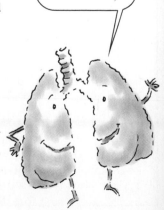

How do we do it? Volume, volume, volume!

Volume, volume, volume

Of the five pulmonary volume tests, tidal volume and expiratory reserve volume are measurements obtained through direct spirography. Minute volume, inspiratory reserve volume, and residual volume are calculated from the results of other pulmonary function tests.

Calculating capacity

Of the pulmonary capacity tests, functional residual capacity, total lung capacity, and maximal midexpiratory flow must be calculat-

---

Interpreting PFTs

This chart lists pulmonary function tests (PFTs) with definitions and implications for each.

Test	Implications
Tidal volume (V_T): amount of air inhaled or exhaled during normal breathing	Decreased V_T may indicate restrictive disease.
Minute volume (MV): total amount of air expired per minute	Normal MV can occur in emphysema; decreased MV may indicate other diseases such as pulmonary edema. Increased MV can occur with acidosis, increased carbon dioxide (CO_2), decreased partial pressure of arterial oxygen (Pao_2), exercise, and low-compliance states.
CO_2 response: increase or decrease in MV after breathing various CO_2 concentrations	Reduced CO_2 response may occur in emphysema, myxedema, obesity, hypoventilation syndrome, and sleep apnea.
Inspiratory reserve volume (IRV): amount of air inspired after normal inspiration	IRV decreases during normal exercise.
Expiratory reserve volume (ERV): amount of air exhaled after normal expiration	ERV decreases in obese people.
Residual volume (RV): amount of air remaining in the lungs after forced expiration	RV greater than 35% of total lung capacity (TLC) after maximal expiratory effort may indicate obstructive disease.
Vital capacity (VC): total volume of air that can be exhaled after maximum inspiration	Normal or increased VC with decreased flow rates may indicate a condition that reduces functional pulmonary tissue such as pulmonary edema. Decreased VC with normal or increased flow rates may indicate decreased respiratory effort resulting from neuromuscular disease, drug overdose, or head injury; decreased thoracic expansion; or limited movement of the diaphragm.
Inspiratory capacity (IC): amount of air that can be inhaled after normal expiration	Decreased IC indicates restrictive disease.

(continued)

Interpreting PFTs *(continued)*

Test	Implications
Thoracic gas volume (TGV): total volume of gas in lungs from both ventilated and non-ventilated airways	Increased TGV indicates air trapping.
Functional residual capacity (FRC): amount of air remaining in lungs after normal expiration	Increased FRC indicates lung overdistention.
TLC: total volume of lungs when maximally inflated	Low TLC indicates restrictive disease; high TLC indicates lung overdistention.
Forced vital capacity (FVC): measurement of the amount of air exhaled forcefully and quickly after maximum inspiration	Decreased FVC indicates flow resistance in the respiratory system from obstructive or restrictive disease.
Flow-volume curve (also called *flow-volume loop*): greatest rate of flow (V_{max}) during FVC maneuvers versus lung volume change	Decreased flow rates at all volumes during expiration indicate obstructive disease. A plateau of expiratory flow near TLC, a plateau of inspiratory flow at mid-VC, and a square wave pattern through most of VC indicate obstructive disease. Normal or increased peak expiratory flow, decreased flow with decreasing lung volumes, and markedly decreased VC indicate restrictive disease.
Forced expiratory volume (FEV): volume of air expired in the 1st, 2nd, and 3rd second of FVC maneuver	Decreased FEV_1 and increased FEV_2 and FEV_3 may indicate obstructive disease; decreased or normal FEV_1 may indicate restrictive disease.
Forced expiratory flow (FEF): average rate of flow during middle half of FVC	Low FEF (25% to 75%) indicates obstructive disease.
Peak expiratory flow rate (PEFR): V_{max} during forced expiration	Decreased PEFR may indicate a mechanical problem. PEFR is usually normal in restrictive disease but decreases in severe cases. Because PEFR is effort-dependent, it's also low in a person who has poor expiratory effort or one who doesn't understand the procedure.
Maximal voluntary ventilation (MVV) (also called *maximum breathing capacity* [MBC]): greatest volume of air breathed per unit of time	Decreased MVV may indicate obstructive disease; normal or decreased MVV may indicate restrictive disease.
Diffusing capacity for carbon monoxide (DLCO): milliliters of carbon monoxide diffused per minute across the alveolocapillary membrane	Decreased DLCO occurs in interstitial pulmonary diseases and emphysema.

ed. Vital capacity and inspiratory capacity may be measured directly or calculated indirectly. Direct spirographic measurements include forced vital capacity, forced expiratory volume, and maximal voluntary ventilation. The amount of carbon monoxide exhaled permits calculation of the diffusing capacity for carbon monoxide.

Nursing considerations

• Before pulmonary function testing, withhold all bronchodilators.
• For some tests, the patient will sit upright and wear a nose clip. For others, he may sit in a small, airtight box called a *body plethysmograph* without a noseclip. In this case, warn him that he may experience claustrophobia. Reassure him that he won't suffocate and that he'll be able to communicate with the technician through the window in the box.
• Explain that he may receive an aerosolized bronchodilator. Administration of the bronchodilator may be repeated in order to evaluate the drug's effectiveness.
• Emphasize that the test will proceed quickly if the patient follows directions, tries hard, and keeps a tight seal around the mouthpiece or tube to ensure accurate results.
• Instruct the patient to loosen tight clothing so he can breathe freely. Tell him he must not smoke or eat a large meal for 4 hours before the test.
• Keep in mind that anxiety can affect test accuracy. Also remember that medications, such as analgesics and bronchodilators, may produce misleading results. You may be asked to withhold bronchodilators and other respiratory treatments before the test. If the patient receives a bronchodilator during the test, don't give another dose for 4 hours.

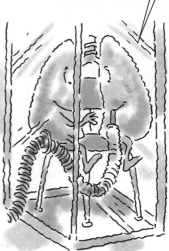

This box will help determine how I'm doing. Relax, release, breathe in, breathe out. I'm going to my happy place...

Pulse oximetry

Pulse oximetry is a continuous noninvasive study of arterial blood oxygen saturation using a clip or probe attached to a sensor site (usually an earlobe or a fingertip). The percentage expressed is the ratio of oxygen to hemoglobin. (See *Pulse oximetry levels*, page 68.)

Nursing considerations

• Explain to the patient that this test assesses the oxygen content in hemoglobin.
• Make sure the patient isn't wearing false fingernails or nail polish.

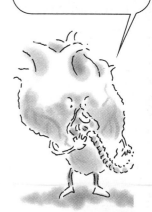

Pulse oximetry monitors oxygenation perioperatively, during an acute illness, and during testing for sleep apnea. It also helps determine bronchodilator effectiveness.

Pulse oximetry levels

Pulse oximetry may be intermittent or continuous, and is used to monitor arterial oxygen saturation. Normal oxygen saturation levels are 95% to 100% for adults and 94% to 100% for full-term neonates. Lower levels may indicate hypoxemia and warrant intervention.

Interfering factors

Certain factors can interfere with accuracy. For example, an elevated bilirubin level may falsely lower oxygen saturation readings, whereas elevated carboxyhemoglobin or methemoglobin levels can falsely elevate oxygen saturation readings.

Certain intravascular substances, such as lipid emulsions and dyes, may also affect readings. Other interfering factors include excessive light (such as from phototherapy or direct sunlight), excessive patient movement, excessive ear pigment, severe peripheral vascular disease, hypothermia, hypotension, and vasoconstriction.

In addition, anemic conditions, vasoconstriction, certain drugs (such as vasopressors), hypotension, vessel obstruction, nail polish or false nails, and lipid emulsions may interfere with test results.

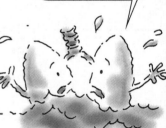

Thoracentesis is also known as *pleural fluid aspiration*. And, hey, I've got plenty of fluid right now. Take all you want!

• Place the probe or clip over the finger or other intended sensor site so that the light beams and sensors are opposite each other.
• Protect the transducer from exposure to strong light. Check the transducer site frequently to make sure the device is in place and examine the skin for abrasion and circulatory impairment.
• Rotate the transducer at least every 4 hours to avoid skin irritation.
• If oximetry has been performed properly, the oxygen saturation readings are usually within 2% of ABG values when saturations range between 84% and 98%.

Thoracentesis

Thoracentesis, also known as *pleural fluid aspiration*, is used to obtain a sample of pleural fluid for analysis, relieve lung compression and, occasionally, obtain a lung tissue biopsy specimen.

Getting serous

The pleural cavity should contain less than 20 ml of serous fluid. Pleural effusion results from the abnormal formation or reabsorption of pleural fluid. Certain characteristics classify pleural fluid as either a transudate or an exudate.

What it means

Pleural fluid may contain blood, chyle, or pus and necrotic tissue. A high percentage of neutrophils suggest septic inflammation. Pleural fluid glucose levels that are 30 to 40 mg/dl (SI, 1.5 to 2 mmol/L) lower than blood glucose levels may indicate cancer, bacterial infection, nonseptic inflammation, or metastasis. Increased amylase levels occur with pleural effusions associated

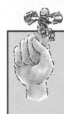

Memory jogger

To remember the difference between transudate and exudate, focus on the prefixes: trans- means "across," as in the transcontinental railroad, and ex- means "out of," as in exhale.

Characteristics of pulmonary transudate and exudate

These characteristics help classify pleural fluid as either a transudate or an exudate.

Characteristic	Transudate	Exudate
Appearance	Clear	Cloudy, turbid
Specific gravity	<1.016	>1.016
Clot (fibrinogen)	Absent	Present
Protein	<3 g/dl (SI, <30 g/L)	>3 g/dl (SI, >30 g/L)
White blood cells	Few lymphocytes	Many lymphocytes; may be purulent
Red blood cells	Few	Variable
Glucose level	Equal to serum level	May be less than serum level
Lactate dehydrogenase	Low	High

Pleural fluid analysis interference

Antimicrobial therapy before aspiration of fluid for culture may decrease the number of bacteria, making isolation of the infecting organism difficult.

with pancreatitis. (See *Characteristics of pulmonary transudate and exudate* and *Pleural fluid analysis interference*.)

Nursing considerations

• Check the patient's history for bleeding disorders, allergies to anesthetics, or anticoagulant therapy.
• Explain that a chest X-ray or ultrasound study may precede the test.
• Tell the patient that his vital signs will be taken and then the area around the needle insertion site will be shaved.

Here comes the burn

• Explain that the doctor will clean the needle insertion site with a cold antiseptic solution and then inject a local anesthetic. The patient may feel a burning sensation as the doctor injects the anesthetic.
• Explain to the patient that, after his skin is numb, the doctor will insert a needle. Tell him that he'll feel pressure during needle insertion and withdrawal and must remain still during the test to avoid the risk of lung injury. He should try to relax and breathe normally during the test and shouldn't cough, breathe deeply, or move. (See *Positioning the patient for thoracentesis*, page 70.)

Positioning the patient for thoracentesis

To prepare a patient for thoracentesis, place him in one of the three positions shown here. These positions serve to widen the intercostal spaces and permit easy access to the pleural cavity. Using pillows (as shown) will make the patient more comfortable.

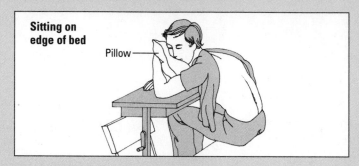

Sitting on edge of bed

Pillow

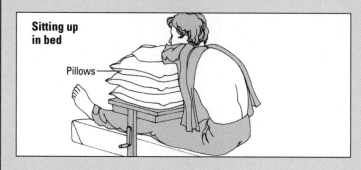

Sitting up in bed

Pillows

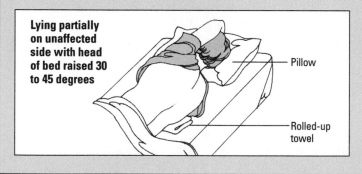

Lying partially on unaffected side with head of bed raised 30 to 45 degrees

Pillow

Rolled-up towel

Recognizing complications of thoracentesis

You can identify complications of thoracentesis by watching for characteristic signs and symptoms:

• *pneumothorax*—apprehension, increased restlessness, cyanosis, sudden breathlessness, tachycardia, chest pain
• *tension pneumothorax*—dyspnea, chest pain, tachycardia, hypotension, absent or diminished breath sounds on the affected side
• *subcutaneous emphysema*—local tissue swelling, crackling on palpation of site
• *infection*—fever, rapid pulse rate, pain
• *mediastinal shift*—labored breathing, cardiac arrhythmias, pulmonary edema.

•   A chest X-ray is usually performed after the procedure to rule out pneumothorax.
• Monitor vital signs every 30 minutes for 2 hours, then every 4 hours until they're stable.
• Watch for signs and symptoms of complications. (See *Recognizing complications of thoracentesis.*)

• Emphasize to the patient that he should tell the doctor if he experiences dyspnea, palpitations, wheezing, dizziness, weakness, or diaphoresis, because these symptoms may indicate respiratory distress. After withdrawing the needle, the doctor will apply slight pressure to the site and then an adhesive bandage.

• Tell the patient to report fluid or blood leakage from the needle insertion site as well as signs and symptoms of respiratory distress.

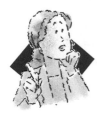

Quick quiz

1. When collecting a nasopharyngeal specimen, position the patient with his head tilted:

    A.   toward the right.

    B.   forward.

    C.   back.

    D.   toward the left.

Answer: C. Ask the patient to cough before you begin collecting the specimen; then position him with his head tilted back.

2. The usual method for collecting a sputum culture is:

    A.   tracheal suctioning.

    B.   expectoration.

    C.   bronchoscopy.

    D.   mediastinoscopy.

Answer: B. The usual method for sputum specimen collection is expectoration; other methods include tracheal suctioning and bronchoscopy.

3. During lung biopsy, monitor the patient for such complications as:

    A.   decreased pulse rate.

    B.   shoulder pain.

    C.   abdominal pain.

    D.   respiratory distress.

Answer: D. During a lung biopsy, monitor the patient for signs of respiratory distress, such as shortness of breath, elevated pulse rate, and cyanosis.

4. After a bronchoscopy that required a biopsy, you should instruct the patient to:

    A.   refrain from clearing his throat and coughing.

    B.   perform deep breathing every 4 hours.

    C.   resume his diet immediately.

    D.   restrict fluid for 24 hours.

Answer: A. The patient must refrain from clearing his throat and coughing because these actions could dislodge the clot at the biopsy site and cause hemorrhaging.

5. A patient's ABG analysis shows a pH less than 7.35, HCO_3^- greater than 26 mEq/L and a $Paco_2$ greater than 45 mm Hg. He's diaphoretic, has tachycardia, and is restless. The condition he probably has is:

    A.   respiratory alkalosis.

    B.   respiratory acidosis.

    C.   metabolic alkalosis.

    D.   metabolic acidosis.

Answer: B. The patient with respiratory acidosis can display all of these signs and symptoms and can also have a headache, confusion, apprehension, and a flushed face.

Scoring

☆☆☆ If you answered all five items correctly, way to go! You can breathe easy about your knowledge of respiratory disorders.

☆☆ If you answered four items correctly, super! Your understanding of respiratory disorders is circulating well!

☆ If you answered fewer than four items correctly, no worries! Take a deep breath, oxygenate those tissues, and review the chapter!

Treatment

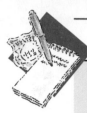

Just the facts

In this chapter, you'll learn:

♦ classes of drugs used to improve respiratory function

♦ surgical procedures used to treat respiratory disorders

♦ how to administer inhalation therapy

♦ how to perform chest physiotherapy.

Understanding respiratory treatments

Respiratory disorders interfere with airway clearance, breathing patterns, and gas exchange. If not corrected, they can adversely affect many other body systems and can be life threatening. Treatments for respiratory disorders include drug therapy, surgery, inhalation therapy, and chest physiotherapy.

Drug therapy

Drugs are used for airway management in patients with such disorders as acute respiratory failure, acute respiratory distress syndrome (ARDS), asthma, emphysema, and chronic bronchitis.

Breathe easy

Drugs used to improve respiratory function include:
- aerosol anti-infectives
- antitussives
- beta$_2$-adrenergic agonists
- corticosteroids
- decongestants
- expectorants
- leukotriene antagonists

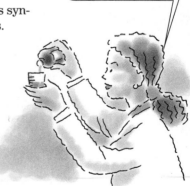

Drugs are used for airway management in patients with certain respiratory disorders.

- mast cell stabilizers
- mucolytics
- xanthines.

Aerosol anti-infectives

Aerosol inhalation provides direct, targeted, local airway delivery of anti-infectives with minimal systemic blood levels.

Go with the flow

Aerosol anti-infectives, especially antibiotics, should be administered with high flow-rate nebulizers that deliver flow rates of 10 to 12 L/minute. The four inhaled anti-infective agents now available are pentamidine (NebuPent), ribavirin (Virazole), tobramycin (TOBI), and zanamivir (Relenza).

Pentamidine to prevent PCP

Pentamidine is an antiprotozoal drug that's recommended as a second line agent for the prevention of *Pneumocystis carinii* pneumonia (PCP) in high-risk human immunodeficiency virus (HIV) infected patients with a history of one or more episodes of PCP or a CD4+ lymphocyte count of less than or equal to 200 μl.

It should be administered in isolation and by using an environmental containment system such as a negative pressure room. The nebulizer system should have one-way valves and scavenging filters that prevent or reduce environmental contamination.

Recommend ribavirin for RSV

Ribavirin is an antiviral drug that's recommended for use in treating respiratory syncytial virus (RSV) or in patients at risk for severe infection. RSV is a common seasonal respiratory infection that occurs in young infants and children. Adverse reactions include bronchospasm, skin rash, eyelid erythema, and conjunctivitis.

Treat with tobramycin

Tobramycin is used for patients with cystic fibrosis for the treatment of *Pseudomonas aeruginosa*. It should be administered after other therapies for cystic fibrosis such as other inhaled drugs.

Inhaled tobramycin should be administered under containment to prevent environmental saturation of the antibiotic into other hospital areas, which helps prevent the development of resistant organisms. Possible adverse reactions include auditory and vestibular damage (with the potential for deafness) and nephrotoxicity. Pregnant women should avoid inhalant exposure because of fetal harm resulting from aminoglycosides.

Influenza and zanamivir

Zanamivir is used in the treatment of cases of influenza in adults and adolescents age 12 or older who have been symptomatic for less than two years. Adverse reactions include diarrhea, vomiting, bronchitis, cough, sinusitis, dizziness, and headaches.

Nursing considerations

• Monitor the patient for bronchospasm and reduction of lung function, especially in patients with asthma or chronic obstructive pulmonary disease (COPD).
• Make sure that the patient understands the proper administration of the aerosol.
• Caution the patient to report possible adverse effects immediately.
• Advise the patient taking inhaled tobramycin that he should report any episodes of tinnitus, voice alteration, or changes in hearing.

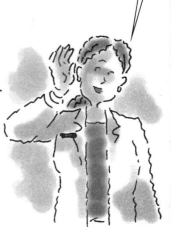

Tell the patient to report any changes in hearing.

Antitussives

Antitussive drugs suppress or inhibit coughing. They're administered orally as a liquid and are typically used to treat dry, nonproductive coughs. The major antitussives include:

 benzonatate (Tessalon Perles)

 codeine

 dextromethorphan (Benylin DM, Suppress, Trocal)

 hydrocodone.

Part of the act

Each of these antitussives acts in a slightly different way. Benzonatate acts by anesthetizing stretch receptors throughout the bronchi, alveoli, and pleura. Codeine, dextromethorphan, and hydrocodone suppress the cough reflex by direct action on the cough center in the medulla of the brain, thus lowering the cough threshold.

Serious use

The uses of these drugs are also slightly variable. However, each treats a serious, nonproductive cough that interferes with a patient's ability to rest or carry out activities of daily living.

Put to the test

In addition, benzonatate relieves coughs caused by pneumonia, bronchitis, the common cold, and chronic pulmonary diseases such as emphysema. It also can be used during bronchial diagnostic tests such as bronchoscopy when the patient must avoid coughing.

Beta$_2$-adrenergic agonists

Beta$_2$-adrenergic agonists are used for the treatment of symptoms associated with asthma and COPD.

Increase the amps

These agents increase levels of cyclic adenosine monophosphate through the stimulation of the beta$_2$-adrenergic receptors in the smooth muscle, resulting in bronchodilation. Inhaled agents are preferred because they act locally in the lung, resulting in fewer adverse effects than systemically absorbed formulations. Agents in this class may be short- or long-acting.

The short of it

The short-acting inhaled beta$_2$-adrenergic agonists, such as albuterol (Proventil) and pirbuterol (Maxair), are used for the fast relief of symptoms in asthmatic patients, including those with exercise-induced asthma. Used primarily on an as-needed basis, they're also effective for COPD; however, some COPD patients may use these agents around-the-clock on a specified schedule.

The long of it

A long-acting agent is best used in combination with anti-inflammatory agents—namely, inhaled corticosteroids—to help control asthma. To date, salmeterol (Serevent) is the only long-acting agent approved in the United States. Serevent is used for maintenance therapy and should be administered on a scheduled basis because its onset is prolonged.

Nursing considerations
• Caution the patient about possible adverse reactions, which may include tremors, nervousness, dizziness, headache, nausea, tachycardia, palpitations, electrocardiogram (ECG) changes, bronchospasm, and cough.

• Make sure that patients taking long-acting beta$_2$-adrenergic agonists know that they can't use them for acute symptoms because the drug's onset is delayed.
• Excessive use of a short-acting beta$_2$-adrenergic agonist may indicate poor asthma control, requiring reassessment of the patient's therapeutic regimen.

Corticosteroids

Corticosteroids are anti-inflammatory agents available in inhaled and systemic formulations for short- and long-term control of asthma symptoms. Many products with different potencies are available.

Reversing obstruction

Corticosteroids are the most effective agents available for the long-term treatment of patients with reversible airflow obstruction. They work by suppressing immune responses and reducing inflammation as well as preventing asthma exacerbations.

It's all in the system

Systemic formulations are commonly reserved for moderate to severe acute exacerbations but are also used in patients with severe asthma that's refractory to other measures.

Lowest and shortest

Systemic corticosteroids should be used at the lowest effective dose and for the shortest period of time possible in order to avoid adverse effects. Systemic drugs, such as dexamethasone (Decadron), methylprednisolone (Medrol), and prednisone, are given to manage an acute respiratory event, such as acute respiratory failure or exacerbation of COPD. These drugs are initially given by I.V. and, when the patient stabilizes, the dosage is tapered and oral dosing may be substituted.

Inhale!

To prevent future exacerbations, inhaled corticosteroids are the mainstay of therapy for most asthmatics with mild to severe disease. Use of inhaled corticosteroids reduces the need for systemic steroids in many patients, thus reducing the risk for serious long-term adverse effects.

Patients with asthma commonly use inhaled steroids, such as beclomethasone (Qvar), budesonide (Pulmicort Turbuhaler), flunisolide (AeroBid), fluticasone (Flovent), and triamcinolone (Azmacort). (See *Understanding corticosteroids*, page 78.)

Systemic drugs are given by I.V. at first, then tapered and delivered orally when the patient stabilizes.

Now I get it!

Understanding corticosteroids

Use this table to learn about the indications, adverse reactions, and practice pointers associated with corticosteroids.

Drug	Indications	Adverse reactions	Practice pointers
Systemic corticosteroids • Dexamethasone • Methylprednisolone • Prednisone	• Anti-inflammatory in acute respiratory failure, acute respiratory distress syndrome, and chronic obstructive pulmonary disease • Anti-inflammatory and immunosuppressor in asthma	• Heart failure, cardiac arrhythmias, edema, circulatory collapse, thromboembolism, pancreatitis, peptic ulcer	• Use cautiously in patients with recent myocardial infarction, hypertension, renal disease, and GI ulcer. • Monitor blood pressure and blood glucose levels.
Inhaled corticosteroids • Beclomethasone • Budesonide • Flunisolide • Fluticasone • Triamcinolone	• Long-term asthma control	• Hoarseness, dry mouth, wheezing, bronchospasm, oral candidiasis	• Do *not* use to treat an acute asthma attack. • Use a spacer to reduce adverse effects. • Rinse mouth after use to prevent oral fungal infection.

Nursing considerations

• To reduce the risk of adverse effects occurring with inhaled agents, use the lowest possible dose to maintain control.
• Advise the patient to rinse his mouth with water after each dose to prevent oropharyngeal fungal infection.
• Caution the patient that inhaled corticosteroids may cause hoarseness, throat and nose irritation, dry mouth, and headache or dizziness.
• Monitor the patient for serious adverse effects, which may include such respiratory symptoms as dyspnea, wheezing, and bronchospasm.

Decongestants

Decongestants may be classified as systemic or topical. Systemic decongestants activate the sympathetic division of the autonomic nervous system to reduce swelling of the respiratory tract's vascular network. Topical decongestants are powerful vasoconstrictors and provide immediate relief from nasal congestion and swollen mucous membranes when applied directly to the nasal mucosa.

Achoooo!

Systemic and topical decongestants are used to relieve the symptoms of swollen nasal membranes resulting from hay fever, allergic rhinitis, vasomotor rhinitis, acute coryza, sinusitis, and the common cold. Topical decongestants act directly on the alpha receptors of the vascular smooth muscle in the nose, causing the arterioles to constrict. As a result of this direct vasoconstriction, absorption of the drug becomes negligible.

Decongestants relieve symptoms of the common cold such as sneezing!

Nursing considerations

• Discourage the use of over-the-counter decongestants in a patient who's hypersensitive to other sympathomimetic amines. Such a patient may also be hypersensitive to decongestants.
• Monitor the patient's blood pressure, pulse, and ECG, as ordered, particularly noting hypertension and an irregular heartbeat or tachycardia.
• Take seizure precautions during decongestant therapy.
• Be aware that drugs the patient is taking may alter urine pH because alkaline urine increases renal tubular reabsorption of sympathomimetic amines.
• Don't administer a monoamine oxidase inhibitor, a beta-adrenergic blocker, methyldopa, reserpine, or guanethidine concomitantly with a topical decongestant.
• Warn the patient that transient burning and stinging of the nasal mucosa may occur during administration of the topical decongestant.
• Inspect the patient receiving a topical decongestant for signs of rebound nasal congestion such as red, swollen, boggy nasal mucosa. If rebound nasal congestion occurs, withhold the drug and notify the prescriber.
• Encourage the patient taking a decongestant to report difficulty urinating, which is especially common in patients with prostatic hypertrophy.

Expectorants

Expectorants thin mucus so it's cleared more easily out of airways. They also soothe mucous membranes in the respiratory tract and result in a more productive cough. The most commonly used oral expectorant is guaifenesin (Robitussin).

Less tension...more T.L.C.

By increasing production of respiratory tract fluids, expectorants reduce the thickness, adhesiveness, and surface tension of mucus, making it easier to clear from the airways. Expectorants also provide a soothing effect on mucous membranes of the respiratory tract.

Nursing considerations

• Caution the patient that the drug may produce vomiting if taken in doses larger than necessary for the expectorant action.
• Monitor the patient for dyspnea or ineffective cough. Keep suction equipment readily available during expectorant therapy.
• Teach the patient about the prescribed agent.
• Monitor the patient for adverse effects, such as diarrhea, drowsiness, nausea, vomiting, and abdominal pain.

Leukotriene receptor antagonists

The leukotriene receptor antagonists zafirlukast (Accolate) and montelukast (Singulair) are primarily used for the prevention and long-term control of mild asthma. They may also be used as steroid sparing agents in some patients.

Smooth and more permeable

Leukotrienes are substances released from mast cells, eosinophils, and basophils. They can result in smooth muscle contraction of the airways, increased permeability of the vasculature, increased secretions, and activation of other inflammatory mediators.

Two to subdue

There are two different mechanisms by which leukotriene is inhibited. The first is by blocking its action of binding to cellular receptors and the second is by inhibiting its production. The leukotriene receptor antagonists (zafirlukast and montelukast) are competitive inhibitors of leukotriene receptors, inhibiting leukotriene from interacting with its receptor, thereby blocking its action. Zileuton (Zyflo) inhibits the production leukotriene.

Nursing considerations

• Accolate's absorption is decreased by food; therefore, the dose should be given 1 hour before or 2 hours after meals.
• The most common adverse reactions experienced with this drug class are headache, abdominal pain, nausea, myalgia, and generalized pain. Elevated liver enzyme levels may also occur.

Give Accolate 1 hour before — or 2 hours after — meals.

• Zafirlukast is associated with airway edema, smooth muscle constriction, and altered cellular activity associated with the inflammatory process.
• Drugs aren't indicated for treatment of acute bronchospasm or for acute exacerbations of the disease.
• Drugs are used in conjunction with corticosteroids and other anti-asthma therapies.
• Zileuton should be used with caution when administered with theophylline and propranolol.
• Zileuton therapy should be continued during acute exacerbations of asthma.
• Patients with liver impairment may require a dosage adjustment if taking Accolate; the patient should be monitored closely for adverse effects, including liver enzyme levels.

Mast cell stabilizers

Mast cell stabilizers are used for the prevention of asthma attacks, particularly in pediatric patients and those with mild disease. They're administered in inhalation form.

Steady the mast, mate

The mechanism of these drugs isn't fully understood; however, these agents inhibit the release of inflammatory mediators by stabilizing the mast cell membrane, possibly through the inhibition of chloride channels. Because these agents control the inflammatory process, they're used for the prevention and long-term control of asthma symptoms. They're also useful for the prevention of exercise-induced asthma.

Adverse reactions may include irritation of the throat, bad taste in the mouth, cough, and nausea.

Nursing considerations

• These drugs shouldn't be used for an acute asthma attack.
• Mast cell stabilizers are used in conjunction with an inhaled beta$_2$-adrenergic agonist or inhaled corticosteroid.
• Reduce dosage gradually to the lowest effective dosage.
• Discontinue the drug if eosinophilic pneumonia or pulmonary infiltrates with eosinophilia occur.

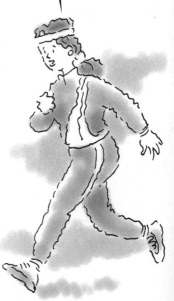

Mast cell stabilizers can help prevent exercise-induced asthma.

Mucolytics

Mucolytics are mucus-controlling agents that are administered by inhalation. They act directly on mucus, breaking down sticky, thick secretions so they're more easily eliminated.

An alteration is in order

The most commonly used mucolytic is acetylcysteine (Mucomyst). It decreases the thickness of respiratory tract secretions by altering the molecular composition of mucus and irritates the mucosa to stimulate clearance.

Send in the clones

Another type of mucolytic, called *dornase alpha* (Pulmozyme), is a genetically engineered clone of natural human pancreatic DNase enzyme. It's a proteolytic enzyme that can break down the deoxyribonucleic acid material found in purulent secretions. For this reason, it has been more effective than acetylcysteine in reducing the viscosity of infected mucous in cystic fibrosis.

In the thick of it

Mucolytics are used with other therapies to treat patients with abnormal or thick mucous secretions and may benefit patients with bronchitis, pulmonary complications related to cystic fibrosis, and atelectasis caused by mucous obstruction, which may occur in pneumonia, bronchiectasis, or chronic bronchitis. Mucolytics may also be used to prepare patients for bronchial studies.

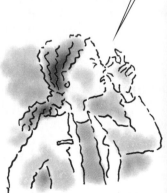

Phew! Remember to prepare the patient for the rotten-egg smell of mucolytics!

Nursing considerations

• Prepare the patient for the drug's "rotten-egg" smell, which may cause nausea.
• Administer acetylcysteine by way of a nebulizer. Because acetylcysteine reacts with iron, copper, and rubber, frequently monitor the patient's nebulizer equipment for reactive effects. The drug doesn't react with glass, plastic, aluminum, or stainless steel.
• Be prepared to administer a beta$_2$-adrenergic agonist by aerosol, as prescribed, if the patient experiences bronchospasm.
• Use 10% and 20% acetylcysteine solutions undiluted as prescribed. If further dilution is needed, use normal saline solution or sterile water for injection.
• Avoid contamination of the solution and refrigerate an opened vial. Discard opened vials after 96 hours.
• Assess the patient's respiratory status before and after administration of each dose, particularly noting any breathing difficulty, ineffective cough, or dyspnea. Follow acetylcysteine administration with chest physiotherapy and postural drainage, as prescribed, and encourage coughing and deep breathing to facilitate removal of respiratory secretions. Suction the patient as needed.

• Have the patient gargle after administration to relieve the unpleasant odor and dryness; wash the patient's face to eliminate stickiness caused by the drug.
• Monitor the patient closely for signs of stomatitis, such as swollen, tender gums that bleed easily; papulovesicular ulcers in the mouth and throat; malaise; irritability; and fever.

Xanthines

Xanthines, also called *methylxanthines*, (theophylline and derivatives) and adrenergics are used to dilate bronchial passages and reduce airway resistance, making it easier for the patient to breathe and allowing sufficient ventilation. They can be administered orally or inhaled.

Relax and breathe deeply

Xanthines decrease airway reactivity and relieve bronchospasm by relaxing bronchial smooth muscle. It's thought that theophylline inhibits phosphodiesterase resulting in smooth muscle relaxation in addition to decreased inflammatory mediators, such as mast cells, T cells, and eosinophils.

Stimulating conversation

In nonreversible obstructive airway disease (chronic bronchitis, emphysema, and apnea), xanthines appear to increase the sensitivity of the brain's respiratory center to carbon dioxide (CO_2) and stimulate respiratory drive.

Pumping you up

In chronic bronchitis and emphysema, these drugs decrease fatigue of the diaphragm, the respiratory muscle that separates the abdomen from the thoracic cavity. They also improve ventricular function and, therefore, the heart's pumping action.

Get in line

Theophylline is used as a second- or third-line agent for the long-term control and prevention of symptoms related to asthma, chronic bronchitis, and emphysema.

Theophylline levels need to be collected to evaluate efficacy and avoid toxicity. Levels must be assessed when a dose is initiated or changed and when drugs are added or removed from the patient's regimen.

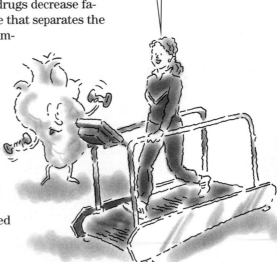

The heart really gets pumping after administration of xanthines!

Kids' korner

Theophylline level in a neonate

When theophylline is administered to a neonate, monitor serum theophylline and caffeine concentration levels because theophylline is metabolized to caffeine in the neonate.

Too much of a good thing

Especially high concentrations of theophylline may cause nausea, vomiting, diarrhea, and such central nervous system effects as irritability, insomnia, anxiety, headache, and seizures (with very high serum concentrations). Adverse effects may also include abdominal cramping, epigastric pain, anorexia, and diarrhea.

Nursing considerations

• Instruct the patient that smoking cigarettes or marijuana increases theophylline elimination, decreasing its serum concentration and effectiveness.
• Advise the patient that taking adrenergic stimulants or drinking beverages that contain caffeine may result in additive adverse reactions to theophylline or signs and symptoms of xanthine toxicity.
• Instruct the patient about possible adverse effects, including tachycardia and palpitations and to notify the doctor if they occur.
• Monitor the patient's serum theophylline concentration during treatment. (See *Theophylline level in a neonate.*)

> *Coffee, or other beverages that contain caffeine, may cause adverse reactions to theophylline.*

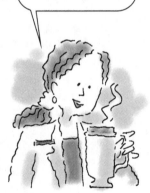

Inhalation therapy

Inhalation therapy employs carefully controlled ventilation techniques to help the patient maintain optimal ventilation in the event of respiratory failure. Techniques include:
• continuous positive airway pressure (CPAP)
• endotracheal (ET) intubation
• end-tidal carbon dioxide ($ETCO_2$) monitoring
• handheld oropharyngeal inhalers
• incentive spirometry
• mechanical ventilation
• nebulizer therapy
• oxygen therapy.

Continuous positive airway pressure

As its name suggests, CPAP ventilation maintains positive pressure in the airways throughout the patient's respiratory cycle. Originally delivered only with a ventilator, CPAP may now be delivered to intubated or nonintubated patients through an artificial airway, a mask, or nasal prongs by means of a ventilator or a separate high-flow generating system. (See *Using CPAP*.)

Goes with the flows

CPAP is available as a continuous-flow system and a demand system. In the continuous-flow system, an air-oxygen blend flows through a humidifier and a reservoir bag into a T-piece. In the demand system, a valve opens in response to the patient's inspiratory flow.

Other talents

In addition to treating ARDS, CPAP has been used successfully to treat pulmonary edema, pulmonary emboli, bronchiolitis, fat emboli, pneumonitis, viral pneumonia, and postoperative atelectasis. In mild to moderate cases of these disorders, CPAP provides an alternative to intubation and mechanical ventilation. It increases the functional residual capacity by distending collapsed alveoli, which improves the partial pressure of arterial oxygen (Pao_2) and decreases intrapulmonary shunting and oxygen consumption. It also

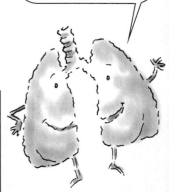

CPAP has successfully treated respiratory distress syndrome, pulmonary edema and emboli, bronchiolitis...and the list goes on. CPAP is my hero!

Using CPAP

The illustration below shows the continuous positive-airway pressure (CPAP) apparatus used to apply positive pressure to the airway to prevent obstruction during inspiration in patients with sleep apnea.

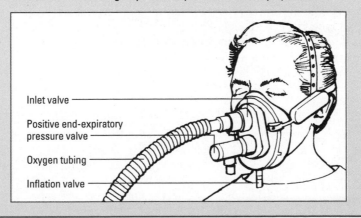

Inlet valve

Positive end-expiratory pressure valve

Oxygen tubing

Inflation valve

reduces the work of breathing. CPAP can also be used to help wean a patient from mechanical ventilation.

Through the nose

Nasal CPAP has proved successful for long-term treatment of obstructive sleep apnea. In this type of CPAP, high-flow compressed air is directed into a mask that covers only the patient's nose. The pressure supplied through the mask serves as a back-pressure splint, preventing the unstable upper airway from collapsing during inspiration.

Not so positive

CPAP may cause gastric distress if the patient swallows air during the treatment (most common when CPAP is delivered without intubation). The patient may feel claustrophobic. Because CPAP via a mask can also cause nausea and vomiting, it shouldn't be used in patients who are unresponsive or at risk for vomiting and aspiration. Rarely, CPAP causes barotrauma or lowers cardiac output.

Nursing considerations

• If the patient is intubated or has a tracheostomy, you can accomplish CPAP with a mechanical ventilator by adjusting the settings. Assess vital signs and breath sounds during CPAP.

• If CPAP is to be delivered through a mask, a respiratory therapist usually sets up the system and fits the mask. The mask should be transparent and lightweight, with a soft, pliable seal. A tight seal isn't required as long as pressure can be maintained. Obtain arterial blood gas (ABG) values and bedside pulmonary function studies to establish a baseline.

• Check for decreased cardiac output, which may result from increased intrathoracic pressure associated with CPAP.

• Watch closely for changes in respiratory rate and pattern. Uncoordinated breathing patterns may indicate severe respiratory muscle fatigue that can't be helped by CPAP. Report this to the doctor; the patient may need mechanical ventilation.

• Check the CPAP system for pressure fluctuations.

• Keep in mind that high airway pressures increase the risk of pneumothorax, so monitor for chest pain and decreased breath sounds.

• Use oximetry, if possible, to monitor oxygen saturation, especially when you remove the CPAP mask to provide routine care.

• If the patient is stable, remove his mask briefly every 2 to 4 hours to provide mouth and skin care along with fluids. Don't apply oils or lotions under the mask—they may react with the mask seal material. Increase the length of time the mask is off as the patient's ability to maintain oxygenation without CPAP improves.

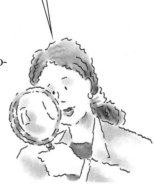

Watch closely for uncoordinated breathing patterns that may indicate severe respiratory muscle fatigue that can't be helped by CPAP.

• Check closely for air leaks around the mask near the eyes (an area difficult to seal); escaping air can dry the eyes, causing conjunctivitis or other problems.
• If the patient is using a nasal CPAP device for sleep apnea, observe for decreased snoring and mouth breathing while he sleeps. If these symptoms don't subside, notify the doctor; either the system is leaking or the pressure is inadequate.

Endotracheal intubation

ET intubation involves insertion of a tube into the lungs through the mouth or nose to establish a patent airway. It protects patients from aspiration by sealing off the trachea from the digestive tract and permits removal of tracheobronchial secretions in patients who can't cough effectively. ET intubation also provides a route for mechanical ventilation.

Conversation stopper

Drawbacks of ET intubation include that it bypasses normal respiratory defenses against infection, reduces cough effectiveness, may be uncomfortable, and prevents verbal communication.
Potential complications of ET intubation include:
• bronchospasm or laryngospasm
• aspiration of blood, secretions, or gastric contents
• tooth damage or loss
• injury to the lips, mouth, pharynx, or vocal cords
• hypoxemia (if attempts at intubation are prolonged or oxygen delivery is interrupted)
• tracheal stenosis, erosion, and necrosis
• cardiac arrhythmias.

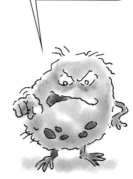

ET intubation bypasses normal respiratory defenses against infection. That's good news for me, but bad news for the patient!

Open up

In orotracheal intubation, the oral cavity is used as the route of insertion. It's preferred in emergency situations because it's easier and faster. However, maintaining exact tube placement is more difficult because the tube must be well secured to avoid kinking and prevent bronchial obstruction or accidental extubation. It's also uncomfortable for conscious patients because it stimulates salivation, coughing, and retching.

Not for everyone

Orotracheal intubation is contraindicated in patients with orofacial injuries, acute cervical spinal injury, and degenerative spinal disorders.

Advice from the experts

Understanding retrograde intubation

When a patient's airway can't be secured using conventional oral or nasal intubation, consider using retrograde intubation. In this technique, a wire inserted through the trachea and out the mouth is used to guide the insertion of an endotracheal (ET) tube (as shown here).

Who may do it

Only doctors, nurses, and paramedics who have been specially trained may perform retrograde intubation. However, the procedure has numerous advantages: It requires little or no head movement; it's less invasive than cricothyrotomy or tracheotomy and doesn't leave a permanent scar; and it doesn't require direct visualization of the vocal cords.

Who shouldn't undergo it

Retrograde intubation is contraindicated in patients with complete airway obstruction, a thyroid tumor, an enlarged thyroid gland that overlies the cricothyroid ligament, or coagulopathy and in those whose mouths can't open wide enough to allow the guide wire to be retrieved. Possible complications include minor bleeding and hematoma formation at the puncture site, subcutaneous emphysema, hoarseness, and bleeding into the trachea.

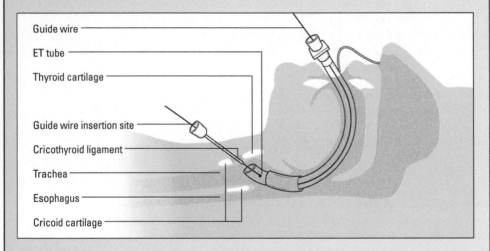

Guide wire
ET tube
Thyroid cartilage
Guide wire insertion site
Cricothyroid ligament
Trachea
Esophagus
Cricoid cartilage

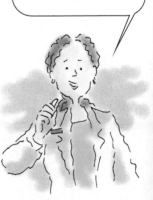

Nasal intubation is preferred when the patient can breathe spontaneously for a short period.

Follow my nose

In nasal intubation, a nasal passage is used as the route of insertion. Nasal intubation is preferred for elective insertion when the patient is capable of spontaneous ventilation for a short period.

A conscious choice

Nasal intubation is more comfortable than oral intubation and is typically used in conscious patients at risk for imminent respiratory arrest or those with cervical spine injuries. It's contraindicated in patients with facial or basilar skull fractures.

Difficult and damaging

Although it's more comfortable than oral intubation, nasal intubation is more difficult to perform. Because the tube passes blindly through the nasal cavity, it causes more tissue damage, increases the risk of infection by nasal bacteria being introduced into the trachea, and increases the risk of pressure necrosis of the nasal mucosa.

When neither orotracheal nor nasotracheal intubation is possible, consider the alternative of retrograde intubation. (See *Understanding retrograde intubation.*)

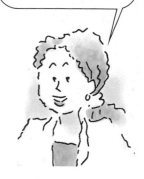

On the downside, nasal intubation is more difficult to do than oral intubation and causes more tissue damage.

Nursing considerations

- If possible, explain the procedure to the patient and his family.
- Obtain the correct size ET tube. The typical size for an oral ET tube is 7.5 mm (indicates the size of the lumen) for women and 8 mm for men.
- Administer medication as ordered to decrease respiratory secretions, induce amnesia or analgesia, and help calm and relax the conscious patient. Remove dentures and bridgework, if present.
- After securing the ET tube, reconfirm tube placement by noting bilateral breath sounds and ETCO_2 readings. (See *Securing an ET tube*, page 90.)
- Auscultate breath sounds and watch for chest movement to ensure correct tube placement and full lung ventilation.
- A chest X-ray may be ordered to confirm tube placement.
- Disposable ETCO_2 detectors are commonly used to confirm tube placement in emergency departments, postanesthesia care units, and critical care units that don't use continual ETCO_2 monitoring. Follow the manufacturer's instructions for proper use of the device. Don't use the detector with a heated humidifier or nebulizer because humidity, heat, and moisture can interfere with the device. (See *Analyzing carbon dioxide levels*, page 91.)
- Follow standard precautions, and suction through the ET tube as the patient's condition indicates, to clear secretions and prevent mucus plugs from obstructing the tube.
- After suctioning, hyperoxygenate the ventilated patient with a handheld resuscitation bag.
- If available, use a closed tracheal suctioning system, which permits the ventilated patient to remain on the ventilator during suctioning. (See *Closed tracheal suctioning*, page 92.)

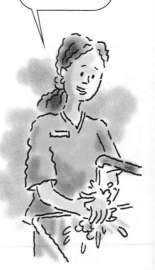

Remember to follow standard precautions when taking care of a patient's ET tube.

Advice from the experts

Securing an ET tube

Before taping an endotracheal (ET) tube in place, make sure the patient's face is clean, dry, and free from beard stubble. If possible, suction his mouth and dry the tube just before taping. Also, check the reference mark on the tube to ensure correct placement. After taping, always check for bilateral breath sounds to ensure that the tube hasn't been displaced by manipulation. To secure the tube, use one of the methods described below.

Method 1

Cut one piece of 1″ cloth adhesive tape long enough to wrap around the patient's head and overlap in front. Then cut an 8″ (20.3-cm) piece of tape and center it on the longer piece, with the sticky sides together. Next, cut a 5″ (12.7-cm) slit in each end of the longer tape (as shown below).

Apply benzoin tincture to the patient's cheeks and under his nose and lower lip. (Don't spray benzoin directly on his face; the vapors can be irritating if inhaled and can harm the eyes.)

Place the top half of one end of the tape under the patient's nose and wrap the lower half around the ET tube. Place the lower half of the other end of the tape along his lower lip, and wrap the top half around the tube (as shown below).

Method 2

ET tube holders are available that can help secure a tracheal tube.

Made of hard plastic or of softer materials, the tube holder is a convenient way to secure an ET tube in place. The tube holder is available in adult and pediatric sizes, and some models may come with bite blocks attached.

The strap is placed around the patient's neck and secured around the tube with Velcro fasteners (as shown below) . Because each model is different, check with the manufacturer's guidelines for correct placement and care.

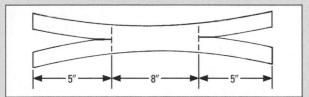

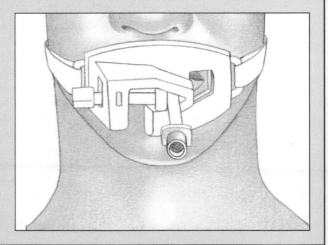

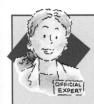

Advice from the experts

Analyzing carbon dioxide levels

Depending on which end-tidal carbon dioxide ($ETCO_2$) detector you use, the meaning of the color changes within the detector dome may differ. Here's a description of one type of detector, the Easy Cap detector, and what the color changes mean:

• The rim of the Easy Cap is divided into four segments—A, B, and C (clockwise from the right) and the CHECK segment at the top, which is solid purple, signifying the absence of carbon dioxide.

• The numbers in sections A, B, and C range from 0.03 to 5, indicating the percentage of exhaled carbon dioxide. The color should fluctuate during ventilation from purple (section A) during inspiration to yellow (section C) at the end of expira-

tion. This indicates that the $ETCO_2$ levels are adequate (above 2%).

• An end-expiratory color change from C to the B range may be the first sign of hemodynamic instability.

• During cardiopulmonary resuscitation (CPR), an end-expiratory color change from the A or B range to the C range may mean the return of spontaneous ventilation.

• During prolonged cardiac arrest, inadequate pulmonary perfusion leads to inadequate gas exchange. The patient exhales little or no carbon dioxide, so the color stays in the purple range even with proper intubation. Ineffective CPR also leads to inadequate pulmonary perfusion.

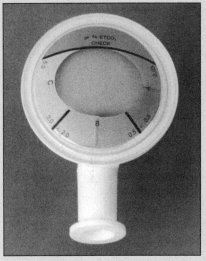

Color indications on detector dome

End-tidal carbon dioxide monitoring

$ETCO_2$ is used to measure the CO_2 concentration at end expiration. An $ETCO_2$ monitor may be a separate monitor or part of the patient's bedside hemodynamic monitoring system. (See *Understanding $ETCO_2$ monitoring*, page 93.)

Indications for $ETCO_2$ monitoring include:

• monitoring patency of the airway in acute airway obstruction and apnea and respiratory function

• detecting changes early in CO_2 production and elimination with hyperventilation therapy or in hypercapnia or hyperthermia

• assessing effectiveness of interventions, such as mechanical ventilation, neuromuscular blockade used with mechanical ventilation, and prone positioning.

In-lightened

In $ETCO_2$ monitoring, a photodetector measures the amount of infrared light absorbed by the airway during inspiration and expiration. (Light absorption increases along with the CO_2 concentra-

(Text continues on page 94.)

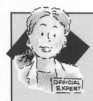

Advice from the experts

Closed tracheal suction

The closed tracheal suction system can ease removal of secretions and reduce patient complications. The system (shown below) permits the patient to remain connected to the ventilator during suctioning.

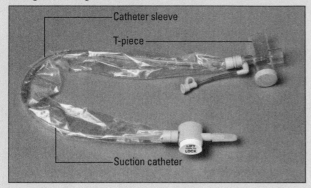

Catheter sleeve

T-piece

Suction catheter

As a result, the patient can maintain the tidal volume, oxygen concentration, and positive end-expiratory pressure delivered by the ventilator while being suctioned. In turn, this reduces the occurrence of suction-induced hypoxemia.

An advantage of this system is a reduced infection risk, even if the same catheter is re-used. The caregiver doesn't touch the catheter and the ventilator circuit remains closed.

Performing the procedure

Gather a closed suction control valve, a T-piece to connect the artificial airway to the ventilator breathing circuit, and a catheter sleeve that encloses the catheter and has connections at each end for the control valve and the T-piece. Then:
• Remove the closed suction system from its wrapping. Attach the control valve to the connecting tubing.
• Depress the thumb suction control valve, and keep it depressed while setting the suction pressure to the desired level.
• Connect the T-piece to the ventilator breathing circuit, making sure the irrigation port is closed; connect the T-piece to the patient's endotracheal or tracheostomy tube (shown above right).
• With one hand keeping the T-piece parallel to the patient's chin, use the thumb and index finger of the other hand to ad-

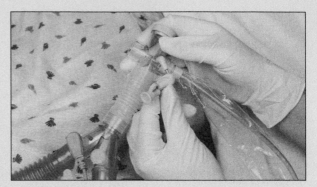

vance the catheter through the tube and into the patient's tracheobronchial tree (as shown below).
• If necessary, gently retract the catheter sleeve as you advance the catheter.

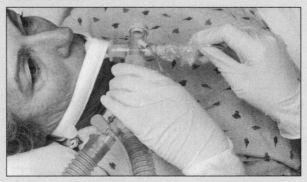

• While continuing to hold the T-piece and control valve, apply intermittent suction and withdraw the catheter until it reaches its fully extended length in the sleeve. Repeat as necessary.
• After suctioning, flush the catheter by maintaining suction while slowly introducing normal saline solution or sterile water into the irrigation port.
• Place the thumb control valve in the off position.
• Dispose of and replace the suction equipment and supplies according to your facility's policy.
• Change the closed suction system every 24 hours to minimize the risk of infection.

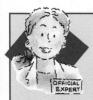

Advice from the experts

Understanding ETco$_2$ monitoring

In ETco$_2$ monitoring, the infrared light passes through the sample chamber and is absorbed in varying amounts, depending on the amount of CO$_2$ the patient just exhaled. The photodetector measures CO$_2$ content and relays this information to the microprocessor in the monitor, which displays the CO$_2$ value and waveform. (See illustration at right.)

Capnogram reading

The CO$_2$ waveform, or capnogram, produced in ETco$_2$ monitoring reflects the course of CO$_2$ elimination during exhalation. A normal capnogram (shown below) consists of several segments, which reflect the stages of exhalation and inhalation.

Normally, any gas eliminated from the airway during early exhalation is dead-space gas that hasn't undergone exchange at the alveolocapillary membrane. Measurements taken during this period contain no CO$_2$. As exhalation continues, CO$_2$ concentration increases sharply and rapidly. The sensor now detects gas that has undergone exchange, producing measurable quantities of CO$_2$.

The final stages of alveolar emptying occur during late exhalation. During the alveolar plateau phase, CO$_2$ concentration increases gradually because alveolar emptying is constant.

The point when the ETco$_2$ value is derived is the end of exhalation, when CO$_2$ concentration peaks. Yet, this value doesn't

accurately reflect alveolar CO$_2$ if no alveolar plateau is present. During inhalation, CO$_2$ concentration declines sharply to zero.

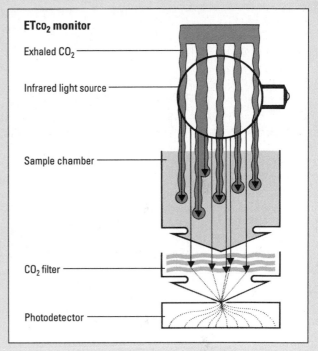

ETco$_2$ monitor

Exhaled CO$_2$

Infrared light source

Sample chamber

CO$_2$ filter

Photodetector

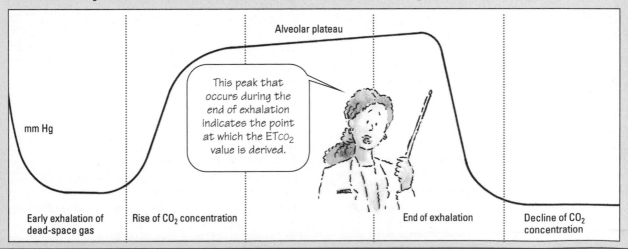

Alveolar plateau

mm Hg

This peak that occurs during the end of exhalation indicates the point at which the ETco$_2$ value is derived.

Early exhalation of dead-space gas

Rise of CO$_2$ concentration

End of exhalation

Decline of CO$_2$ concentration

tion.) The monitor converts these data to a CO_2 value and a corresponding waveform, or a capnogram if capnography is used.

Crunching the numbers

$ETco_2$ values are obtained by monitoring samples of expired gas from an ET tube or an oral or nasopharyngeal airway. Although the values are similar, the $ETco_2$ values are usually 2 to 5 mm Hg lower than the partial pressure of arterial carbon dioxide ($Paco_2$) value. In addition, $ETco_2$ monitoring reduces the need for frequent ABG sampling.

Nursing considerations

• Explain the procedure to the patient and his family.
• Assess the patient's respiratory status, vital signs, oxygen saturation, and $ETco_2$ readings.
• Observe waveform quality and trends of $ETco_2$ readings and observe for suddenly increased readings (which may indicate hypoventilation, partial airway obstruction, or respiratory depression from drugs) or decreased readings (due to complete airway obstruction, dislodged ET tube, or ventilator malfunction). Notify the doctor of a 10% increase or decrease in readings.

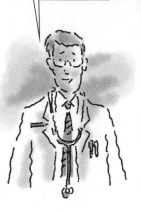

Notify the doctor if there's a 10% increase or decrease in $ETco_2$ readings.

Handheld oropharyngeal inhalers

Handheld oropharyngeal inhalers include the metered-dose inhaler (MDI), the turbo-inhaler, and the diskus. These devices deliver topical medications to the respiratory tract, producing local and systemic effects. The mucosal lining of the respiratory tract absorbs the inhalant almost immediately.

The use of these inhalers may be contraindicated in patients who can't form an airtight seal around the device and in patients who lack the coordination or clear vision necessary to assemble a turbo-inhaler. Specific inhalant drugs may also be contraindicated. For example, bronchodilators are contraindicated if the patient has tachycardia or a history of cardiac arrhythmias associated with tachycardia.

Common inhalants include:
• bronchodilators, used to improve airway patency and facilitate mucous drainage
• mucolytics, which attain a high local concentration to liquify tenacious bronchial secretions
• corticosteroids, used to decrease inflammation.

Compact, portable, and easy

MDIs are handheld inhalers that use air under pressure to produce a mist containing medication. Drugs delivered in this form, such as bronchodilators and mucolytics, can travel deep into the lungs. MDIs are portable, compact, and relatively easy to use. (See *Types of handheld inhalers*, page 96.)

> MDIs use air under pressure. Kind of like me... Whoa!

Keep us in suspense

The pressurized MDI canister contains a micronized powder form of a medication that is either dissolved or suspended in one or more liquid propellants along with oily, viscous substances called *surfactants* that are used to keep the drug suspended in the propellants. The surfactant also lubricates the valve mechanism of the MDI.

Go with the flow

In the past, MDIs required hand-breath coordination to successfully deliver the aerosol during the patient's inhalation. However, newer devices called *flow-triggered MDIs* eliminate the need for this hand-breath coordination. They automatically trigger the medication in response to the patient's inspiratory effort.

Give me more space

Inhalers with a special attachment called a *spacer provider* allow greater therapeutic benefit for children and patients with poor coordination. The spacer attachment, an extension to the inhaler's mouthpiece, provides more dead-air space for mixing medication.

Brummmm, brrummm

Other MDIs called *turbo-inhalers* administer dry powder medication without the use of propellants and also don't require hand-breath coordination. Used to dispense terbutaline (Brethine) or budesonide (Pulmicort), these inhalers are stocked with 200 doses of medication.

Let's do the twist

The patient holds the turbo-inhaler in the upright position and twists the lower ring to load the medication. He then exhales and places his mouth over the dispenser and inhales the medication. The dispenser has a dose counter so that the patient knows when he has 20 doses remaining.

Types of handheld inhalers

Handheld inhalers use air under pressure to produce a mist containing tiny droplets of medication. Drugs delivered in this form (such as mucolytics and bronchodilators) can travel deep into the lungs.

Metered-dose inhaler

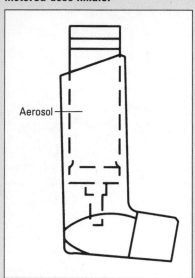

Aerosol

Turbo-inhaler

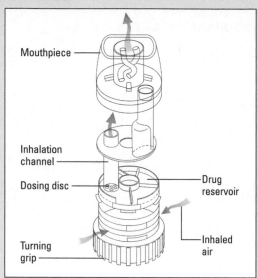

Mouthpiece

Inhalation channel

Dosing disc

Drug reservoir

Turning grip

Inhaled air

Inhaler with built-in spacer

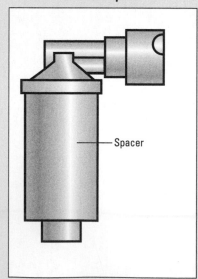

Spacer

Diskus dry powder inhaler

Strip lid peeled from pockets

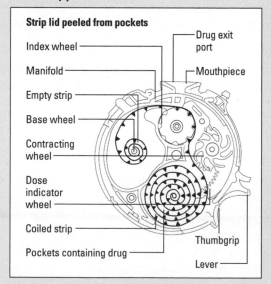

Index wheel

Manifold

Empty strip

Base wheel

Contracting wheel

Dose indicator wheel

Coiled strip

Pockets containing drug

Drug exit port

Mouthpiece

Thumbgrip

Lever

The diskus

Another device, called the *diskus*, incorporates a disk that contains 60 sealed pockets on an aluminum foil strip within the disk. A lever that the patient activates advances the strip. As the drug pocket reaches the mouthpiece, the cover is peeled away and the medication is dispensed and ready for inhalation.

Nursing considerations

• Instruct the patient how to use the device and encourage him to practice before actually using it to develop hand-breath coordination.
• Inform the patient of possible adverse reactions to each drug.
• Instruct the patient to rinse his mouth after drug administration to prevent stomatitis.
• If the patient is using a steroid inhaler along with a bronchodilator, instruct him to use the bronchodilator first, wait 5 minutes, and then use the steroid inhaler.
• Instruct the patient to exhale completely before using the inhaler. This increases his inspiratory effort allowing him better drug administration.
• Monitor the effectiveness of the medication.
• Assess the patient's ability to use the equipment correctly to ensure delivery of the proper dosage.
• Assess the patient's breath sounds before and after medication administration.

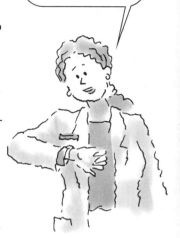

Tell the patient to use the steroid inhaler 5 minutes after the bronchodilator.

Incentive spirometry

Incentive spirometry involves using a breathing device to help the patient achieve maximal ventilation. The device measures respiratory flow or respiratory volume and induces the patient to take a deep breath and hold it for several seconds. This deep breath:
• increases lung volume
• boosts alveolar inflation
• promotes venous return.

This exercise also establishes alveolar hyperinflation for a longer time than is possible with a normal deep breath, thus preventing and reversing the alveolar collapse that causes atelectasis and pneumonitis.

What you see is what you get

Devices used for incentive spirometry provide a visual incentive to breathe deeply. Some are activated when the patient inhales a certain volume of air; the device then estimates the amount of air inhaled. Others contain plastic floats, which rise according to the amount of air the patient pulls through the device when he inhales.

The lows and highs

Patients at low risk for developing atelectasis may use a flow incentive spirometer. Patients at high risk may need a volume incentive spirometer, which measures lung inflation more precisely.

Incentive spirometry benefits the patient on prolonged bed rest, especially the postoperative patient who may regain his normal respiratory pattern slowly due to such predisposing factors as abdominal or thoracic surgery, advanced age, inactivity, obesity, smoking, and decreased ability to cough effectively and expel lung secretions.

Nursing considerations

• Explain the procedure to the patient, making sure that he understands the importance of performing incentive spirometry regularly to maintain alveolar inflation.
• Help the patient into a comfortable sitting or semi-Fowler's position to promote optimal lung expansion. If you're using a flow incentive spirometer and the patient is unable to assume or maintain this position, he can perform the procedure in any position as long as the device remains upright. Tilting a flow incentive spirometer decreases the effort required and, thus, the exercise's effectiveness.
• Auscultate the patient's lungs to provide a baseline for comparison with posttreatment auscultation.
• Instruct the patient to insert the mouthpiece and close his lips tightly around it because a weak seal may alter flow or volume readings.
• Instruct the patient to exhale normally and then to inhale as slowly and as deeply as possible. If he has difficulty with this step, tell him to suck as he would through a straw but slower. Ask the patient to retain the entire volume of air he inhaled for 3 seconds or, if you're using a device with a light indicator, until the light turns off. This deep breath creates sustained transpulmonary pressure near the end of inspiration and is sometimes called a *sustained maximal inspiration*.
• Tell the patient to remove the mouthpiece and exhale normally. Allow him to relax and take several normal breaths before attempting another breath with the spirometer. Repeat this sequence 5 to 10 times during every waking hour. Note tidal volumes.
• Evaluate the patient's ability to cough effectively, and encourage him to cough after each effort because deep lung inflation may

I'll use an incentive spirometer to record the volumes you achieve now, so we can compare later.

loosen secretions and facilitate their removal. Observe any expectorated secretions.
• Auscultate the patient's lungs and compare findings with the first auscultation.

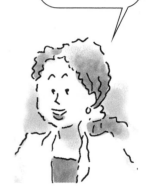

Mechanical ventilation corrects profoundly impaired ventilation.

Mechanical ventilation

Mechanical ventilation corrects profoundly impaired ventilation, evidenced by hypercapnia and symptoms of respiratory distress (such as nostril flaring, intercostal retractions, decreased blood pressure, and diaphoresis). It typically requires an ET or tracheostomy tube and delivers up to 100% room air under positive pressure or oxygen-enriched air in concentrations up to 100%.

Positive, negative, and high

The main types of mechanical ventilation systems are positive-pressure, negative-pressure, and high-frequency ventilation (HFV). Positive-pressure systems, the most commonly used, can be volume-cycled or pressure-cycled. During a cycled breath, inspiration ceases when a preset pressure or volume is met. Negative-pressure systems provide ventilation for patients who can't generate adequate inspiratory pressures. HFV systems provide high ventilation rates with low peak airway pressures, synchronized to the patient's own inspiratory efforts.

In control

Mechanical ventilators can be programmed to assist, control, or assist-control. In *assist* mode, the patient initiates inspiration and receives a preset tidal volume from the machine, which augments his ventilatory effort while letting him determine his own rate. In *control* mode, a ventilator delivers a set tidal volume at a prescribed rate, using predetermined inspiratory and expiratory times. This mode can fully regulate ventilation in a patient with paralysis or respiratory arrest. In *assist-control* mode, the patient initiates breathing and a backup control delivers a preset number of breaths at a set volume. (See *Ventilator modes*, page 100.)

SIMV helps condition respiratory muscles.

Synchronicity

In synchronized intermittent mandatory ventilation (SIMV), the ventilator delivers a set number of specific-volume breaths; however, the patient may breathe spontaneously between the SIMV breaths at volumes that differ from those on the machine. Commonly used as a weaning tool, SIMV may also be used for ventilation and helps to condition respiratory muscles.

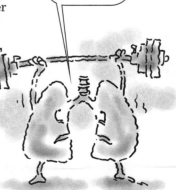

Advice from the experts

Ventilator modes

Positive pressure ventilators are categorized as volume or pressure ventilators and have various modes and options.

Volume modes

Volume modes include controlled ventilation (CV) or controlled mandatory ventilation (CMV), assist-control (A/C) or assisted mandatory ventilation (AMV), and intermittent mandatory ventilation (IMV) and synchronized intermittent mandatory ventilation (SIMV).

CV or CMV

In the CV or CMV mode, the ventilator supplies all ventilation for the patient. The respiratory rate, tidal volume (V_T), inspiratory time, and positive end expiratory pressure (PEEP) are preset. This mode is usually used when a patient can't initiate spontaneous breaths, such as when he's paralyzed from a spinal cord injury or neuromuscular disease or chemically paralyzed with neuromuscular blocking agents.

A/C or AMV

In the A/C or AMV mode, the basic respiratory rate is set along with the V_T, inspiratory time, and PEEP; however, the patient is allowed to breathe faster than the preset rate. The sensitivity is set so that when the patient initiates a spontaneous breath, a full V_T is delivered, so that all breaths are the same V_T, whether triggered by the patient or delivered at the set rate. If the patient tires and his drive to breathe is negated, the ventilator continues to deliver breaths at the preset rate.

IMV or SIMV

IMV and SIMV modes require preset respiratory rate, V_T, inspiratory time, sensitivity, and PEEP. Mandatory breaths are delivered at a set rate and V_T. In between the mandatory breaths, the patient can breathe spontaneously at his own rate and V_T. The V_T of these spontaneous breaths can vary because the breaths are determined by the patient's ability to generate negative pressure in his chest. With SIMV, the ventilator synchronizes the mandatory breaths with the patient's own inspirations.

Pressure modes

Pressure modes include pressure support ventilation (PSV), pressure controlled ventilation (PCV), and pressure-controlled/inverse ratio ventilation (PC/IRV).

PSV

The PSV mode augments inspiration for a spontaneously breathing patient. The inspiratory pressure level, PEEP, and sensitivity are preset. When the patient initiates a breath, the breath is delivered at the preset pressure level and is maintained throughout inspiration. The patient determines the V_T, respiratory rate, and inspiratory time.

PCV

In PCV mode, inspiratory pressure, inspiratory time, respiratory rate, and PEEP are preset. V_T varies with the patient's airway pressure and compliance.

PC/IVR

PC/IVR combines pressure-limited ventilation with an inverse ratio of inspiration to expiration. In this mode, the inspiratory pressure, respiratory rate, inspiratory time (1:1, 2:1, 3:1, or 4:1), and PEEP are preset. PCV and PC/IRV modes may be used in patients with acute respiratory distress syndrome.

Nursing considerations

• Set up a communication system with the patient (such as a letter board) and reassure him that a nurse will always be nearby. Keep in mind that an apprehensive patient may fight the machine, defeating its purpose.
• Obtain baseline vital signs and ABG readings.
• If the patient doesn't have an ET or tracheostomy tube in place, he may start on a noninvasive form of mechanical ventilation to

avoid intubation or tracheotomy. If more conservative measures fail, the patient may be intubated to establish an artificial airway.
• A bite block is commonly used with an oral ET tube to prevent the patient from biting the tube. Arrange for a chest X-ray after intubation to evaluate tube placement. Make sure he has a communication device and a call bell within reach.
• Check ABG levels as ordered. Overventilation may cause respiratory alkalosis from decreased CO_2 levels. Inadequate alveolar ventilation or atelectasis from an inappropriate tidal volume may cause respiratory acidosis.

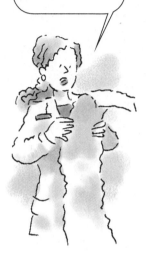

Check ABG levels as ordered to detect respiratory alkalosis or acidosis.

Follow, follow, follow

Perform these steps every 1 to 2 hours and as needed:
• Check all connections between the ventilator and the patient. Make sure critical alarms are turned on. Ensure that the patient can reach his call bell.
• Verify that ventilator settings are correct and that the ventilator is operating at those settings. (See *Understanding manual ventilation*, page 102.)
• Check the humidifier and refill it if necessary. Check the corrugated tubing for condensation; drain collected water into a container and discard. Don't drain condensation into the humidifier because it may be contaminated with bacteria. Also be careful not to drain condensation into the patient's airway.
• If ordered, give the patient several deep breaths (usually two or three) each hour by setting the sigh mechanism on the ventilator or by using a handheld resuscitation bag.
• Check oxygen concentration every 8 hours and ABG values whenever ventilator settings are changed. Assess respiratory status at least every 2 hours in the acute patient and every 4 hours in the stable chronic patient to detect the need for suctioning and to evaluate the response to treatment. Suction the patient as necessary, noting the amount, color, odor, and consistency of secretions. Auscultate for decreased breath sounds on the left side — an indication of tube slippage into the right mainstem bronchus.

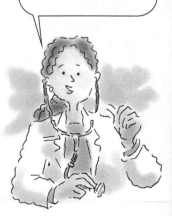

To detect tube slippage in a patient receiving mechanical ventilation, auscultate for decreased breath sounds on the left side of the chest.

Other steps

• Monitor the patient's fluid intake and output and his electrolyte balance. Weigh him as ordered.
• Using sterile technique, change the humidifier, nebulizer, and ventilator tubing according to facility protocol.
• Reposition the patient frequently, and perform chest physiotherapy as necessary.
• Provide emotional support to reduce stress, and give antacids and other medications as ordered, to reduce gastric acid production and to help prevent GI complications.
• Monitor for decreased bowel sounds and abdominal distention, which may indicate paralytic ileus.

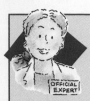

Advice from the experts

Understanding manual ventilation

A handheld resuscitation bag is an inflatable device that can be attached to a face mask or directly to a tracheostomy or an endotracheal (ET) tube to allow manual delivery of oxygen or room air to the lungs of a patient who can't breathe by himself.

Although usually used in an emergency, manual ventilation can also be performed while the patient is temporarily disconnected from a mechanical ventilator, such as during a tubing change, during transport, or before suctioning. In such instances, the use of the handheld resuscitation bag maintains ventilation. Oxygen administration with a resuscitation bag can help improve a compromised cardiorespiratory system.

Ventilation guidelines

To manually ventilate a patient with an ET or tracheostomy tube, follow these guidelines:
• If oxygen is readily available, connect the handheld resuscitation bag to the oxygen. Attach one end of the tubing to the bottom of the bag and the other end to the nipple adapter on the flowmeter of the oxygen source.
• Turn on the oxygen and adjust the flow rate according to the patient's condition.

• Before attaching the handheld resuscitation bag, suction the ET or tracheostomy tube to remove any secretions that may obstruct the airway.
• Remove the mask from the ventilation bag and attach the handheld resuscitation bag directly to the tube.
• Keeping your nondominant hand on the connection of the bag to the tube, exert downward pressure to seal the mask against his face. For an adult patient, use your dominant hand to compress the bag every 5 seconds to deliver approximately 1 L of air.

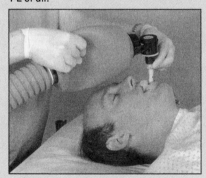

• Deliver breaths with the patient's own inspiratory effort if any is present. Don't attempt to deliver a breath as the patient exhales.

• Observe the patient's chest to ensure that it rises and falls with each compression. If ventilation fails to occur, check the connection and patency of the patient's airway; if necessary, reposition his head and suction.
• Be alert for possible underventilation, which commonly occurs because the handheld resuscitation bag is difficult to keep positioned while ensuring an open airway. In addition, the volume of air delivered to the patient varies with the type of bag used and the hand size of the person compressing the bag. An adult with a small- or medium-sized hand may not consistently deliver 1 L of air. For these reasons, have someone assist with the procedure if possible.
• Keep in mind that air is forced into the patient's stomach with manual ventilation, placing the patient at risk for aspiration of vomitus (possibly resulting in pneumonia) and gastric distention.
• Record the date and time of the procedure, the reason and length of time the patient was disconnected from mechanical ventilation and received manual ventilation, complications and the nursing action taken, and the patient's tolerance of the procedure.

• If the patient is receiving high-pressure ventilation, assess for signs of a pneumothorax (absent or diminished breath sounds on the affected side, acute chest pain and, possibly, tracheal deviation or subcutaneous or mediastinal emphysema).
• If he's receiving a high oxygen concentration, watch for signs of toxicity (substernal chest pain, increased coughing, tachypnea, decreased lung compliance and vital capacity, and decreased $Paco_2$ without a change in oxygen concentration).

Advice from the experts

Criteria for weaning

Successful weaning from a ventilator depends on the patient's ability to breathe independently. To meet this requirement, the patient must have a spontaneous respiratory effort that can maintain ventilation, a stable cardiovascular system (as evidenced by the absence of arrhythmias and hemodynamically stable vital signs), and sufficient respiratory muscle strength and level of consciousness to sustain spontaneous breathing.

Pulmonary function criteria
Pulmonary function criteria (that indicate a respiratory effort that can maintain ventilation) include:
• minute ventilation less than or equal to 10 L/minute, indicating that the patient is breathing at a stable rate with adequate tidal volume
• negative inspiratory force greater than or equal to –20 cm H_2O, indicating the patient's ability to initiate respirations independently
• maximum voluntary ventilation greater than or equal to twice the resting minute volume, indicating the patient's ability to sustain maximal respiratory effort
• tidal volume of 5 to 10 ml/kg, indicating the patient's ability to ventilate lungs adequately
• partial pressure of arterial oxygen (PaO_2) greater than or equal to 60 mm Hg (if the patient has chronic lung disease, 50 mm Hg or the ability to maintain baseline levels)
• partial pressure of arterial carbon dioxide ($PaCO_2$) less than or equal to 45 mm Hg (or normal for the patient)

• arterial pH ranging from 7.35 to 7.45 (or normal for the patient)
• fractional concentration of inspired oxygen less than or equal to 0.4.

Other criteria
Other criteria include:
• adequate natural airway or functioning tracheostomy
• ability to cough and mobilize secretions
• successful withdrawal of any neuromuscular blocker, such as pancuronium bromide or vecuronium
• clear or clearing chest X-ray
• absence of infection, acid-base or electrolyte imbalance, hyperglycemia, arrhythmia, renal failure, anemia, fever, and excessive fatigue.

After weaning
After being weaned, the patient should ultimately demonstrate:
• respiratory rate less than 24 breaths/minute
• heart rate and blood pressure within 15% of his baseline
• tidal volume of at least 3 to 5 ml/kg
• arterial pH greater than 7.35
• PaO_2 maintained at greater than 60 mm Hg
• $PaCO_2$ maintained at less then 45 mm Hg
• oxygen saturation maintained at greater than 90%
• absence of cardiac arrhythmias
• absence of accessory muscle use.

Have emergency equipment available in case there's a problem.

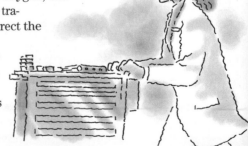

• Make sure that emergency equipment is readily available in case the ventilator malfunctions or the patient is accidentally extubated . If there's a problem with the ventilator, disconnect the patient from the ventilator and manually ventilate with 100% oxygen; use a handheld resuscitation bag connected to the ET or tracheostomy tube, troubleshoot the ventilator, and correct the problem.
• Successful weaning depends on a strong spontaneous respiratory effort, a stable cardiovascular system, and sufficient respiratory muscle strength and level of consciousness (LOC) to sustain spontaneous breathing. (See *Criteria for weaning*.)

No place like home

Home ventilator therapy

If the patient requires a ventilator at home, conduct thorough patient teaching with him and a family member. Be sure to include these points:

• Show him how to check the device and its settings for accuracy and the nebulizer and oxygen equipment for proper functioning. Tell him to do so at least once per day.

• Tell him to be sure to refill his humidifier as necessary.

• Explain that his arterial blood gas levels will be measured periodically to evaluate his therapy.

• Demonstrate how to count his pulse rate and tell him to report changes in rate or rhythm as well as chest pain, fever, dyspnea, or swollen extremities.

• Tell him to bring his ventilator with him if he needs to be treated for an acute problem because it may be possible to stabilize him without hospitalization. However, be sure to explain that, if hospitalization is required, he may not be able to use his own ventilator.

• Tell him to call his doctor or respiratory therapist if he has questions or problems.

• If the patient requires a ventilator at home, teach him and a family member how to care for the patient and the ventilator. (See *Home ventilator therapy.*)

Nebulizer therapy

An established component of respiratory care, nebulizer therapy aids bronchial hygiene by restoring and maintaining mucous blanket continuity; hydrating dried, retained secretions; promoting expectoration of secretions; humidifying inspired oxygen; and delivering medications. The therapy may be administered through nebulizers that have a large or small volume, are ultrasonic, or are placed inside ventilator tubing. (See *Comparing nebulizers.*)

It's electric!

Ultrasonic nebulizers are electrically driven. They use high-frequency vibrations to break up surface water into particles. The resultant dense mist can penetrate smaller airways and is useful for hydrating secretions and inducing a cough.

Comparing nebulizers

Nebulizer	Characteristics

Ultrasonic

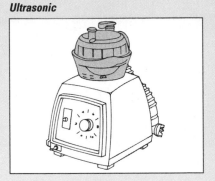

Uses high-frequency sound waves to create an aerosol mist

Advantages
- Provides 100% humidity
- About 20% of its particles reach the lower airways
- Loosens secretions

Disadvantages
- May cause bronchospasm in patients with asthma
- Increases risk of overhydration (in infants)

Large volume (Venturi jet)

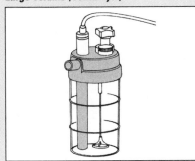

Works by passing air through a Venturi opening, drawing liquid up through feeding tubes, and nebulizing the solution

Advantages
- Provides 100% humidity with cool or heated devices
- Provides oxygen and aerosol therapy
- Can be used for long-term therapy

Disadvantages
- Increases the risk of bacterial growth (in reusable units)
- Causes a collection of condensate in large-bore tubing
- May cause mucosal irritation from breathing hot, dry air (if water level isn't maintained correctly in reservoir)
- Increases the risk of overhydration from mist (in infants)
- Uses a handheld device to deliver aerosolized medication

Small volume (Mini-nebulizer, Maxi-Mist)

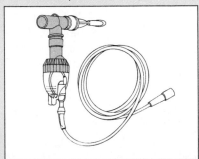

Handheld device that disperses a moisturizing agent medication into microscopic droplets and delivers it to the lungs with inhalation

Advantages
- Allows the patient to inhale and exhale on his own
- Can cause less air trapping than drug administered by intermittent positive-pressure breathing
- May be used with compressed air, oxygen, or compressor pump
- Allows for portability and disposability

Disadvantages
- Increases the time of the procedure if the patient needs your assistance
- Distributes medication unevenly if the patient doesn't breathe properly

It's not the heat, it's...

Large-volume nebulizers are used to provide humidity for an artificial airway such as a tracheostomy, and small-volume nebulizers are used to deliver medications such as bronchodilators. In-line nebulizers are used to deliver medications to patients who are being mechanically ventilated. In this case, the nebulizer is placed in the inspiratory side of the ventilatory circuit as close to the ET tube as possible.

Nursing considerations

• Explain the procedure to the patient.
• Take the patient's vital signs, and auscultate his lung fields to establish a baseline. If possible, place the patient in a sitting or high Fowler's position to encourage full lung expansion and promote aerosol dispersion. Encourage the patient to take slow, even breaths during the treatment.
• Before using an ultrasound nebulizer, administer an inhaled bronchodilator (MDI or small-volume nebulizer) to prevent bronchospasm.
• Check the patient frequently during the procedure to observe for adverse reactions. Watch for labored respirations because ultrasonic nebulizer therapy may hydrate retained secretions and obstruct airways. Take the patient's vital signs, and auscultate his lung fields.
• Encourage the patient to cough and expectorate, or suction as needed.
• Check the water level in a large-volume nebulizer at frequent intervals and refill or replace as indicated. When refilling a reusable container, discard the old water to prevent infection from bacterial or fungal growth, and refill the container to the indicator line with sterile distilled water.
• Change the nebulizer unit and tubing according to your facility's policy to prevent bacterial contamination.

Okay, now it's the heat...

• If the nebulizer is heated, tell the patient to report warmth, discomfort, or hot tubing because these may indicate a heater malfunction.
• Auscultate the patient's lungs to evaluate the effectiveness of therapy.
• Be especially careful when using an ultrasonic nebulizer in children; monitor their weight and note any changes. (See *Nebulizer therapy in children*.)

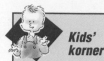

Kids' korner

Nebulizer therapy in children

When using high-output nebulizers, such as an ultrasonic nebulizer on pediatric patients or patients with a delicate fluid balance, be alert for signs of overhydration (exhibited by unexplained weight gain occurring over several days after the beginning of therapy), pulmonary edema, crackles, and electrolyte imbalance.

Young children may be frightened by the mask used to deliver the medication and may become fatigued from fighting. Because of this, they may appear worse after the medication has been dispensed. Allow the child time to calm down before assessing his breath sounds after the treatment.

• Nebulized particulates can irritate the mucosa in some patients and cause bronchospasm and dyspnea. Other complications include airway burns (when heating elements are used), infection from contaminated equipment (although rare), and adverse reactions from medications.

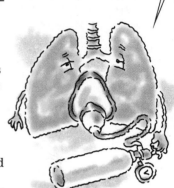

Oxygen therapy prevents or reverses hypoxemia and reduces the work of breathing. Thank you!

Oxygen therapy

In oxygen therapy, oxygen is delivered by mask, nasal prongs, nasal catheter, or transtracheal catheter to prevent or reverse hypoxemia and reduce the work of breathing. Possible causes of hypoxemia include emphysema, pneumonia, Guillain-Barré syndrome, heart failure, and myocardial infarction. (See *Oxygen delivery systems*, pages 108 and 109.)

Fully equipped

The equipment depends on the patient's age and condition and the required fraction of inspired oxygen (FIO_2). High-flow systems, such as a Venturi mask and ventilators, deliver a precisely controlled air-oxygen mixture. Low-flow systems, such as nasal prongs, a nasal catheter, a simple mask, a partial rebreather mask, and a nonrebreather mask, allow variation in the oxygen percentage delivered, based on the patient's respiratory pattern. Children and infants don't tolerate masks well. (See *Oxygen delivery in children*, page 110.)

Compare and contrast

Nasal catheters can deliver low-flow oxygen at somewhat higher concentrations, but aren't commonly used because of discomfort and drying of the mucous membranes. Masks deliver up to 100% oxygen concentrations but can't be used to deliver controlled oxygen concentrations. In addition, they may fit poorly, causing discomfort, and must be removed to eat.

Nasal prongs deliver oxygen at flow rates from 0.5 to 6 L/minute. Inexpensive and easy to use, the prongs permit talking, eating, and suctioning—interfering less with the patient's activities than other devices. However, the prongs may cause nasal drying and can't deliver high oxygen concentrations.

Transtracheal oxygen catheters, used for patients requiring chronic oxygen therapy, permit highly efficient oxygen delivery and increased mobility with portable oxygen systems and avoid the adverse effects of nasal delivery systems. However, they may

Oxygen delivery systems

Patients may receive oxygen through one of several administration systems, including a nasal cannula, simple mask, partial re-breather mask, nonrebreather mask, Venturi mask, CPAP mask, aerosols, and transtracheal oxygen.

Nasal cannula

Oxygen is delivered in concentrations of less than 40% through a plastic cannula in the patient's nostrils.

Simple mask

Oxygen flows through an entry port at the bottom of the mask and exits through large holes on the sides of the mask. It delivers oxygen in concentrations of 40% to 60%.

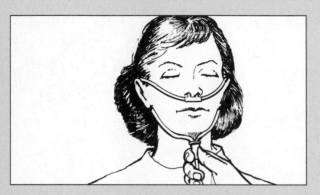

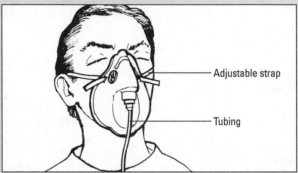

Partial rebreather mask

The patient inspires oxygen from a reservoir bag along with at-mospheric air and oxygen from the mask. The first third of ex-haled tidal volume enters the bag; the rest exits the mask. Be-cause air entering the reservoir bag comes from the trachea and bronchi where no gas exchange occurs, the patient re-breathes the oxygenated air he just exhaled. Oxygen can be ad-ministered in concentrations of 40% to 60%.

Nonrebreather mask

On inhalation, the one-way inspiratory valve opens, directing oxygen from a reservoir bag into the mask. On exhalation, gas exits the mask through the one-way expiratory valves and en-ters the atmosphere. The patient breathes air only from the bag. It delivers the highest possible oxygen concentration (60% to 90%), short of intubation and mechanical ventilation.

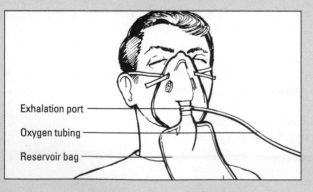

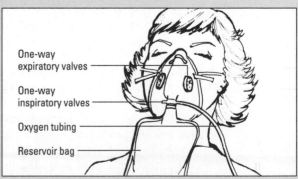

Oxygen delivery systems *(continued)*

Venturi mask

The mask is connected to a Venturi device, which mixes a specific volume of air and oxygen. It delivers highly accurate oxygen concentration despite the patient's respiratory pattern.

CPAP mask

This system allows the spontaneously breathing patient to receive continuous positive airway pressure (CPAP) with or without an artificial airway.

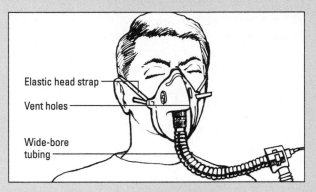

Elastic head strap
Vent holes
Wide-bore tubing

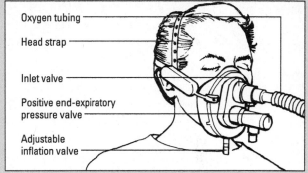

Oxygen tubing
Head strap
Inlet valve
Positive end-expiratory pressure valve
Adjustable inflation valve

Aerosols

A face mask, hood, tent, or tracheostomy tube or collar is connected to wide-bore tubing that receives aerosolized oxygen from a jet nebulizer. It delivers high-humidity oxygen.

Transtracheal oxygen

The patient receives oxygen through a catheter inserted into the base of his neck in a simple outpatient procedure.

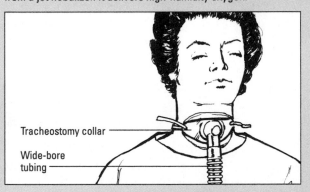

Tracheostomy collar
Wide-bore tubing

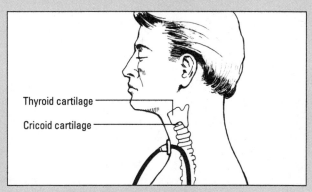

Thyroid cartilage
Cricoid cartilage

become a source of infection and require close monitoring and follow-up after insertion as well as daily maintenance care.

Nursing considerations

• Instruct the patient, his roommates, and visitors not to use improperly grounded radios, televisions, electric razors, or other

Kids' korner

Oxygen delivery in children

Oxygen delivery to children can be accomplished using an oxygen hood, nasal cannula or prongs, or a mist tent.

Oxygen hood

Oxygen delivery to an infant is best tolerated by administering it through an oxygen hood, as shown below.

   High as well as low concentrations of oxygen can be delivered by an oxygen hood. Remember not to allow the oxygen to flow directly on the infant's face. This cold stimulation can trigger the diving reflex, which results in bradycardia and shunting of blood to the central circulation. Older infants and children can also use a nasal cannula or nasal prongs.

Mist tent

For children beyond infancy, an oxygen tent or mist tent, shown below, is another option. The drawback is that the concentration of the oxygen within the tent is very difficult to regulate and hard to control.

   Remember to remove all toys that may produce a spark, including those that are battery-operated. Oxygen supports combustion, and the smallest spark can cause a fire.

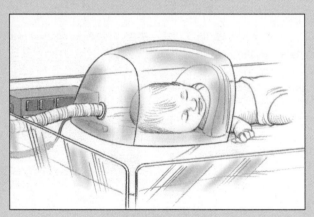

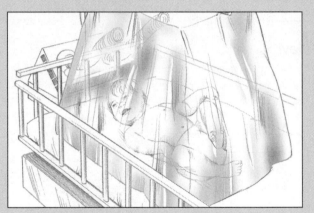

equipment. Place an OXYGEN PRECAUTIONS sign on the outside of the patient's door.
- Perform a cardiopulmonary assessment, and check that baseline ABG or oximetry values have been obtained.
- Check the patency of the patient's nostrils (he may need a mask if they're blocked). Consult the doctor if a change in administration route is necessary.
- Assemble the equipment, check the connections, and turn on the oxygen source. Make sure the humidifier bubbles and oxygen flows through the prongs, catheter, or mask.
- Set the flow rate as ordered. If necessary, have the respiratory care practitioner check the flowmeter for accuracy.
- Periodically perform a cardiopulmonary assessment on the patient receiving any form of oxygen therapy.

No place like home

Home oxygen therapy

If your patient will receive oxygen therapy after discharge, make sure he's familiar with the types of oxygen therapy, the services available, and the service schedules offered by local home suppliers. Together with the doctor and patient, help choose the device that's best suited to the patient.

If the patient receives transtracheal oxygen therapy, teach him how to clean the catheter. Advise him to keep the skin around the insertion site clean and dry to prevent infection.

Safety and supplies

No matter which device the patient uses, you'll need to evaluate his and his caregivers' ability and motivation to administer oxygen therapy at home. Make sure they understand the reason he's receiving oxygen and the safety issues involved. Teach them how to properly use and clean the equipment.

Paperwork points

If the patient will be discharged with oxygen for the first time, make sure his health insurance covers home oxygen. If it doesn't, find out what criteria he must meet to obtain coverage. Without a third-party payer, he may not be able to afford home oxygen therapy.

To every thing turn, turn, turn

- If the patient is on bed rest, change his position frequently to ensure adequate ventilation and circulation.
- Provide good skin care to prevent irritation and breakdown caused by the tubing, prongs, or mask. (See *Home oxygen therapy.*)
- Be sure to humidify oxygen flow exceeding 3 L/minute to help prevent drying of mucous membranes. However, humidity isn't added with a Venturi mask because water can block the jets.
- Assess for signs of hypoxia, including decreased LOC, tachycardia, arrhythmias, diaphoresis, restlessness, altered blood pressure or respiratory rate, clammy skin, and cyanosis. If these occur, notify the doctor, obtain a pulse oximetry reading, and check the oxygen delivery equipment to see if it's malfunctioning. Be especially alert for changes in respiratory status when you change or discontinue oxygen therapy.

Check those valves

- If your patient is using a nonrebreather mask, periodically check the valves to see if they're functioning properly. If the valves stick closed, the patient is re-inhaling CO_2 and not receiving adequate oxygen. Replace the mask if necessary.
- If the patient receives high oxygen concentrations (exceeding 50%) for more than 24 hours, ask about symptoms of oxygen toxicity, such as burning, substernal chest pain, dyspnea, and dry cough. Atelectasis and pulmonary edema may also occur.

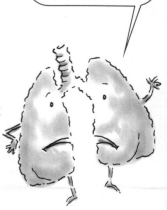

If the valves of the nonrebreather mask stick, I get more carbon dioxide instead of the oxygen I need.

Take a deep breath and cough

- Encourage coughing and deep breathing to help prevent atelectasis. Monitor ABG levels frequently and reduce oxygen concentrations as soon as ABG values indicate this is feasible.
- Use a low flow rate if your patient has chronic pulmonary disease. However, don't use a simple face mask because low flow rates won't flush CO_2 from the mask, and the patient will rebreathe CO_2. Watch for alterations in LOC, heart rate, and respiratory rate.

Go home with the flow

- If the patient needs oxygen at home, the doctor will order the flow rate, the number of hours per day to use it, and the conditions of use. Several types of delivery systems are available, including a tank, concentrator, and liquid oxygen system. The chosen system depends on the patient's needs and the availability and cost of each system. Make sure the patient can use the prescribed system safely and effectively. He'll need follow-up care to evaluate his response to therapy.

Surgery

If drugs or other therapeutic approaches fail to maintain airway patency and protect healthy tissues from disease, surgical intervention may be necessary. Respiratory surgeries include:
- chest tube insertion
- lung transplant
- thoracotomy
- tracheotomy.

Chest tube insertion

A chest tube may be required to help treat pneumothorax, hemothorax, empyema, pleural effusion, or chylothorax. Inserted into the pleural space, the tube allows blood, fluid, pus, or air to drain and allows the lung to reinflate. (See *Chest tubes in children.*)

In pneumothorax, the tube restores negative pressure to the pleural space through an underwater-seal drainage system. The water in the system prevents air from being sucked back into the pleural space during inspiration. If a leak occurs through the bronchi and can't be sealed, suction applied to the underwater-seal system removes air from the pleural space faster than it can collect.

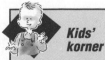

Closed chest-drainage system

One-piece, disposable plastic drainage systems, such as the Pleur-evac (shown right), contain three chambers. The drainage chamber is on the right and has three calibrated columns that display the amount of drainage collected. When the first column fills, drainage carries over into the second and, when that fills, into the third. The water-seal chamber is located in the center. The suction-control chamber on the left is filled with water to achieve various suction levels. Rubber diaphragms are provided at the rear of the device to change the water level or remove samples of drainage. A positive-pressure relief valve at the top of the water-seal chamber vents excess pressure into the atmosphere, preventing pressure buildup.

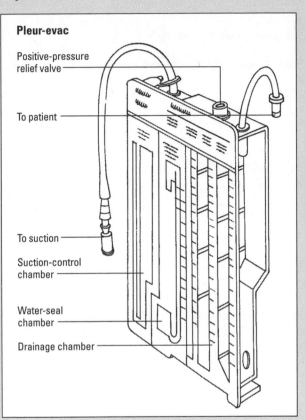

Pleur-evac

Positive-pressure relief valve

To patient

To suction

Suction-control chamber

Water-seal chamber

Drainage chamber

Chest tubes in children

In a child, chest tube drainage greater than 3 ml/kg/hour for 3 hours or longer is considered excessive drainage. Such drainage may indicate hemorrhage and is more likely to occur in the postoperative phase. Notify the doctor immediately as cardiac tamponade may develop from hemorrhaging and could result in death.

The chest tube is typically placed in the sixth or seventh intercoastal space, in the auxillary region. An underwater system is usually used. The water in the system prevents air from being pulled back into the pleural space during inspiration. (See *Closed chest-drainage system.*)

Nursing considerations

• If time permits, the doctor will obtain a signed consent form after explaining the procedure. Reassure the patient that chest tube insertion will help him breathe more easily.
• Obtain baseline vital signs and administer a sedative as ordered.
• Collect necessary equipment, including a thoracotomy tray and an underwater-seal drainage system. Prepare lidocaine (Xylo-

Advice from the experts

Combating tension pneumothorax

A tension pneumothorax, the entrapment of air within the pleural space, can be fatal without prompt treatment.

What causes it?

An obstructed or dislodged chest tube is a common cause of tension pneumothorax. Other causes include blunt chest trauma or high-pressure mechanical ventilation. In such cases, increased positive pressure within the patient's chest cavity compresses the affected lung and the mediastinum, shifting them toward the opposite lung. This impairs venous return and cardiac output and may cause the lung to collapse.

Telltale signs

Suspect tension pneumothorax if the patient develops dyspnea, chest pain, an irritating cough, vertigo, syncope, or anxiety after a blunt chest trauma or if the patient has a chest tube in place. Is his skin cold, pale, and clammy? Are his respiratory and pulse rates unusually rapid? Does the patient have equal bilateral chest expansion?

If you note these signs and symptoms, palpate his neck, face, and chest wall for subcutaneous emphysema and palpate his trachea for deviation from midline. Auscultate the lungs for decreased or absent breath sounds on one side. Then percuss them for hyperresonance. If you suspect tension pneumothorax, immediately notify the doctor and help identify the cause.

caine) for local anesthesia as directed. The doctor will clean the insertion site with povidone-iodine solution. Set up the underwater-seal drainage system according to the manufacturer's instructions and place it at the bedside, below the patient's chest level. Stabilize the unit to avoid knocking it over.

• When the patient's chest tube is stabilized, instruct him to take several deep breaths to inflate his lungs fully and help push pleural air out through the tube.

• Obtain vital signs immediately after tube insertion and every 15 minutes thereafter, according to facility policy (for about 1 hour).

• Routinely assess chest-tube function. Describe and record the amount of drainage on the intake and output sheet.

• Ensure all connections in the sysem are tightly secured with tape over the insertion site. Never clamp the chest tube, especially if you see air bubbles in the water-seal chamber.

• Add water to the suction system when necessary. Monitor changes in suction pressure.

• After most of the air has been removed, the drainage system should bubble only during forced expiration unless the patient has a bronchopleural fistula. Constant bubbling in the system may indicate that a connection is loose or that the tube has advanced slightly out of the patient's chest. Promptly correct any loose connections to prevent complications. (See *Chest tube dislodgement.*)

• Change the dressing daily (or per facility policy) to clean the site and remove drainage.

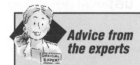

Advice from the experts

Chest tube dislodgment

If a chest tube becomes dislodged, cover the opening immediately with petroleum gauze; apply pressure to prevent negative inspiratory pressure from sucking air into the patient's chest.

Call the doctor and have an assistant obtain the necessary equipment for tube reinsertion while you continue applying pressure.

• Reassure the patient and monitor him closely for signs of tension pneumothorax. (See *Combating tension pneumothorax.*)
• The doctor will remove the patient's chest tube after the lung is fully reexpanded. As soon as the tube is removed, apply an airtight, sterile petroleum dressing.
• Typically, a patient is discharged with a chest tube only if it's used to drain a loculated empyema, which doesn't require an underwater-seal drainage system.

Lung transplantation

Lung transplantation involves the replacement of one or both lungs with that from a donor. Cystic fibrosis is the most common underlying disease that necessitates lung transplantation; others include bronchopulmonary dysplasia, pulmonary hypertension, and pulmonary fibrosis.

In some cases, only one lobe may be involved in transplantation. Single lung transplantation is considered for patients with end-stage COPD. Typically, the patient has a life expectancy of less than 2 years. One-year survival rates after transplantation range from 75% to 85%, decreasing to 50% after 5 years.

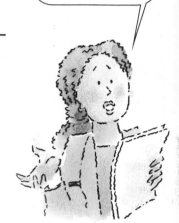

Before lung transplantation, your patient must meet specific criteria.

Must-haves

To be a candidate for lung transplantation, a patient must:
• have forced vital capacity less than 40%
• have forced expiratory volume less than 30% of predicted value
• have PaO_2 less than 60 mm Hg on room air at rest
• exhibit evidence of major pulmonary complications
• demonstrate increased antibiotic resistance.

Not gonna happen

In addition to relative contraindications, which include symptomatic osteoporosis, lung transplantation is absolutely contraindicated in cases of:
• major organ dysfunction, especially involving the renal or cardiovascular system
• HIV infection
• active malignancy
• hepatitis C with positive biopsy for liver damage
• progressive neuromuscular disease.

Pass me by!

Cardiopulmonary bypass is common during lung transplantation.

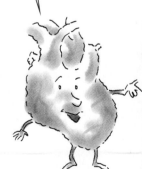
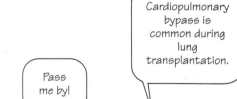

TKO for transplant

Lung transplantation is performed under general anesthesia. Bilateral anterior thoracotomy incisions and a transverse sternotomy provide access to the thoracic cavity. After removal of the patient's lungs, the donor lungs are implanted with anastomoses to the same areas as for a single lung transplant. Cardiopulmonary bypass is commonly used during the transplantation procedure.

Major snags

The major complication after lung transplantation is organ rejection, which occurs because the recipient's body responds to the implanted tissue as a foreign body and triggers an immune response. This leads to fibrosis and scar formation.

Secondary snags

Another major complication after lung transplantation is infection due to immunosuppressive therapy. Other possible complications include hemorrhage and reperfusion edema. Long-term complications (typically occurring after 3 years) include obliterative bronchiolitis and posttransplant lymphoproliferative disorder. Either may be fatal.

Nursing considerations

• Answer all questions about the transplant procedure and what the patient can expect. Explain postoperative care (intubation, for example), equipment used in the acute postoperative phase, and availability of analgesics for pain.
• Administer medications and obtain laboratory testing as ordered.
• Assess cardiopulmonary status frequently (every 5 to 15 minutes in the immediate postoperative period) until the patient is stabilized. Be alert for cardiac index less than 2.2, hypotension, fever higher than 99.5° F (37.5° C), crackles or rhonchi, and decreased oxygen saturation.

Keep on assessing

• Assess respiratory status and ventilatory equipment frequently and suction secretions as necessary. Expect frequent ABG analyses and daily chest X-rays to evaluate the patient's readiness to be weaned from the ventilator.
• Assess chest-tube drainage for amount, color, and characteristics. Assess for bleeding. Notify the doctor according to the hospital's and surgeon's parameters for normal drainage.

What goes in and out

• Closely monitor fluid intake and output. If the patient becomes hemodynamically unstable, administer vasoactive and inotropic agents as ordered and titrate the dose to achieve the desired response.

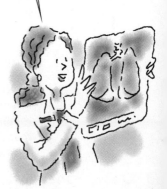

Check the patient's ABG levels and chest X-rays daily to decide whether he can be weaned from the ventilator.

• After extubation, assess the patient often for shortness of breath, tachypnea, dyspnea, malaise, and increased sputum production, which suggest acute rejection.
• After a single-lung transplantation, the newly implanted lung is denervated but the patient's original lung continues to send messages to the brain indicating poor oxygenation. The patient may complain of shortness of breath and dyspnea even with arterial oxygen saturation levels greater than 90%.
• Maintain strict infection control precautions such as meticulous hand washing.
• Inspect surgical dressings for bleeding in the early postoperative phase. Inspect the surgical incisions later for redness, swelling, and other signs of infection.

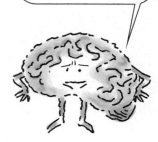

After a single-lung transplantation, the original lung tells the brain it's oxygen-starved, even with oxygen saturation greater than 90%.

Thoracotomy

A *thoracotomy* is the surgical removal of all or part of a lung; it aims to spare healthy lung tissue from disease. Lung excision may involve a pneumonectomy, lobectomy, segmental resection, or wedge resection.

Whole shebang

A *pneumonectomy* is the excision of an entire lung. It's usually performed to treat bronchogenic carcinoma but may also be used to treat tuberculosis (TB), bronchiectasis, or a lung abscess. It's used only when a less radical approach can't remove all diseased tissue. Chest cavity pressures stabilize after a pneumonectomy and, over time, fluid enters the cavity where lung tissue was removed, preventing significant mediastinal shift.

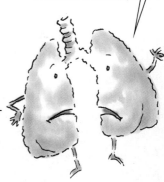

Thoracotomy surgically removes all or part of a lung to spare healthy tissue from disease. Oh, dear.

One lobe out of five ain't bad

A *lobectomy* is the removal of one of the five lung lobes; it's used to treat bronchogenic carcinoma, TB, a lung abscess, emphysematous blebs or bullae, benign tumors, and localized fungal infections. After this surgery, the remaining lobes expand to fill the entire pleural cavity.

Segments and wedges

A *segmental resection* is the removal of one or more lung segments; it preserves more functional tissue than lobectomy and is commonly used to treat bronchiectasis. A *wedge resection* is the removal of a small portion of the lung without regard to segments; it preserves the most functional tissue of all the surgeries but can treat only a small, well-circumscribed lesion. Remaining lung tissue must be reexpanded after both types of resection.

No place like home

Post-thoracotomy home care

• Tell the patient to continue his coughing and deep-breathing exercises to prevent complications. Advise him to report changes in sputum characteristics to his doctor.
• Instruct the patient to continue performing range-of-motion exercises to maintain mobility of his shoulder and chest wall.
• Tell the patient to avoid contact with people who have upper respiratory tract infections and to refrain from smoking.
• Provide instructions for wound care and dressing changes as necessary.

Nursing considerations

• Explain the anticipated surgery to the patient and inform him that he'll receive a general anesthetic.
• Inform the patient that postoperatively he may have chest tubes in place and may receive oxygen.
• Teach him deep-breathing techniques and explain that he'll perform these after surgery to facilitate lung reexpansion. Also teach him to use an incentive spirometer; record the volumes he achieves to provide a baseline.
• After a pneumonectomy, the patient should lie only on the operative side or on his back until stabilized. This prevents fluid from draining into the unaffected lung if the sutured bronchus opens.
• Make sure the chest tube is functioning, if present, and observe for signs of tension pneumothorax.
• Provide analgesics as ordered.
• Have the patient begin coughing and deep-breathing exercises as soon as his condition is stable. Auscultate his lungs, place him in semi-Fowler's position, and have him splint his incision to facilitate coughing and deep breathing.

Night moves

• Perform passive range-of-motion (ROM) exercises the evening of surgery and two or three times daily thereafter. Progress to active ROM exercises.
• Provide discharge instructions for the patient going home after a thoracotomy. (See *Post-thoracotomy home care*.)

Tracheotomy

A tracheotomy provides an airway for an intubated patient who needs prolonged mechanical ventilation and helps remove lower tracheobronchial secretions in a patient who can't clear them. It's also performed in emergencies when ET intubation isn't possible, to prevent an unconscious or paralyzed patient from aspirating food or secretions, and to bypass upper airway obstruction due to trauma, burns, epiglottiditis, or a tumor.

After the doctor creates the surgical opening, he inserts a tracheostomy tube to permit access to the airway. He may select from several tube styles, depending on the patient's condition. (See *Comparing tracheostomy tubes*, page 120.)

> A tracheotomy helps remove lower tracheobronchial secretions in a patient who can't clear them. Phew!

Nursing considerations

• For an emergency tracheotomy, briefly explain the procedure to the patient as time permits and quickly obtain supplies or a tracheotomy tray.
• For a scheduled tracheotomy, explain the procedure and the need for general anesthesia to the patient and his family. If possible, mention whether the tracheostomy will be temporary or permanent.
• Set up a communication system with the patient (letter board or flash cards), and practice it with him to ensure he'll be able to communicate comfortably while his speech is limited.
• Ensure that samples for ABG analysis and other diagnostic tests have been collected and that the patient or a responsible family member has signed a consent form.
• Auscultate breath sounds every 2 hours after the procedure. Note crackles, rhonchi, or diminished breath sounds.
• Turn the patient every 2 hours to avoid pooling tracheal secretions. As ordered, provide chest physiotherapy to help mobilize secretions, and note their quantity, consistency, color, and odor.

Skip the nose

• Replace humidity lost in bypassing the nose, mouth, and upper airway mucosa to reduce the drying effects of oxygen on mucous membranes. Humidification will also help to thin secretions. Oxygen administered through a T-piece or tracheostomy mask should be connected to a nebulizer or heated cascade humidifier.
• Monitor ABG values and compare them with baseline values to check adequacy of oxygenation and CO_2 removal. Also monitor the patient's oximetry values as ordered.
• Suction the tracheostomy using sterile technique to remove excess secretions when necessary. Avoid suctioning a patient for

> Avoid suctioning a patient for longer than 10 seconds at a time and stop if the patient develops respiratory distress.

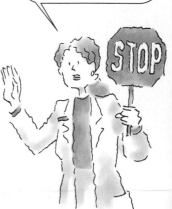

Advice from the experts

Comparing tracheostomy tubes

Tracheostomy tubes are made of plastic or metal and come in uncuffed, cuffed, or fenestrated varieties. Tube selection depends on the patient's condition and the doctor's preference.

Make sure you're familiar with the advantages and disadvantages of these commonly used tracheostomy tubes.

Uncuffed
(plastic or metal)

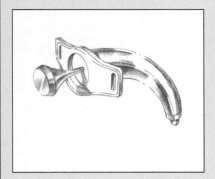

Plastic cuffed
(low pressure and high volume)

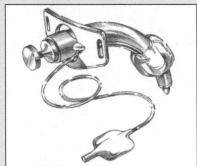

Fenestrated

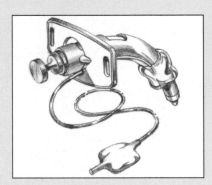

Advantages
- Free flow of air around tube and through larynx
- Reduced risk of tracheal damage
- Mechanical ventilation possible in patient with neuromuscular disease

Disadvantages
- Increased risk of aspiration in adults due to lack of cuff
- Adapter possibly needed for ventilation

Advantages
- Disposable
- Cuff bonded to tube (won't detach accidentally inside trachea)
- Low cuff pressure that's evenly distributed against tracheal wall (no need to deflate periodically to lower pressure)
- Reduced risk of tracheal damage

Disadvantages
- Possibly more expensive than other tubes

Advantages
- Speech possible through upper airway when external opening is capped and cuff is deflated
- Breathing by mechanical ventilation possible with inner cannula in place and cuff inflated
- Easy removal of inner cannula for cleaning

Disadvantages
- Possible occlusion of fenestration
- Possible dislodgment of inner cannula
- Cap removal necessary before inflating cuff

longer than 10 seconds at a time and discontinue the procedure if the patient develops respiratory distress.
• Make sure the tracheostomy ties are secure but not too tight. To prevent accidental tube dislodgment or expulsion, avoid changing the ties until the stoma track is stable. Report any tube pulsation

to the doctor; this may indicate the tube is close to the innominate artery, which predisposes the patient to hemorrhage.
• Change the tracheostomy dressing when soiled or once per shift, using sterile technique, and check the color, odor, amount, and type of drainage. Also check for swelling, crepitus, erythema, and bleeding at the site and report excessive bleeding or unusual drainage immediately. Wear goggles, gloves, and mask when changing tracheostomy tubes.
• Keep a sterile tracheostomy tube (with obturator) at the patient's bedside and be prepared to replace an expelled or contaminated tube. Also keep available a sterile tracheostomy tube (with obturator) that's one size smaller than the tube currently being used. The smaller tube may be necessary if the trachea begins to close after tube expulsion, making insertion of the same size tube difficult.

Miscellaneous treatments

Other miscellaneous treatments for respiratory disorders include:
• chest physiotherapy
• extracorporeal membrane oxygenation (ECMO)
• mucus clearing devices
• prone positioning.

Chest physiotherapy

Chest physiotherapy is usually performed with other treatments, such as suctioning, incentive spirometry, and the administration of such medications as small-volume nebulizer aerosol treatments and expectorants. (See *Chest physiotherapy*, page 122.) Recent studies indicate that percussion and vibration aren't effective treatments for most diseases; exceptions include cystic fibrosis and bronchiectasis. Improved breath sounds, increased PaO_2, sputum production, and improved airflow suggest successful treatment.

Nursing considerations

• Administer pain medication before the treatment as ordered, and teach the patient to splint his incision.
• Auscultate the lungs to determine baseline status, and check the doctor's order to determine which lung areas require treatment.
• Obtain pillows and a tilt board if necessary.
• Don't schedule therapy immediately after a meal; wait 2 to 3 hours to reduce the risk of nausea and vomiting.

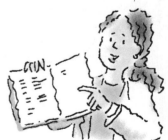

Except in bronchiectasis and cystic fibrosis, recent studies show percussion and vibration aren't effective treatments for most diseases.

Advice from the experts

Chest physiotherapy

Especially important for the bedridden patient, chest physiotherapy improves secretion clearance and ventilation and helps prevent or treat atelectasis and pneumonia.

Types of chest physiotherapy

Chest physiotherapy procedures include:
• postural drainage, which uses gravity to promote drainage of secretions from the lungs and bronchi into the trachea
• percussion, which involves cupping the hands and fingers together and clapping them alternately over the patient's lung fields to loosen secretions (also achieved with vibration)
• vibration, which can be used with percussion or as an alternative to it in a patient who's frail, in pain, or recovering from thoracic surgery or trauma
• deep-breathing exercises, which help loosen secretions and promote more effective coughing
• coughing, which helps clear the lungs, bronchi, and trachea of secretions and prevents aspiration.

Performing chest physiotherapy

Chest physiotherapy may be performed using postural drainage, percussion, or vibration.

Postural drainage

• Position the patient as ordered. (The doctor usually determines a position sequence after auscultation and chest X-ray review.) Be sure to position the patient so drainage is always oriented toward larger, more central airways.
• If the patient has a localized condition such as pneumonia in a specific lobe, expect to start with that area first to avoid infecting uninvolved areas. If he has a diffuse disorder expect to start with the lower lobes and work toward the upper ones.

Percussion

• Place your cupped hands against the patient's chest wall and rapidly flex and extend your wrists, generating a rhythmic, popping sound (a hollow sound helps verify correct performance of the technique).
• Percuss each segment for a minimum of 3 minutes. The vibrations you generate pass through the chest wall and help loosen secretions from the airways.
• Perform percussion throughout inspiration and expiration and encourage the patient to take slow, deep breaths.
• Don't percuss over the spine, sternum, liver, kidneys, or the female patient's breasts because you may cause trauma, especially in elderly patients.
• Percussion is painless when done properly, and the impact is diminished by a cushion of air formed in the cupped palm. This technique requires practice.

Vibration

• Ask the patient to inhale deeply, then exhale slowly through pursed lips.
• During exhalation, firmly press your fingers and the palms of your hands against the chest wall. Tense the muscles of your arms and shoulders in an isometric contraction to send fine vibrations through the chest wall.
• Repeat vibration for five exhalations on each chest segment.
• When the patient says "ah" on exhalation, you should hear a tremble in his voice.

• Make sure the patient is adequately hydrated to facilitate removal of secretions.
• If ordered, administer bronchodilator and mist therapies before the treatment.
• Provide tissues, an emesis basin, and a cup for sputum.
• Set up suction equipment if the patient doesn't have an adequate cough to clear secretions.
• If he needs oxygen therapy or is borderline hypoxemic without it, provide adequate flow rates of oxygen during therapy.

- Evaluate the patient's tolerance for therapy, and make adjustments as needed. Watch for fatigue and remember that the patient's ability to cough and breathe deeply diminishes as he tires.
- Assess for difficulty expectorating secretions. Use suction if the patient has an ineffective cough or a diminished gag reflex.
- Provide oral hygiene after therapy; secretions may taste foul or have an unpleasant odor.
- Be aware that postural drainage positions can cause nausea, dizziness, dyspnea, and hypoxemia.
- The patient with chronic bronchitis, bronchiectasis, or cystic fibrosis may need chest physiotherapy at home.

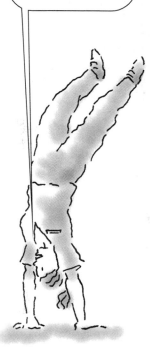

Be aware that postural drainage positions can cause nausea, dizziness, dyspnea, and hypoxemia. This is another dizzying position!

Extracorporeal membrane oxygenation

ECMO, one of a group of supportive therapies called extracorporeal life support, involves the oxygenation of blood outside of the body. It exposes a patient's lungs to low pressures as well as providing a means for oxygen delivery and CO_2 removal. When ECMO is used, lower FIO_2 concentrations and volumes can be delivered through mechanical ventilation, thereby reducing the risk of oxygen toxicity and barotrauma. Even so, ECMO doesn't cure the underlying disease.

Historically, ECMO was used to treat neonates who experienced severe respiratory distress. Today, ECMO is used to treat severe acute respiratory failure in neonates and adults. (See *ECMO in neonates.*)

The primary indication for using ECMO is severe respiratory failure. It also maybe indicated in other situations, such as:
- ARDS

Kids' korner

ECMO in neonates

In neonates, extracorporeal membrane oxygenation (ECMO) is considered the standard treatment for severe respiratory distress. However, in adults, ECMO is used only after other modes of ventilation have been used without success. These modes include:
- low tidal volume ventilation and high-level, positive end-expiratory pressure to facilitate mechanical ventilation
- pharmacologic therapy, such as neuromuscular blocking agents, sedatives, and opiates, to minimize oxygen consumption.

- perioperative cardiac failure
- primary myocardial failure
- bridge to transplantation.

There are two basis types of ECMO: venoarterial ECMO (VAECMO) and venovenous ECMO (VV-ECMO).

The arteries have it

VA-ECMO, the standard type used for neonates, involves the insertion of a catheter into the internal jugular or femoral veins for blood removal. Blood is returned to the patient and arterial circulation via the carotid or femoral arteries. This type of ECMO provides partial to complete cardiopulmonary bypass and is used most commonly when the patient has severe cardiac failure in addition to pulmonary failure.

Unfortunately, this type of ECMO increases the risk of air or a blood clot being directly introduced into the arterial circulation causing emboli. In addition, neurologic complications can occur with ligation of the carotid artery when therapy is discontinued.

The veins have it

VV-ECMO involves the insertion of a catheter to remove and return blood to the right atrium via the right internal jugular or femoral veins. Often a double lumen catheter is used. This type of ECMO is used for patients requiring only respiratory support, as with ARDS. It doesn't provide cardiac support to assist systemic circulation. Pulmonary blood flow is maintained and the lungs are perfused with oxygenated blood. As blood leaves the patient's body, it's pumped through a membrane oxygenator, which acts as an artificial lung, supplying oxygen to the blood. (See *ECMO set up*.)

The circuit also has numerous safety and pressure monitors located throughout. A roller pump regulates the blood flow to the oxygenator, turning off whenever the pump flow is greater than blood return to the patient. In this way, excessive pressure on the right atrium or major vessels is averted. The pump automatically restarts when the flow rate balances.

Nursing considerations

- Assess cardiopulmonary and hemodynamic status closely, including central venous pressure, pulmonary artery pressure, and cardiac output, at least every 15 minutes immediately after the procedure and then hourly or more frequently as indicated by the patient's condition or your facility's policy.
- Assess ET tube and mechanical ventilation.
- Monitor oxygen saturation levels and ABG values as ordered. Suction as necessary.

Advice from the experts

ECMO setup

Extracorporeal membrane oxygenation (ECMO) is managed by either a critical care nurse or respiratory therapist with special training in its operation. Illustrated below and described here is a typical ECMO setup:

• The *arterial filter* removes air bubbles and clots from the blood as it travels through the ECMO circuit.

• The *cannula* is a catheter through which blood travels to and from the patient.

• The *control desk module* continuously monitors pressure throughout the circuit and regulates blood flow rate as needed in response to changing pressures in the system.

• The *heater* generates heat needed to keep blood at a constant temperature.

• The *heat exchanger* uses heat generated by a heater to maintain the temperature of the blood as it's oxygenated.

• The *hemochron* monitors blood clotting.

• The *I.V. pump* allows injection of medications such as antibiotics into the cannula of the ECMO circuit.

• The *membrane oxygenator* serves as the artificial lung supplying oxygen to the blood.

• The *transonic blood flowmeter* measures the amount of blood flowing through the cannula at various places along the ECMO circuit.

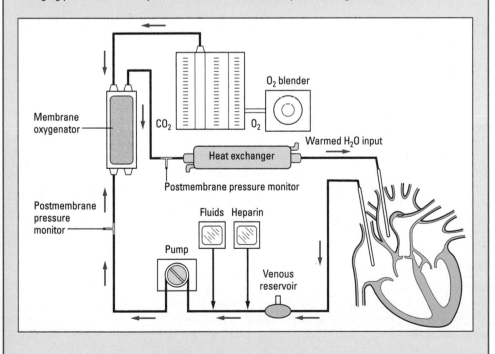

• After ECMO is initiated and the patient's gas exchange shows signs of improvement, expect to lower the ventilator settings.

- Be alert for changes in tidal volumes, which should increase as the lungs improve.
- Perform chest physiotherapy as needed.

From anticipation to oxygenation

- Change the patient's position frequently. Anticipate placing the patient with ARDS in the prone position, which helps to improve oxygenation.
- Administer sedatives and analgesics as ordered to aid the patient's tolerance of the procedure, maximize oxygen delivery and patient comfort, and decrease the risk of catheter dislodgement. If necessary, apply soft restraints as ordered to reduce the risk of the patient touching the catheter.
- Monitor intake and output at least hourly. Assess daily weight. Monitor blood urea nitrogen levels and serum creatinine levels closely for renal dysfunction.
- Assess for signs and symptoms of acute renal failure.
- Monitor activated clotting times as indicated and assist with adjustments to heparin infusion.
- Expect to administer blood transfusions. Obtain hematocrit, hemoglobin levels, and platelet counts every 4 hours and as needed.

Oozing observations

- Inspect catheter insertion sites for oozing or hematoma at least every 4 hours. Observe ECMO catheter insertion sites hourly; change dressings as needed to keep site clean and dry. If necessary, weigh saturated dressings to determine fluid volume loss.
- Assess neurologic status frequently, at least every 2 to 4 hours.
- Assess the affected extremity distal to the ECMO catheter insertion site for pulses, color, and temperature at least every 2 hours to prevent ischemia.
- Throughout the patient's care, explain all procedures and treatments, even if the patient is sedated. Offer emotional support to the patient's family; encourage them to visit and interact with the patient.

Remember to assess neurologic status frequently!

Mucus clearance device

Patients with chronic respiratory disorders, such as cystic fibrosis, bronchitis, and bronchiectasis, require therapy to mobilize and remove mucus secretions from the lungs. A handheld mucus clearance device, also known as the *flutter*, can help such patients cough up secretions more easily. This device is basically a ball valve that vibrates as the patient exhales vigorously through it. The vibrations propagate throughout the airways during expiration, thereby loosening the mucus.

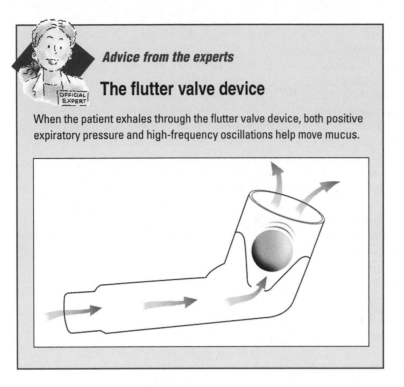

Advice from the experts

The flutter valve device

When the patient exhales through the flutter valve device, both positive expiratory pressure and high-frequency oscillations help move mucus.

As the patient repeats this process, the mucus progressively moves up the airways until it can be coughed out easily. The frequency and duration with which this device can be used should be determined by a licensed practitioner. (See *The flutter valve device.*)

Nursing considerations

• Explain the procedure to the patient. Tell him that this device will help move the mucus through his airways so that he can eventually expectorate it.
• Tell the patient to hold the device so that the stem is parallel to the floor.
• Tell the patient to keep his cheeks as flat and hard as possible while exhaling. Suggest that he hold his cheeks lightly with his other hand.
• To help the patient achieve the best fluttering effect, you may need to place one hand on his back and the other on his chest as he exhales through the device. If he's achieving the maximum effect, you'll feel the vibrations in his lungs as he exhales. If results are unsatisfactory at first, tell the patient to adjust the angle at which he's holding the device until optimal fluttering occurs.

Huffing and puffing

- If the patient's final cough doesn't seem to work, he can try repeated, controlled, short, rapid exhalations ("huffing"), as though he were trying to cough a bread crumb out of his throat, to aid mucus removal.
- Make sure the patient cleans the device after each use to remove mucus from the internal components. Instruct him to clean it more thoroughly every 2 days. All parts should be washed in a solution of mild soap or detergent. Tell him not to use bleach or other chlorine-containing products. After thorough cleaning, all parts should be rinsed under a stream of hot tap water, wiped with a clean towel, and reassembled and stored in a clean, dry place.
- Auscultate for the patient's breath sounds to determine the effectiveness of his coughing.

Prone positioning

Prone positioning is a therapeutic maneuver to improve oxygenation and pulmonary mechanics in patients with acute lung injury or ARDS. Also known as *proning*, prone positioning involves physically turning a patient from his back (supine position) to a face-down position. This positioning improves oxygenation in patients by shifting blood flow to regions of the lung that are less severely injured and better aerated. The criteria for prone positioning commonly include:

- acute onset of respiratory signs and symptoms
- hypoxemia, specifically a PaO_2 to FIO_2 ratio of 300 or less for acute lung injury and a PaO_2 to FIO_2 ratio of 200 or less for ARDS
- radiologic evidence of diffuse bilateral pulmonary infiltrates
- no evidence of left atrial hypertension.

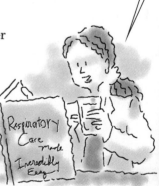

It says here that proning may facilitate better movement of the diaphragm.

Get that diaphragm movin'

With the appropriate equipment, proning may also facilitate better movement of the diaphragm by allowing the abdomen to expand more fully. It's usually performed for 6 or more hours per day, for as long as 10 days, until the requirement for a high concentration of inspired oxygen resolves. Patients who respond to the prone position by an increase in the PaO_2 to FIO_2 ratio of more than 20% within 2 hours of the patient being turned from supine to prone are classified as responders to prone positioning.

Prone positioning is indicated to support mechanically ventilated patients with ARDS who require high concentrations of inspired oxygen. It also corrects severe hypoxemia and maintains adequate oxygenation (PaO_2 greater than 60%) in patients with acute lung injury, while avoiding ventilator-induced lung injury. Prone positioning improves systemic oxygenation in patients with acute lung injury or ARDS.

Don't look down

Prone positioning is contraindicated in patients whose heads can't be supported in a face-down position or those who can't tolerate a head-down position. Hemodynamically unstable patients (systolic blood pressure less than 90 mm Hg), despite aggressive fluid resuscitation and vasopressors, shouldn't be placed in the prone position. It's also contraindicated in patients who are extremely obese (typically, more than 300 lb [136 kg]), with cerebral hypertension unresponsive to therapy, unstable bone fractures, left ventricular failure (nonpulmonary respiratory failure), and in patients with an active intra-abdominal process.

Nursing considerations

• Assess the patient's hemodynamic status to determine if he'll be able to tolerate the prone position.
• Assess the patient's mental status before prone positioning. Although agitation isn't a contraindication for prone positioning, it must be effectively managed.

Size matters

• Determine whether the patient's size and weight will allow turning him on a generally narrow critical care bed.
• Explain the purpose of and procedure for prone positioning to the patient and his family.
• Remove anterior chest wall ECG monitoring leads but make sure the patient's cardiac rate and rhythm can be monitored. These leads will be repositioned onto the patient's back after he's in the prone position.

Wearin' the shades

• Provide eye care, if indicated, including lubrication and horizontal taping of eyelids.
• Ensure the patient's tongue is inside his mouth; if it's edematous or protruding, insert a bite block.
• Secure the patient's ET or tracheotomy tube to prevent dislodgment.

Apply the brakes

• Make sure that the brake of the bed is engaged. Attach the surface of the prone positioner to the bed frame, as recommended by the manufacturer.

• Position staff appropriately. A minimum of three people is required: one on either side of the bed and one at the head of the bed.
• Adjust all patient tubing and invasive monitoring lines to prevent dislodgment, kinking, disconnection, or contact with the patient's body during the turning procedure and while the patient remains in the prone position.
• Adjust the pelvic piece of the device so that it rests ½″ (1.3 cm) above the iliac crest.

Monitoring response

• Monitor the patient's response to prone positioning through his vital signs, pulse oximetry, and mixed venous oxygen saturation. During the initial positioning, ABG levels should be obtained within ½ hour of prone positioning and within ½ hour before returning the patient to the supine position.
• Reposition the patient's head hourly while in the prone position to prevent facial breakdown. As one person lifts the patient's head, the second person should move the headpieces to provide head support in a different position.
• Provide ROM exercises to arms and legs every 2 hours.
• Proning is discontinued when the patient no longer demonstrates improved oxygenation with the position change.

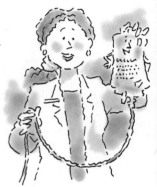

Adjust all equipment to prevent dislodgement during the turning procedure and when the patient is in the prone position.

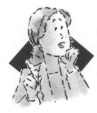

Quick quiz

1. Which ventilator mode supplies all ventilation for the patient?
    A.   Intermittent mandatory ventilation
    B.   Pressure support ventilation
    C.   Pressure-controlled ventilation
    D.   Controlled mandatory ventilation

Answer: D. Controlled mandatory ventilation is used when the patient can't initiate spontaneous breaths such as with a patient paralyzed because of a spinal cord injury.

2. ET tubes have inflatable cuffs to:
    A.   measure pressure on tracheal tissues.
    B.   drain gastric contents.
    C.   prevent backflow of oxygen.
    D.   treat laryngeal edema.

Answer: C. ET tube cuffs prevent backflow of oxygen so that it's delivered fully to the lungs.

3. When suctioning a patient you should:
   A.   apply suction intermittently as you insert the catheter.
   B.   suction the patient for longer than 10 seconds at a time.
   C.   oxygenate the patient's lungs before and after suctioning.
   D.   apply suction continuously as you insert the catheter.

Answer: C. Oxygenate the patient before and after suctioning to reduce the risk of hypoxemia. In addition, you should avoid suctioning for longer than 10 seconds and apply suction intermittently as you withdraw the catheter.

4. After oropharyngeal airway insertion, you should:
   A.   tape the tube in place.
   B.   position the patient on his side.
   C.   leave the airway in and perform mouth care every 2 to 4 hours.
   D.   insert a bite block.

Answer: B. After oropharyngeal airway insertion, position the patient on his side to decrease the risk of aspirating vomitus.

5. If a patient with a nasopharyngeal airway coughs or gags, you should:
   A.   explain that this is normal and the patient will get used to it.
   B.   encourage the patient to cough to help clear secretions.
   C.   remove the airway and insert a shorter one.
   D.   use a spray anesthetic to stop the irritation.

Answer: C. If the patient coughs or gags, the tube may be too long. If so, remove the airway and insert a shorter one.

6. Which device is used to help the patient achieve maximal ventilation?
   A.   Incentive spirometer
   B.   MDI
   C.   Diskus
   D.   Turbo-inhaler

Answer: A. An incentive spirometer is a breathing device used to help the patient achieve maximal ventilation by inducing the patient to take a deep breath and hold it.

7. Which type of tracheostomy tube permits speech through the upper airway?
  A. Uncuffed tube
  B. Cuffed tube
  C. Fenestrated tube
  D. Two-piece tube

Answer: C. The fenestrated tube permits speech through the upper airway when the external opening is capped and the cuff is deflated.

Scoring

☆☆☆ If you answered all seven items correctly, way to go! You can breathe easily about your knowledge of respiratory treatments.

☆☆ If you answered six items correctly, great! You're A-OK with airways and oxygen.

☆ If you answered fewer than six items correctly, no need to hyperventilate. Just take a deep breath and give this chapter another try.

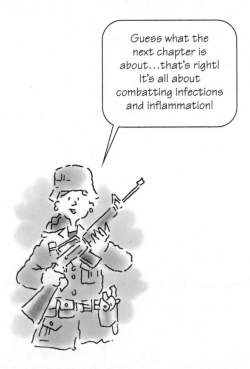

Guess what the next chapter is about...that's right! It's all about combatting infections and inflammation!

Infection and inflammation

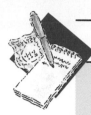

Just the facts

In this chapter, you'll learn:

♦ common acute and chronic respiratory infections and in-flammatory disorders

♦ causes, pathophysiology, and signs and symptoms

♦ diagnostic test results for respiratory infections

♦ treatment options.

Understanding respiratory infection and inflammation

This chapter discusses common respiratory infections and inflammatory disorders, along with their causes, pathophysiology, signs and symptoms, diagnostic test findings, treatments, and nursing interventions. These disorders may be acute or chronic.

BOOP, idiopathic

Idiopathic bronchiolitis obliterans with organizing pneumonia (BOOP), also known as *cryptogenic organizing pneumonia*, is one of several types of bronchiolitis obliterans. *Bronchiolitis obliterans* is a generic term used to describe an inflammatory disease of the small airways. *Organizing pneumonia* refers to unresolved pneumonia, in which inflammatory alveolar exudate persists and eventually leads to fibrosis. Most patients with BOOP are between ages 40 and 70; however, BOOP has been reported in children. Incidence is equally divided between men and women. A history of cigarette smoking doesn't seem to increase the risk of developing this chronic disorder.

C'mon, rookie. This is OUR chapter. Here we go ...!

The scoop on BOOP

BOOP was first described in 1901, but confusing terminology and pathology that overlapped other small airway diseases kept it from being sufficiently recognized until the mid-1980s. Since then, BOOP has been diagnosed with increasing frequency, although the various pathologies and classifications of bronchiolitis obliterans are still debated.

What causes it

BOOP has no known cause. However, other forms of bronchiolitis obliterans and organizing pneumonia may be associated with specific diseases or situations, such as bone marrow, heart, or heart-lung transplantation; collagen vascular diseases, such as rheumatoid arthritis and systemic lupus erythematosus; inflammatory diseases, such as Crohn's disease, ulcerative colitis, and polyarteritis nodosa; bacterial, viral, or mycoplasmal respiratory infections; inhalation of toxic gases; and drug therapy with amiodarone (Cordarone, Pacerone), bleomycin (Blenoxane), penicillamine (Cuprimine, Depen), or lomustine (CeeNU, CCNU).

How it happens

BOOP is a nonspecific reaction to bronchiolar injury. It's characterized by the proliferation of granulation tissue polyps that fill the lumens of terminal and respiratory bronchioles. Granulation tissue forms within the small airways, alveolar ducts, and airspaces. The surrounding tissues become inflamed.

What to look for

The presenting symptoms of BOOP are usually subacute, with a flulike syndrome of:
- fever
- persistent and nonproductive cough
- dyspnea (especially with exertion)
- malaise
- anorexia
- weight loss lasting for several weeks to several months.

Physical assessment findings may reveal dry crackles as the only abnormality. Less common signs and symptoms include a productive cough, hemoptysis, chest pain, generalized aching, and night sweats.

What tests tell you

- *Chest X-ray* usually shows patchy, diffuse airspace opacities with a ground-glass appearance that may migrate from one location to another. High-resolution computed tomography (CT) scans show areas of consolidation. Except for the migrating opacities, these findings are nonspecific and present in many other respiratory disorders.
- *CT scan findings* are also nonspecific but are more informative than chest X-ray in assessing distribution of the disease.
- *Open thoracotomy and biopsy* are usually required for a definitive diagnosis of BOOP.
- *Arterial blood gas (ABG) analysis* usually shows mild to moderate hypoxemia at rest, which worsens with exercise.
- *Blood tests* reveal an increased erythrocyte sedimentation rate, increased C-reactive protein level, increased white blood cell (WBC) count with a somewhat increased proportion of neutrophils, and a minor rise in eosinophils. Immunoglobulin (Ig) G and IgM levels are normal or slightly increased, and the IgE level is normal.
- *Bronchoscopy* reveals normal or slightly inflamed airways. Bronchoalveolar lavage fluid obtained during bronchoscopy shows a moderate elevation in lymphocytes and, sometimes, elevated neutrophil and eosinophil levels. Foamy-looking alveolar macrophages may also be found.

How it's treated

Oxygen is used to correct hypoxemia. The patient may need no oxygen or a small amount of oxygen at rest and a greater amount when he exercises. Other treatments vary, depending on the patient's symptoms, and may include inhaled bronchodilators, cough suppressants, and bronchial hygiene therapies.

Corticosteroids are the current treatment for BOOP, although the ideal dosage and treatment duration are sources of ongoing debate. Relapse is common when corticosteroids are tapered off or stopped. This usually can be reversed when steroids are increased or resumed. Occasionally, a patient may need to continue corticosteroids indefinitely. BOOP is very responsive to treatment and usually can be completely reversed with corticosteroid therapy.

Immunosuppressive-cytotoxic drugs such as cyclophosphamide (Cytoxan, Neosar) have been used in the few cases of intolerance or unresponsiveness.

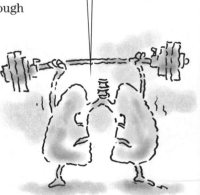

Patients with hypoxemia may need oxygen when they're working out.

What to do

• Explain all diagnostic tests to the patient. He may experience anxiety and frustration because of the length of time and number of tests needed to establish the diagnosis.
• Explain the diagnosis to the patient and his family. This uncommon diagnosis may cause confusion and anxiety.
• The patient may need to be referred to a pulmonologist for treatment.

Moon and mood

• Monitor the patient for adverse effects of corticosteroid therapy, including weight gain, "moon face," glucose intolerance, fluid and electrolyte imbalance, mood swings, cataracts, peptic ulcer disease, opportunistic infections, and osteoporosis leading to bone fractures. These effects leave many patients unable to tolerate the treatment. Teach the patient and his family about these adverse effects, emphasizing which reactions they should report to the doctor.
• Monitor oxygenation, both at rest and with exertion. The doctor will probably prescribe an oxygen flow rate for use when the patient is at rest and a higher one for exertion. Teach the patient how to increase the oxygen flow rate to the appropriate level for exercise.
• Teach the patient and his family about the adverse effects of the medications prescribed, emphasizing which reactions they should report.
• Teach measures that may help prevent complications related to treatment, such as infection control and improved nutrition.
• Teach breathing, relaxation, and energy conservation techniques to help the patient manage his symptoms.
• If the patient needs oxygen at home, ensure continuity of care by making appropriate referrals to discharge planners, respiratory care practitioners, and home equipment vendors.

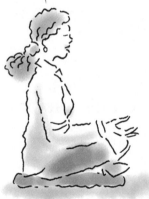

Teach relaxation exercises to help manage symptoms.

Bronchiectasis

An irreversible condition marked by chronic abnormal dilation of bronchi and destruction of bronchial walls, bronchiectasis can occur throughout the tracheobronchial tree or can be confined to one segment or lobe. However, it's usually bilateral, involving the basilar segments of the lower lobes. This chronic disorder affects people of both sexes and all ages.

Forms of bronchiectasis

The different forms of bronchiectasis may occur separately or simultaneously:
• In *cylindrical bronchiectasis,* the bronchi expand unevenly, with little change in diameter, and end suddenly in a squared-off fashion.
• In *varicose bronchiectasis,* abnormal, irregular dilation and narrowing of the bronchi give the appearance of varicose veins.
• In *saccular bronchiectasis,* many large dilations end in sacs. These sacs balloon into pus-filled cavities as they approach the periphery and are then called *saccules.*

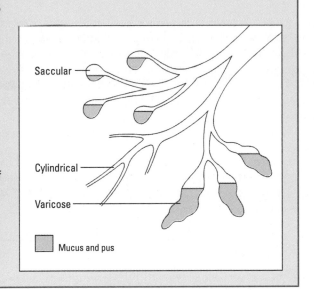

Saccular

Cylindrical

Varicose

Mucus and pus

What causes it

Bronchiectasis results from repeated damage of bronchial walls and abnormal mucociliary clearance that causes the breakdown of supportive tissue adjacent to the airways. This disease has three forms:

 cylindrical (fusiform)

 varicose

 saccular (cystic). (See *Forms of bronchiectasis.*)
Bronchiectasis may be caused by such conditions as:
• mucoviscidosis (cystic fibrosis of the pancreas)
• immunologic disorders such as agammaglobulinemia
• recurrent, inadequately treated bacterial respiratory tract infections such as tuberculosis (TB)
• measles, pneumonia, pertussis, or influenza
• obstruction by a foreign body, tumor, or stenosis associated with recurrent infection
• inhalation of corrosive gas or repeated aspiration of gastric juices into the lungs.

How it happens

Hyperplastic squamous epithelium, denuded of cilia, replace ulcerated columnar epithelia. Abscess formation occurs, involving all layers of the bronchial walls, which produces inflammatory cells and fibrous tissue, resulting in dilation and narrowing of the airways. Sputum stagnates in the dilated bronchi and leads to secondary infection, characterized by inflammation and leukocytic accumulations.

Debris disasters

Additional debris collects in the bronchi and occludes them. Building pressure from the retained secretions induces mucosal injury. Extensive vascular proliferation of bronchial circulation occurs and produces frequent hemoptysis.

What to look for

Initially, bronchiectasis may not produce symptoms. Assess the patient for a chronic cough that produces copious, foul-smelling, mucopurulent secretions, possibly totaling several cupfuls daily (classic symptom).

Other characteristic findings include:
• coarse crackles during inspiration over involved lobes or segments
• occasional wheezes
• dyspnea
• weight loss, malaise
• clubbing
• recurrent fever, chills, and other signs of infection.

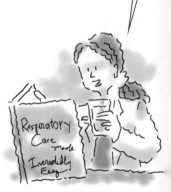

Watch for a chronic cough that produces up to several cupfuls of foul-smelling, mucopurulent secretions. Suddenly, I'm not thirsty.

What tests tell you

In addition to aiding diagnosis, these tests also help determine the physiologic severity of the disease and the effects of therapy, and they help in the evaluation of the patient for surgery:
• *Bronchography* is the most reliable diagnostic test and reveals the location and extent of disease.
• *Chest X-rays* show peribronchial thickening, areas of atelectasis, and scattered cystic changes.
• *Bronchoscopy* helps identify the source of secretions or the site of bleeding in hemoptysis.
• *Sputum culture* and *Gram stain* identify predominant organisms.

• *Complete blood count* and *WBC differential* identify anemia and leukocytosis.
• *Pulmonary function tests* detect decreased vital capacity and decreased expiratory flow.
• *ABG analysis* shows hypoxemia.

How it's treated

Treatment of bronchiectasis includes:
• antibiotics given by mouth or I.V. for 7 to 10 days or until sputum production decreases
• bronchodilators, with postural drainage and chest percussion, to help remove secretions if the patient has bronchospasm and thick, tenacious sputum
• bronchoscopy used occasionally to aid removal of secretions
• oxygen therapy for hypoxemia
• lobectomy or segmental resection for severe hemoptysis.

What to do

• Provide a warm, quiet, comfortable environment, and urge the patient to rest as much as possible.
• Administer antibiotics as ordered.
• Perform chest physiotherapy several times per day (early morning and bedtime are best); include postural drainage and chest percussion for involved lobes. Have the patient maintain each position for 10 minutes; then perform percussion and ask him to cough.

Eating right

• Encourage balanced, high-protein meals to promote good health and tissue healing and plenty of fluids to aid expectoration.
• Provide frequent mouth care to remove foul-smelling sputum.
• Evaluate the patient. His secretions should be thin and clear or white. (See *Teaching the patient with bronchiectasis*, page 140.)

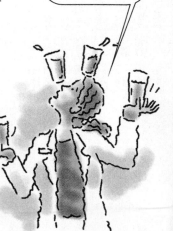

Encourage plenty of fluids to aid expectoration.

No place like home

Teaching the patient with bronchiectasis

• Explain all diagnostic tests.
• Show the patient's family members how to perform postural drainage and percussion. Also, teach the patient coughing and deep-breathing techniques to promote good ventilation and the removal of secretions.
• Advise the patient to stop smoking, which stimulates secretions and irritates the airways. Refer the patient to a local self-help group for smoking cessation.

• Teach the patient to properly dispose of secretions.
• Tell the patient to avoid air pollutants and people with upper respiratory tract infections.
• Instruct him to take medications (especially antibiotics) exactly as ordered.
• To help prevent this disease, vigorously treat bacterial pneumonia and stress the need for immunization to prevent childhood diseases.

Croup

Croup is a severe inflammation and obstruction of the upper airway. This acute childhood disease affects boys more commonly than girls.

A family affair

Croup usually occurs in the winter as acute laryngotracheobronchitis (the most common form), laryngitis, or acute spasmodic laryngitis and must be distinguished from epiglottiditis. Usually mild and self-limiting, acute laryngotracheobronchitis appears most commonly in children ages 3 months to 3 years. Acute spasmodic laryngitis affects children between ages 1 and 3, particularly those with allergies and a family history of croup. Overall, up to 15% of patients have a family history of croup; recovery is usually complete.

What causes it

Croup usually results from a viral infection. Parainfluenza viruses cause about two-thirds of such infections; adenoviruses, respiratory syncytial virus (RSV), influenza viruses, measles viruses, and bacteria (pertussis and diphtheria) account for the rest. Airway obstruction, respiratory failure, and dehydration are complications of croup. Latent complications are ear infection and pneumonia.

How it happens

Inflammatory swelling and spasms constrict the larynx, thereby reducing airflow. Inflammatory changes almost completely obstruct the larynx (which includes the epiglottis) and significantly narrow the trachea.

What to look for

Typically, the child or his parents report a recent upper respiratory tract infection preceding croup. On inspection, you may observe the use of accessory muscles with nasal flaring during breathing. You typically hear the child's sharp, barking cough and hoarse or muffled vocal sounds. As croup progresses, the patient may display further upper airway obstruction with severely compromised ventilation. (See *Croup and the upper airways*.) Auscultation may disclose inspiratory stridor and diminished breath sounds. These signs and symptoms may last for only a few hours, or they may persist for 1 to 2 days.

Now I get it!

Croup and the upper airways

In croup, inflammatory swelling and spasms constrict the larynx, thereby reducing airflow. This cross-sectional drawing (from chin to chest) shows the upper airway changes caused by croup. Inflammatory changes almost completely obstruct the larynx (which includes the epiglottis) and significantly narrow the trachea.

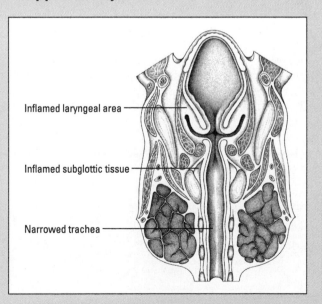

Inflamed laryngeal area

Inflamed subglottic tissue

Narrowed trachea

Each form of croup has additional characteristics:

• In *laryngotracheobronchitis*, the patient may complain of fever and breathing problems that occur more commonly at night. Typically, the child becomes frightened because he can't breathe out (because inflammation causes edema in the bronchi and bronchioles). During auscultation, you may hear diffusely decreased breath sounds, expiratory rhonchi, and scattered crackles.

• In *laryngitis*, which results from vocal cord edema, the patient usually reports mild signs and symptoms and no respiratory distress. If the patient is an infant, some respiratory distress may occur. In children, the history may include such signs and symptoms as a sore throat and cough that, rarely, may progress to marked hoarseness. Inspection may disclose suprasternal and intercostal retractions, inspiratory stridor, dyspnea, diminished breath sounds, restlessness and, in later stages, severe dyspnea and exhaustion.

Hoarses and clams

• In *acute spasmodic laryngitis*, the patient history may reveal mild to moderate hoarseness and nasal discharge, followed by the characteristic cough and noisy inspiration that often awaken the child at night. As the child understandably becomes anxious, this leads to increasing dyspnea and transient cyanosis. Inspection may disclose labored breathing with retractions and clammy skin. Palpation may reveal a rapid pulse rate. These severe signs diminish after several hours but reappear in a milder form on the next one or two nights.

What tests tell you

In evaluating the patient with croup, diagnosis should rule out the possibility of masses, cysts, and foreign body obstruction—common causes of croupy cough in young children. Tests used to diagnose croup include:

• *Throat cultures* can identify infecting organisms and their sensitivity to antibiotics when bacterial infection is the cause. Throat cultures can also rule out diphtheria.

• *Blood cultures* can distinguish between bacterial and viral infections.

• *X-ray studies* of the neck may show upper airway narrowing and edema in subglottic folds.

• *Laryngoscopy* may reveal inflammation and obstruction in epiglottal and laryngeal areas.

How it's treated

For most children with croup, home care with rest, cool humidification during sleep, and antipyretic drugs such as acetaminophen relieve signs and symptoms. However, respiratory distress that interferes with oral hydration usually requires hospitalization and parenteral fluid replacement to prevent dehydration. If the patient has croup from a bacterial infection, he needs antibiotic therapy. Oxygen therapy may also be required.

Bring the swelling down

For moderately severe croup, aerosolized racemic epinephrine may temporarily reduce airway swelling. Intubation is performed only if other means of preventing respiratory failure are unsuccessful. Several studies support the practice of prescribing corticosteroids for acute laryngotracheobronchitis.

What to do

• Monitor cough and breath sounds, hoarseness, severity of retractions, inspiratory stridor, cyanosis, respiratory rate and character (especially prolonged and labored respirations), restlessness, fever, and heart rate.

Pillow talk

• Keep the child as quiet as possible but avoid sedation, which may depress respiration. If the patient is an infant, position him in an infant seat or prop him up with a pillow; place an older child in Fowler's position. If an older child requires a cool-mist tent to help him breathe, describe it to him and his parents and explain why it's needed.
• Change bed linens as necessary to keep the patient dry.
• Control the patient's energy output and oxygen demand by providing age-appropriate diversional activities to keep him quietly occupied.
• If possible, isolate patients suspected of having RSV and parainfluenza infections. Wash your hands carefully before leaving the room, to avoid transmitting germs to other patients, particularly infants.
• Control fever with sponge baths and antipyretics. Keep a hypothermia blanket on hand if the patient's temperature rises above 102° F (38.9° C). Watch for seizures in infants and young children with high fevers. Give I.V. antibiotics as ordered.

> Provide age-appropriate activities to keep the child occupied without exerting too much energy.

No place like home

Home care for croup

• If the child has croup at home, tell the parents that bed rest is essential to conserve energy and limit oxygen needs.
• To ease the child's breathing, advise the parents to use pillows to prop him into a sitting or semi-sitting (semi-Fowler's) position. Warn the parents never to rest a child or an infant with croup flat on his back.
• Advise the child's parents that keeping the child quiet and comfortable reduces his oxygen needs. Holding him as often as possible soothes and comforts him. If the child is hospitalized, explain that the same measures apply.
• Urge the parents to ensure adequate hydration by giving the child plenty of fluids. Suggest fluid electrolyte replacement (such as Pedialyte, flavored gelatin dissolved in water, or gin-

ger ale with the bubbles stirred out). Fluids should be room temperature. Instruct them to avoid thicker, milk-based fluids.
• To relieve sore throat, suggest fruit sorbet or ice pops. Instruct the parents to withhold solid food until the child can breathe and swallow more easily. The child may have little or no appetite until he feels better.
• Warn parents not to give aspirin to reduce fever because of its link to Reye's syndrome.
• Suggest using a cool-mist humidifier (vaporizer) in the home, and then teach the parents how to use one, if necessary. To relieve acute croup spells at home, instruct the parents to carry the child to the bathroom, shut the door, turn on the hot water, and allow steam to fill the room. Breathing warm, moist air should quickly ease an acute croup spell.

Popsicle?

• Relieve sore throat with soothing, water-based ices, such as fruit sorbet and ice pops. Avoid thicker, milk-based fluids if the patient has thick mucus or swallowing difficulties. Apply petroleum jelly or another ointment around the nose and lips to decrease irritation from nasal discharge and mouth breathing.
• Institute measures to prevent the child's crying, which increases respiratory distress. As necessary, adapt treatment to conserve the child's energy and to include parents, who can provide reassurance.

Kudos to parents

• Reassure parents that they made the right decision by bringing their child to the emergency department — especially at night when the evening air may improve the child's breathing significantly, leaving the parents wondering if they overreacted. (The doctor may ask the nurse to take the child outside for a few minutes to relieve the patient's croupiness.)
• Watch for signs of complete airway obstruction, such as increased heart and respiratory rates, use of respiratory accessory muscles in breathing, nasal flaring, and increased restlessness.
• Because croup may be treated at home or in a health care facility, you need to tailor your teaching accordingly. Because this disease primarily affects young children, patient teaching usually centers on the parents. (See *Home care for croup*.)

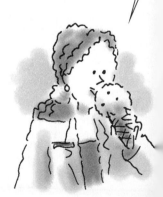

Ice cream may not be the best thing for patients with swallowing difficulties. Instead, offer ice pops or sorbet.

• If the child is hospitalized, advise the parents that he may be placed in a cool-mist tent (with or without oxygen) to provide high humidity.

• Explain that the hospitalized child may require hydration with I.V. fluids if he can't be hydrated orally.

• Warn parents that ear infections and pneumonia may complicate croup. These disorders may follow croup about 5 days after recovery. Urge the parents to seek immediate medical attention if the patient has an earache, productive cough, high fever, or increased shortness of breath.

Epiglottiditis

Acute epiglottiditis is an acute inflammation of the epiglottis that tends to cause airway obstruction. It typically strikes children between ages 2 and 8. A critical emergency, epiglottiditis can prove fatal in 8% to 12% of patients unless it's recognized and treated promptly.

What causes it

Epiglottiditis usually results from infection with *Haemophilus influenzae* type B and, occasionally, pneumococci and group A streptococci. Since the advent of the *H. influenzae* type B (Hib) vaccine, epiglottiditis is becoming more rare.

How it happens

An infection of the epiglottis and surrounding area leads to intense inflammation of the supraglottal region. Swelling of the epiglottis, aryepiglottic folds, arytenoid cartilage, and ventricular bands leads to acute airway obstruction.

What to look for

Sometimes preceded by an upper respiratory tract infection, epiglottiditis may rapidly progress to complete upper airway obstruction within 2 to 5 hours. Laryngeal obstruction results from inflammation and edema of the epiglottis. Accompanying symptoms include high fever, stridor, sore throat, dysphagia, irritability, restlessness, and drooling.

Sit up, lean forward

To relieve severe respiratory distress, the child with epiglottiditis may hyperextend his neck, sit up, and lean forward with his mouth open, tongue protruding, and nostrils flaring as he tries to breathe. He may develop inspiratory retractions and rhonchi. The barking cough of croup is notably absent.

What tests tell you

In acute epiglottiditis, throat examination reveals a large, edematous, bright red epiglottis. Such examination should follow lateral neck X-rays and, generally, should *not* be performed if the suspected obstruction is great. Special equipment (laryngoscope and endotracheal [ET] tubes) should be available because a tongue blade can cause sudden complete airway obstruction.

Leave your mark

Trained personnel (such as an anesthesiologist) should be on hand during the throat examination to secure an emergency airway. On the lateral soft tissue X-ray of the neck, a large, thick but indistinct ("thumbprint") epiglottis will be seen.

How it's treated

- A child with acute epiglottiditis and airway obstruction requires emergency hospitalization; he may need emergency ET intubation or a tracheotomy with subsequent monitoring in an intensive care unit.
- Respiratory distress that interferes with swallowing necessitates parenteral fluid administration to prevent dehydration.
- A child with acute epiglottiditis should always receive a complete course of antibiotics—usually a parenteral second- or third-generation cephalosporin. (If the child is allergic to penicillin, a quinolone or sulfa drug may be substituted.)

What to do

- Keep these pieces of equipment available in case of sudden complete airway obstruction: a tracheotomy tray, ET tubes, hand-held resuscitation bag, oxygen equipment, and a laryngoscope, with blades of various sizes. Monitor ABG levels for hypoxemia and hypercapnia.

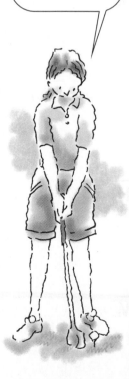

Patients with acute epiglottiditis should always receive a complete course of antibiotics.

- Watch for increasing restlessness, rising heart rate, fever, dyspnea, and retractions, which may indicate the need for an emergency tracheotomy.

Anticipation

- After a tracheotomy, anticipate the patient's needs because he won't be able to cry or call out; provide emotional support. Reassure the patient and his family that the tracheotomy is a short-term intervention (usually 4 to 7 days). Monitor the patient for rising temperature and pulse rate and hypotension—signs of secondary infection.

Laryngitis

Laryngitis, a common disorder, is an acute or chronic inflammation of the vocal cords. Acute laryngitis may occur as an isolated infection or as part of a generalized bacterial or viral upper respiratory tract infection. Repeated attacks of acute laryngitis produce inflammatory changes associated with chronic laryngitis.

What causes it

Acute laryngitis usually results from infection (primarily viral) or excessive use of the voice, which is an occupational hazard in such vocations as teaching, public speaking, and singing. It may also result from leisure activities, such as cheering at a sports event, inhalation of smoke or fumes, or aspiration of caustic chemicals. Chronic laryngitis may be caused by chronic upper respiratory tract disorders (sinusitis, bronchitis, nasal polyps, or allergy), breathing through the mouth, smoking, constant exposure to dust or other irritants, and alcohol abuse.

How it happens

Inflammatory response to cell damage by viruses results in hyperemia and fluid exudation. Irritant receptors are triggered. Kinins and other inflammatory mediators may induce spasm of upper airway smooth muscle.

What to look for

Acute laryngitis typically begins with hoarseness, ranging from mild to complete loss of voice. In chronic laryngitis, persistent hoarseness is usually the only symptom. Associated clinical features of acute laryngitis include:

- pain (especially when swallowing or speaking)
- persistent dry cough
- fever
- laryngeal edema
- malaise.

What tests tell you

Indirect laryngoscopy is used to confirm the diagnosis by revealing red, inflamed and, occasionally, hemorrhagic vocal cords, with rounded rather than sharp edges and exudate. Bilateral swelling may be present.

    In severe cases or if toxicity is a concern, obtain a culture of the exudate. Consider 24-hour pH probe testing in chronic laryngitis and gastroesophageal reflux disease. Also consider biopsy in chronic laryngitis in an adult with a history of smoking or alcohol abuse.

How it's treated

- The primary treatment for laryngitis is resting the voice.
- Steam inhalation may be beneficial as well as smoking cessation, reducing alcohol intake, and changing or modifying the patient's job.
- Severe, acute laryngitis may necessitate hospitalization.
- In chronic laryngitis, effective treatment must eliminate the underlying cause.
- Medication used to treat a patient with laryngitis depends on the cause.
- When laryngeal edema causes airway obstruction, a tracheostomy may be necessary.

Steam inhalation can help treat your laryngitis. Whew, it's hot in here.

What to do

- Explain to the patient and his family why he shouldn't talk.
- For the patient with a bacterial infection, stress the importance of completing the full course of antibiotic therapy.
- Suggest that the patient maintain adequate humidification by using a vaporizer or humidifier during the winter, avoiding air conditioning during the summer (because it dehumidifies), using medicated throat lozenges, and not smoking.

Pharyngitis

Pharyngitis is an acute or chronic inflammation of the pharynx. It's the most common throat disorder and is widespread among adults who live or work in dusty or very dry environments; use their voices excessively; habitually use tobacco or alcohol; or suffer from chronic sinusitis, persistent coughs, or allergies. It typically accompanies the common cold.

What causes it

Pharyngitis is usually caused by a virus. The most common bacterial cause is group A beta-hemolytic streptococci. Other common causes include *Mycoplasma* and *Chlamydia*.

How it happens

Cellular damage caused by a virus or bacteria causes an inflammatory response, which results in hyperemia and fluid exudation.

What to look for

Pharyngitis produces a sore throat and slight difficulty in swallowing. Swallowing saliva is usually more painful than swallowing food. Pharyngitis can also cause the sensation of a lump in the throat as well as a constant, aggravating urge to swallow. Associated features can include:

- mild fever
- headache
- muscle and joint pain
- coryza
- rhinorrhea.

Over 90% of cases of sore throat and fever in children are of viral origin. Associated symptoms usually include a runny nose and nonproductive cough. Uncomplicated pharyngitis usually subsides in 3 to 10 days.

Physical examination of the pharynx reveals generalized redness and inflammation of the posterior wall and red, edematous mucous membranes studded with white or yellow patches of exudate.

What tests tell you

Bacterial pharyngitis usually produces a large amount of exudate. A throat culture may be performed to identify bacterial organisms that may be the cause of the inflammation.

How it's treated

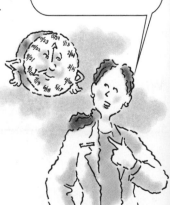

Encourage patients with pharyngitis to quit smoking.

• Treatment for a patient with acute viral pharyngitis is usually symptomatic and consists mainly of rest, warm saline gargles, throat lozenges containing a mild anesthetic, and plenty of fluids.
• If the patient can't swallow fluids, I.V. hydration may be required. Chronic pharyngitis necessitates the same supportive measures as acute pharyngitis but with greater emphasis on eliminating the underlying cause such as an allergen.

Hot vs. cold

• Preventive measures include adequate humidification and avoidance of excessive exposure to air conditioning. In addition, the patient should be urged to stop smoking.
• Medication used to treat a patient with pharyngitis may include acetaminophen (Anacin-3 Maximum Strength, Children's Tylenol, Tylenol, Tylenol Extra Strength) and penicillin (Beepen-VK, Ledercillin VK, V-cillin K, Veetids) or erythromycin (E-Base, E-Mycin) for bacterial pharyngitis.

What to do

Children with pharyngitis should receive at least 24 hours of therapy before returning to school.

• If treatment isn't successful, the patient may need to be referred to an otolaryngologist.
• Refer the patient to a self-help group to stop smoking if appropriate.
• Encourage the patient to drink plenty of fluids.
• If the patient has acute bacterial pharyngitis, emphasize the importance of completing the full course of antibiotic therapy.

Humidify to clarify

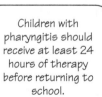

• Teach the patient with chronic pharyngitis how to minimize sources of throat irritation in the environment such as using a bedside humidifier.
• Children attending school should receive at least 24 hours of therapy before returning to school.

• If a patient has exhibited three or more documented infections within 6 months, consider daily penicillin prophylaxis during the winter months. Also, consider treatment for carriers who live in closed or semiclosed communities.

Pneumonia

Pneumonia is an acute infection of the lung parenchyma that commonly impairs gas exchange. More than 3 million cases of pneumonia are diagnosed yearly in the United States. Pneumonia is the seventh leading cause of death in the United States, and in 2003, severe acute respiratory syndrome (SARS), a new, deadly type of pneumonia, emerged. (See *SARS*.) Pneumonia is classified according to the infectious agent, location, or other factors.

Infectious agents may be bacterial, viral, mycoplasmal, rickettsial, fungal, protozoal, or mycobacterial.

What's your type?

Types of pneumonia based on location of the infection include:
• *bronchopneumonia*, involving distal airways and alveoli
• *lobular pneumonia*, involving part of a lobe
• *lobar pneumonia*, involving an entire lobe.

Pneumonia may be classified as community-acquired, hospital-acquired (nosocomial), or aspiration pneumonia. (See *Types of pneumonia*, pages 152 and 153.)

Shared with the community

As the name implies, community-acquired pneumonia occurs in the community setting or within the first 48 hours of admission to a health care facility because of community exposure.

Not-so-comical pneumonia

Nosocomial pneumonia refers to the development of pneumonia 48 hours after admission to a health care facility. For example, development of pneumonia after ET intubation and placement on a ventilator can be a type of nosocomial pneumonia.

When location doesn't matter

In addition to pneumonia acquired in a specific setting, aspiration pneumonia can occur in the community or health care facility setting.

(Text continues on page 154.)

SARS

The Centers for Disease Control and Prevention and the World Health Organization are investigating the disease called *severe acute respiratory syndrome* (SARS).

SARS typically begins with a fever greater than 100.4° (38°C), headache, general discomfort and body aches and, in some patients, mild respiratory symptoms. After 2 to 7 days, patients with SARS may develop a dry cough and difficulty breathing. The disease, which is highly contagious, is spread by droplets and through contact with contaminated objects. It's also possible that SARS can be spread more broadly through the air or by other ways that aren't currently known. A new type of coronavirus is the suspected cause.

Current treatment for SARS is mostly palliative. Antivirals, such as oseltamivir and ribavirin, and steroids in combination with antivirals have been used in patients with SARS. However, the efficacy of these treatments is unknown.

Advice from the experts

Types of pneumonia

Here's an overview of the various types of pneumonia, including their causative agents and common assessment findings.

Type	Causative agent	Assessment findings
Aspiration pneumonia	Aspiration of gastric or oropharyngeal contents into trachea or lungs	• Fever • Crackles • Dyspnea • Hypotension • Tachycardia • Cyanosis • Chest X-ray with infiltrates
Community-acquired pneumonias		
Streptococcal pneumonia (pneumococcal pneumonia)	*Streptococcus pneumoniae*	• Sudden onset of single shaking chill • Fever of 102° to 104° F (38.9° to 40° C) • History of previous upper respiratory infection • Pleuritic chest pain • Severe cough • Rust-colored sputum • Areas of consolidation on chest X-ray (usually lobar) • Elevated white blood cell (WBC) count • Sputum culture possibly positive for gram-positive *S. pneumoniae*
Hemophilus influenza	*Haemophilus influenzae*	• Insidious onset • History of upper respiratory tract infection 2 to 6 weeks earlier • Fever

Type	Causative agent	Assessment findings
Community-acquired pneumonias *(continued)*		
Hemophilus influenza *(continued)*		• Chills • Dyspnea • Productive cough • Nausea and vomiting • Chest X-ray with infiltrates in one or more lobes
Mycoplasma pneumonia	*Mycoplasma pneumoniae*	• Insidious onset • Sore throat • Nasal congestion • Ear pain • Headache • Low-grade fever • Pleuritic pain • Erythematous rash • Pharyngitis
Viral pneumonia	Influenza virus, type A	• Initially beginning as upper respiratory infection • Cough (initially nonproductive; later purulent sputum) • High fever • Chills • Malaise • Dyspnea • Substernal pain • Moist crackles • Cyanosis • Frontal headache

Types of pneumonia *(continued)*

Type	Causative agent	Assessment findings
Community-acquired pneumonias *(continued)*		
Viral pneumonia *(continued)*		• Chest X-ray with diffuse bilateral bronchopneumonia radiating from hilus • Normal to slightly elevated WBC
Legionnaires' disease	*Legionella pneumophila*	• Flulike symptoms • Malaise • Headache within 24 hours • Fever • Shaking chills • Progressive dyspnea • Mental confusion • Anorexia • Nausea, vomiting • Myalgia • Chest X-ray with patchy infiltrates, consolidation, and possible effusion
Hospital-acquired pneumonias		
Klebsiella pneumonia	*Klebsiella pneumoniae*	• Fever • Recurrent chills • Rusty, bloody, viscous sputum • Cyanosis of lips and nail beds • Shallow grunting respirations • Severe pleuritic chest pain

Type	Causative agent	Assessment findings
Hospital-acquired pneumonias *(continued)*		
Klebsiella pneumonia *(continued)*		• Chest X-ray typically with consolidation in upper lobe • Elevated WBC • Sputum culture and Gram stain possibly positive for gram-negative cocci, Klebsiella
Pseudomonas pneumonia	*Pseudomonas aeruginosa*	• Fever • Chills • Confusion • Delirium • Green, foul-smelling sputum • Chest X-ray with diffuse consolidation
Staphylococcal pneumonia (may also be community acquired)	*Staphylococcus aureus*	• Cough • Chills • High fever of 102° to 104° F • Pleuritic pain • Progressive dyspnea • Bloody sputum • Tachypnea • Hypoxemia • Chest X-ray with multiple abscesses and infiltrates; empyema • Elevated WBC • Sputum culture and Gram stain possibly positive for gram-positive staphylococci

Those at risk

The prognosis is good for patients with pneumonia who are otherwise healthy. Debilitated patients are at much greater risk; bacterial pneumonia is a leading cause of death among such individuals. Pneumonia occurs in both sexes and in all ages, but older adults are at greater risk for developing it.

What causes it

Primary pneumonia results from inhalation of a pathogen, such as bacteria or a virus. Examples are pneumococcal and viral pneumonia.

Secondary pneumonia may follow initial lung damage from a noxious chemical or other insult (superinfection) or may result from hematogenous spread of bacteria from a distant area.

Aspiration pneumonia results from inhalation of foreign matter — such as vomitus or food particles — into the bronchi. It's more common in elderly or debilitated patients; those receiving nasogastric (NG) tube feedings; and those with an impaired gag reflex, poor oral hygiene, or a decreased level of consciousness.

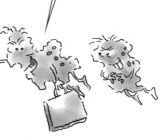

We get around! Bacterial pneumonia can move through the bloodstream to the lungs.

How it happens

The disease process varies depending on the type of pneumonia:
• In *bacterial pneumonia*, which can affect any part of the lungs, an infection initially triggers alveolar inflammation and edema. Capillaries become engorged with blood, causing stasis. As the alveolocapillary membrane breaks down, the alveoli fill with blood and inflammatory exudates, resulting in atelectasis.
• *Viral pneumonia* more commonly attacks bronchiolar epithelial cells, causing interstitial inflammation and desquamation. It then spreads to the alveoli.
• *Aspiration pneumonia* triggers similar inflammatory changes in the affected area and also inactivates surfactant over a large area, leading to alveolar collapse. Acidic gastric contents may directly damage the airways and alveoli, and small particles may cause obstruction. The resulting inflammation makes the lungs susceptible to secondary bacterial pneumonia.

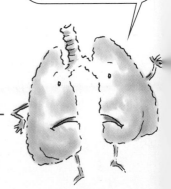

Bacterial pneumonia can affect any part of the lungs. Viral pneumonia attacks bronchiolar epithelial cells and spreads to the alveoli.

What to look for

Signs and symptoms of pneumonia include pleuritic chest pain, cough, fever, fatigue, and adventitious lungs sounds. Older adults may lack typical symptoms, such as fever or cough, and may have atypical symptoms, such as confusion and behavior changes.

Sounds, sights, and sensations

The patient's cough may be dry, as in mycoplasma pneumonia, or very productive. The sputum may be creamy yellow, green, or rust-colored. In advanced cases of all types of pneumonia, palpation and percussion reveal dullness and increased tactile fremitus over the affected area of the lung. Auscultation may disclose crackles, wheezes, or rhonchi over the affected areas as well as decreased breath sounds and increased voice sounds.

What tests tell you

- *Chest X-rays* disclose infiltrates, confirming the diagnosis.
- Sputum specimen for *Gram stain and culture and sensitivity testing* may reveal inflammatory cells as well as bacterial cells.
- *WBC count and differential* may indicate the presence and type of infection. Elevated polymorphonucleocytes may indicate bacterial infection in viral or mycoplasmal pneumonia, although the WBC count may not be elevated.
- *ABG analysis* is performed to determine the extent of respiratory compromise due to alveolar inflammation.
- *Bronchoscopy* or *transtracheal aspiration* allows the collection of material for cultures to identify the specific infectious organism. Pleural fluid may also be sampled for culture and Gram stain.
- *Pulse oximetry* may show a reduced arterial oxygen saturation level and indicate the need for oxygen supplementation.

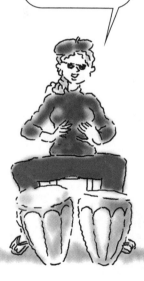

Percussion performed. Dullness revealed. Advanced pneumonia is what I feel.

How it's treated

Anti-infective agents, which are specific to the causative infectious organism, are used to treat pneumonia. In the case of aspiration pneumonia, steps are taken to reduce or eliminate the risk of aspiration. Prophylactic agents may be used to combat secondary infections or for specific cases such as in patients with human immunodeficiency virus (HIV) infection at risk for *Pneumocystis carinii* pneumonia (PCP).

More oxygen, please

The patient may receive oxygen supplementation, including ET intubation and mechanical ventilation in severe cases when respiratory arrest is imminent. In severe cases, positive end-expiratory pressure (PEEP) may also be necessary to prevent alveolar collapse.

Add-ons

Other treatment measures include:
- bronchodilator therapy
- antitussives for cough
- high-calorie diet and adequate fluid intake
- bed rest
- analgesics to relieve pleuritic chest pain.

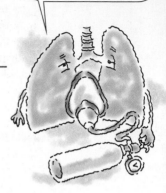

In severe cases of pneumonia, PEEP may be needed to prevent alveolar collapse.

What to do

- Maintain a patent airway and oxygenation. Place the patient in Fowler's position to maximize chest expansion and give supplemental oxygen as ordered. Monitor oxygen saturation and ABG levels as ordered.
- Assess respiratory status often, at least every 2 hours. Auscultate the lungs for abnormal breath sounds, such as crackles, wheezes, or rhonchi. Encourage coughing and deep breathing.
- If the patient's respiratory status deteriorates, anticipate the need for intubation and mechanical ventilation.
- Adhere to standard precautions and institute appropriate transmission-based precautions, depending on the causative organism.
- Institute cardiac monitoring to detect the development of arrhythmias secondary to hypoxemia.

Get comfortable

- Reposition the patient to maximize chest expansion, allow rest, and reduce discomfort and anxiety.
- Obtain ordered diagnostic tests, and report results promptly.
- Administer drug therapy as ordered.
- Carefully monitor the patient's intake and output to allow early identification of dehydration, fluid overload, and accurate tracking of nutritional status.
- To prevent aspiration during NG tube feedings, elevate the patient's head, check the position of the tube, and administer feedings slowly. Don't give large volumes at one time because this could cause vomiting. If the patient has a tracheostomy or an ET tube, inflate the tube cuff. Keep his head elevated for at least 30 minutes after feeding.

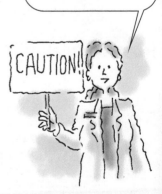

Adhere to standard precautions and other appropriate safety measures, depending on the causative organism.

Growing concerns

- Be aware that antimicrobial agents used to treat cytomegalovirus, PCP, and RSV pneumonia may be hazardous to fetal development. Pregnant health care workers or those attempting to conceive should minimize exposure to these agents (such as acyclovir [Zovirax], ribavirin [Virazole], and pentamidine [NebuPent]).

No place like home

Teaching the patient with pneumonia

• Teach the patient how to cough and perform deep-breathing exercises to clear secretions, and encourage him to do so often.
• Urge all bedridden and postoperative patients to perform deep-breathing exercises frequently. Position patients properly to promote full ventilation and drainage of secretions.
• Encourage annual influenza and pneumococcal vaccination for high-risk patients, such as those with chronic obstructive pulmonary disease, chronic heart disease, or sickle cell disease.
• To prevent pneumonia, advise the patient to avoid using antibiotics indiscriminately during minor viral infections because this may result in upper airway colonization with antibiotic-resistant bacteria. If the patient then develops pneumonia, the infecting organisms may require treatment with more toxic antibiotics.

• Evaluate the patient. His chest X-rays should be normal and his ABG levels should show a partial pressure of arterial oxygen of 50 to 60 mm Hg. (See *Teaching the patient with pneumonia.*)

Respiratory syncytial virus

RSV infection results from a subgroup of the myxoviruses that resemble paramyxovirus. Antibody titers seem to indicate that few children under age 4 escape contracting some form of RSV, even if it's mild. In fact, RSV is the only viral disease that has its maximum impact during the first few months of life (incidence of RSV bronchiolitis peaks at age 2 months).

'Tis the season

RSV, an acute virus, occurs in annual epidemics during the late winter and early spring in temperate climates and during the rainy season in the tropics. RSV may cause death in infants; however, in older children and adults, the disease may only be mild. (See *RSV in children,* page 158.)

It gets complicated

Complications of RSV include:
• pneumonia

- sudden infant death syndrome
- otitis media
- bronchiolitis
- croup
- residual lung damage
- tonsillitis.

What causes it

The organism that causes RSV is transmitted from person to person by respiratory secretions and has an incubation period of 4 to 5 days. School-age children, adolescents, and young adults with mild reinfections are probably the source of infection for infants and young children.

How it happens

The virus attaches to cells, eventually resulting in necrosis of the bronchiolar epithelium; in severe infection, peribronchiolar infiltrate of lymphocytes and mononuclear cells occurs. The result is intra-alveolar thickening and filling of the alveolar spaces with fluid.

What to look for

Clinical features of RSV infection vary in severity from mild, cold-like symptoms to bronchiolitis or bronchopneumonia and, in a few patients, severe, life-threatening lower respiratory tract infections. Reinfection is common, producing milder symptoms than the primary infection.

RSV has been identified in patients with a variety of central nervous system (CNS) disorders, such as meningitis and myelitis. Symptoms of RSV usually include:
- coughing
- wheezing
- malaise
- pharyngitis
- dyspnea
- inflamed mucous membranes (nose and throat).

Kids' korner

RSV in children

Respiratory syncytial virus (RSV) is the leading cause of lower respiratory tract infections in infants and young children. It's the major cause of pneumonia, tracheobronchitis, and bronchiolitis in this age-group and a suspected cause of the fatal respiratory diseases of infancy.

School-age children with mild reinfections are among the sources of infection for infants and young children.

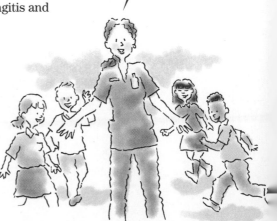

What tests tell you

Diagnosis of RSV is usually based on clinical findings and epi-
demiologic information:
- *Cultures* of nasal and pharyngeal secretions may show RSV;
however, the virus is labile, so cultures aren't always reliable.
- *Serum antibody titers* may be elevated; however, before age 6
months, maternal antibodies can impair test results.
- *Chest X-rays* help to detect pneumonia.

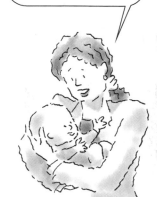

It's important for
parents to hold and
cuddle the infant who
has RSV.

How it's treated

- Goals of treatment are to support respiratory function, maintain
fluid balance, and relieve symptoms.
- Medication used to treat a patient with RSV may include ribavirin (may be administered to severely ill patients or those at
high risk for complications), albuterol nebulizer and, for high-risk
infants, RSV immunoglobulin.

What to do

- Tell family members to continue to hold and cuddle infants and
talk to and play with toddlers. Tell them to offer diversionary activities that are appropriate for the child's condition and age.
- Teach good hand-washing technique to family members to prevent spreading the illness.

Tonsillitis

Tonsillitis, or inflammation of the tonsils, can be acute or chronic.
The uncomplicated acute form usually lasts 4 to 6 days and commonly affects children between ages 5 and 10. The presence of
proven chronic tonsillitis justifies tonsillectomy, the only effective
treatment. Tonsils tend to hypertrophy during childhood and atro-
phy after puberty.

What causes it

Tonsillitis generally results from infection with group A beta-
hemolytic streptococci but can result from other bacteria or viruses or from oral anaerobes.

How it happens

The inflammatory response to cell damage by viruses or bacteria result in hyperemia and fluid exudation.

What to look for

Acute tonsillitis commonly begins with a mild to severe sore throat. A very young child, unable to describe a sore throat, may stop eating. Tonsillitis may also produce:
- dysphagia
- fever
- swelling and tender lymph glands in the submandibular area
- muscle and joint pain
- chills
- malaise
- headache
- pain (frequently referred to the ears).

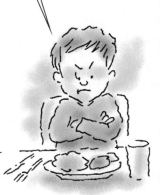

I can't eat, it hurts to swallow, and I have a headache. When will they realize I have tonsillitis!

Blocked and constricted

Excess secretions can cause a constant urge to swallow; the back of the throat may feel constricted. Such discomfort usually subsides after 72 hours. However, chronic tonsillitis produces a recurrent sore throat and purulent drainage in the tonsillar crypts. Frequent attacks of acute tonsillitis may also occur.

What tests tell you

Culture may be used to determine the infecting organism and appropriate antibiotic therapy for tonsillitis. Leukocytosis is usually present.

Definitive diagnosis requires a thorough *throat examination* that reveals:
- generalized inflammation of the pharyngeal wall
- swollen tonsils project from between the tonsillar pillars and the uvula with patchy white or yellow exudate
- purulent drainage when pressure is applied to the tonsillar pillars
- possible edematous and inflamed uvula.

How it's treated

- Treatment for acute tonsillitis requires rest, adequate fluid intake, and administration of analgesics and antibiotics.
- Chronic tonsillitis or complications (obstructions from tonsillar hypertrophy, peritonsillar abscess) may necessitate a tonsillecto-

my but only after the patient has been free from tonsillar or respiratory tract infections for 3 to 4 weeks.

What to do

- Urge the patient to drink plenty of fluids, especially if he has a fever. Parents may offer a child ice cream, flavored drinks, and ices.
- Make sure that the patient and his parents understand the importance of completing the prescribed course of antibiotic therapy.
- After surgery, tell the patient and his parents to expect a white scab to form in the throat between 5 and 10 days postoperatively and to report bleeding, ear discomfort, or a fever that lasts longer than 3 days.

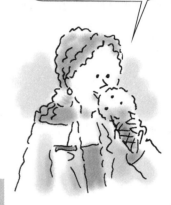

Keep your freezer stocked with ice cream for the child with tonsillitis.

Tuberculosis

TB is an acute or chronic infection characterized by pulmonary infiltrates and by the formation of granulomas with caseation, fibrosis, and cavitation. The main site of infection is the lung, but approximately 15% of mycobacterium infections are extrapulmonary.

Typical TB

The disease is twice as common in men as in women and four times as common in nonwhites as in whites. However, incidence is highest in people who live in crowded, poorly ventilated, unsanitary conditions, such as in some prisons, tenement houses, and homeless shelters. The typical newly diagnosed TB patient is a single, homeless, nonwhite man. With proper treatment, the prognosis is usually excellent.

What causes it

TB results from exposure to *Mycobacterium tuberculosis* and, sometimes, other strains of mycobacteria. Transmission occurs when an infected person coughs or sneezes, spreading infected aerosolized droplets. These droplets are inhaled. Contact with the infected person isn't necessary. The risk of infection increases with increased duration and intensity of exposure. (See *Understanding TB*, page 162.)

Dormant disease

Most individuals who contact the infection don't develop active TB. Only about 2% of normal healthy individuals develop early disease. The disease becomes dormant and may activate later in life when the individual becomes aged or otherwise immunocompromised. However, about 90% of persons infected will never develop active TB.

In HIV infected individuals, the rate of initial development of early disease is approximately 40% and the development of dormant disease into reactivated disease is 20% to 50%.

Populations that incur a high incidence of TB with presenting symptoms include:
- Black and Hispanic men between ages 25 and 44
- persons in close contact with a newly diagnosed TB patient
- persons who have had TB before
- persons with multiple sexual partners
- recent immigrants from Africa, Asia, Mexico, and South America
- gastrectomy patients
- persons affected with silicosis, diabetes, malnutrition, cancer, Hodgkin's disease, or leukemia

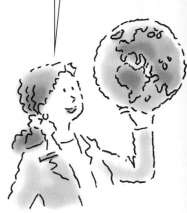

Recent immigrants may have a higher incidence of TB than other populations.

Advice from the experts

Understanding TB

When a person without immunity inhales droplets infected with *Mycobacterium tuberculosis*, the bacilli lodge in the alveoli, causing irritation. The immune system responds by sending leukocytes, lymphocytes, and macrophages to surround the bacilli, and the local lymph nodes swell and become inflamed.

Rupture and spread

If the encapsulated bacilli (tubercles) and the inflamed nodes rupture, the infection contaminates the surrounding tissue and may spread through the blood and lymphatic circulation to distant sites—a process called *hematogenous dissemination.* This same phagocytic cycle occurs whenever the bacilli spread. Sites of ex-

trapulmonary tuberculosis (TB) include the pleura, meninges, joints, lymph nodes, peritoneum, and GI tract.

TB exposure

After exposure to *M. tuberculosis,* roughly 5% of infected people develop active TB within 1 year. In the remainder, microorganisms cause a latent infection. The host's immunologic defense system usually destroys the bacillus or walls it up in a tubercle. However, the live, encapsulated bacilli may lie dormant within the tubercle for years, reactivating later to cause active infection. In this respect, the disease is an opportunistic infection.

- drug and alcohol abusers
- patients in mental health facilities

Elderly risks

- nursing home residents, who are ten times more likely to contract TB than anyone in the general population
- persons receiving treatment with immunosuppressants or corticosteroids
- persons with weak immune systems or diseases that affect the immune system, especially those with acquired immunodeficiency syndrome
- prisoners
- homeless persons.

It gets worse...

TB can cause massive pulmonary tissue damage, with inflammation and tissue necrosis eventually leading to respiratory failure. Bronchopleural fistulas can develop from lung tissue damage, resulting in pneumothorax. The disease can also lead to hemorrhage, pleural effusion, and pneumonia. Small mycobacterial foci can infect other body organs, including the kidneys, the CNS, and the skeletal system. The patient may also develop liver complications from drug therapy.

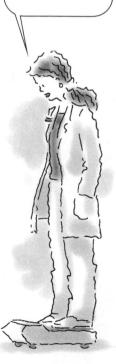

Weight loss is a common symptom of TB.

How it happens

Multiplication of the bacillus *M. tuberculosis* causes an inflammatory process where deposited. A cell-mediated immune response follows, usually containing the infection within 4 to 6 weeks. The T-cell response results in the formation of granulomas around the bacilli making them dormant. This confers immunity to subsequent infection. Bacilli within granulomas may remain viable for many years, resulting in a positive purified protein derivative (PPD) or other skin test for TB.

TB on the move

Active disease develops in 5% to 15% of those infected. Transmission occurs when an infected person coughs or sneezes, spreading infected droplets.

What to look for

The most common symptoms are fatigue, cough, fever, night sweats, anorexia, and weight loss. Patients may report chest pain or blood tinged sputum.

When you percuss, you may note dullness over the affected area, a sign of consolidation or the presence of pleural fluid. On auscultation, you may hear crepitant crackles, bronchial breath sounds, wheezes, and whispered pectoriloquy.

What tests tell you

It may be necessary to conduct several diagnostic tests to distinguish TB from other diseases that may mimic it, such as lung carcinoma, lung abscess, pneumoconiosis, and bronchiectasis.

These tests include:

• *Chest X-rays* show nodular lesions, patchy infiltrates (mainly in upper lobes), cavity formation, scar tissue, and calcium deposits. They may not help distinguish between active and inactive TB.

Sampling the skin

• A *tuberculin skin test* reveals that the patient has been exposed to *M. tuberculosis* at some point but it doesn't indicate active disease. In this test, intermediate-strength PPD or 5 tuberculin units (0.1 ml) are injected intradermally on the forearm and read in 48 to 72 hours. A positive reaction (equal to or more than a 10-mm induration) develops within 2 to 10 weeks after infection with the tubercle bacillus in both active and inactive TB. Persons who have been vaccinated with BCG (Bacille, Calmette-Guérin) may exhibit a positive skin test.

• *Stains and cultures* of sputum, cerebrospinal fluid, urine, drainage from an abscess, or pleural fluid show heat-sensitive, nonmotile, aerobic, acid-fast bacilli.

• *CT scanning* and *magnetic resonance imaging* allow the evaluation of lung damage or confirm a difficult diagnosis.

• *Bronchoscopy* may be performed if the patient can't produce an adequate sputum specimen.

How it's treated

Latent TB is treated with isoniazid (Laniazid) daily or twice weekly for 9 months. Treatment regimen requires alterations based upon co-morbid conditions, age, drug resistance, and strains of TB. Patients with a weakened immune system will be treated with multiple-drug therapy. Bacteria that causes TB can also become resistant to antibiotics used to kill or control the organism causing this disease and will require a change in the drug regimen. Active TB is treated with a combination of drugs — usually 3 to 4 drugs daily for 2 months, followed by 2 drugs for another 4 months.

First line of defense

First line treatment drugs are isoniazid, rifampin (Rifadin), ethambutol (Myambutol), and pyrazinamide. After 2 to 4 weeks of treatment, the disease is no longer infectious and the patient can resume normal activities while continuing to take medication.

The patient with atypical mycobacterial disease or drug-resistant TB may require second-line drugs, such as capreomycin (Capastat), streptomycin (Streptomycin), para-aminosalicylic acid, pyrazinamide, and cycloserine.

What to do

• Administer ordered antibiotics and antitubercular agents.
• Isolate the infectious patient in a quiet, properly ventilated room, as per guidelines from the Centers for Disease Control and Prevention, and maintain TB precautions. Provide diversional activities and check on him frequently. Make sure the call button is nearby.

Talking trash

• Place a covered trash can nearby, or tape a plastic bag to the bed for used tissues. Tell the patient to wear a mask when outside his room. Visitors and health care personnel should also take proper precautions while in the patient's room.
• Make sure the patient gets plenty of rest. Provide for periods of rest and activity to promote health as well as conserve energy and reduce oxygen demand.
• Provide the patient with well-balanced, high-calorie foods — preferably in small, frequent meals to conserve energy. (Small, frequent meals may also encourage the anorexic patient to eat more.) Record the patient's weight weekly. If he needs oral supplements, consult with the dietitian.
• Watch for adverse reactions to the medications.
• Administer isoniazid with food. This drug can cause hepatitis or peripheral neuritis, so monitor levels of aspartate aminotransferase and alanine aminotransferase. To prevent or treat peripheral neuritis, give pyridoxine (vitamin B_6) as ordered.

Visual effects

• If the patient receives ethambutol, give the medication with food. Check the patient's vision monthly, and watch for signs of optic neuritis. If these signs occur, report them to the doctor, who's likely to discontinue the drug.
• If the patient receives rifampin, watch for signs of hepatitis, purpura, and a flulike syndrome as well as other complications such as hemoptysis. Monitor liver and kidney function tests throughout therapy.
• Perform chest physiotherapy, including postural drainage and chest percussion, several times per day.

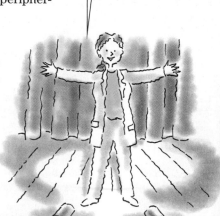

Provide diversional activities for the patient with TB. Just try to keep it quiet!

Preventing TB

Explain respiratory and standard precautions to the hospitalized patient with tuberculosis (TB). Before discharge, tell him that he must take precautions to prevent spreading the disease, such as wearing a mask around others, until his doctor tells him that he's no longer contagious. He should tell all health care providers he sees, including his dentist and eye doctor, that he has TB so that they can institute infection-control precautions.

Teach the patient other specific precautions to avoid spreading the infection. Tell him to cough and sneeze into tissues and to dispose of the tissues properly. Stress the importance of washing his hands thoroughly in hot, soapy water after handling his own secretions. Also instruct him to wash his eating utensils separately in hot, soapy water.

Teaching the patient with TB

- Show the patient and his family members how to perform postural drainage and chest percussion. Also teach the patient coughing and deep-breathing techniques. Instruct him to maintain each position for 10 minutes and then to perform percussion and cough.
- Teach the patient the adverse effects of his medication and tell him to report them immediately. Emphasize the importance of follow-up examinations, and instruct the patient and his family members concerning the signs and symptoms of recurring tuberculosis (TB). Stress the need to follow long-term treatment faithfully.

- Give the patient supportive care and help him adjust to the changes he may have to make during his illness. Include the patient in care decisions and let his family take part in the patient's care whenever possible. (See *Teaching the patient with TB*.)
- DOT, directly observed therapy, requires the patient be directly observed taking the medications. Even with good health education adherence to medication regimens is unreliable. DOT helps assure compliance and is usually coordinated by public health departments.
- Advise anyone exposed to an infected patient to receive tuberculin tests and, if a positive reaction occurs, chest X-rays and prophylactic isoniazid. (See *Preventing TB*.)

Color concerns

- Warn the patient taking rifampin that the drug temporarily makes body secretions appear orange; reassure him that this effect is harmless. If the patient is a woman, warn her that oral contraceptives may be less effective while she's taking rifampin.
- Teach the patient the signs and symptoms that require medical assessment, including increased cough, hemoptysis, unexplained weight loss, fever, and night sweats.
- Stress the importance of eating high-calorie, high-protein, balanced meals.

Tell the patient to eat high-calorie, high-protein meals. De-lish!

• Emphasize the importance of scheduling and keeping follow-up appointments.

• Refer the patient to such support groups as the American Lung Association.

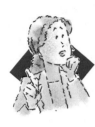

Quick quiz

1. The five cardinal signs and symptoms of early bacterial pneumonia are:

    A.   dry cough, shaking chills, fever, sweating, pleuritic chest pain.

    B.   sharp, stabbing chest pain; pleural friction rub; fever; chills; sweating.

    C.   coughing, sputum production, pleuritic chest pain, shaking chills, fever.

    D.   dry cough, shaking chills, fever, sweating, sharp, stabbing chest pain.

Answer: C. Coughing, sputum production, pleuritic chest pain, shaking chills, and fever are the five cardinal signs and symptoms of early bacterial pneumonia.

2. TB is transmitted through:

    A.   inhalation of infected aerosolized droplets.

    B.   contact with blood.

    C.   the fecal-oral route.

    D.   skin-to-skin contact.

Answer: A. TB spreads by inhalation of aerosolized droplet nuclei when an infected person coughs or sneezes.

3. A patient with clinically active TB is prescribed isoniazid, rifampin, pyrazinamide, and ethambutol. Which findings best indicate the effectiveness of drug therapy?

    A.   Cavities are no longer evident on chest X-ray.

    B.   Tuberculin skin test is negative.

    C.   The patient is afebrile and no longer coughing.

    D.   The sputum culture converts to negative.

Answer: D. A change in sputum culture from positive to negative is the best indication of the effectiveness of antitubercular medications.

4.   Which of these characteristics best describes croup?
   A.   Inflammation of the palatine tonsils
   B.   A highly contagious respiratory infection
   C.   Infection of the supraglottic area with involvement of the epiglottis
   D.   Clinical syndrome of laryngitis and laryngotracheobronchitis

Answer: D. Croup is a general term referring to acute infections affecting varying degrees of the larynx, trachea, and bronchi.

5.   Which of these signs is most characteristic in a child with croup?
   A.   Barking cough
   B.   Fever
   C.   Low heart rate
   D.   Respiratory distress

Answer: A. A resonant cough described as *barking* is the most characteristic sign of croup.

Scoring

☆☆☆   If you answered all five items correctly, way to go! You can breathe easy about your knowledge of respiratory disorders.

☆☆   If you answered four items correctly, super! Your understanding of respiratory disorders is circulating well!

☆   If you answered fewer than four items correctly, no worries! Take a deep breath, oxygenate those tissues, and review the chapter!

6

Obstructive disorders

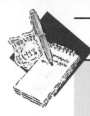

Just the facts

In this chapter, you'll learn:

♦ common obstructive disorders

♦ potential causes of obstructive disorders of the respiratory tract

♦ how to recognize an obstructive disorder affecting the respiratory tract

♦ treatment for a variety of obstructive respiratory conditions.

Understanding obstructive disorders

Among chronic obstructive disorders of the lung, chronic obstructive pulmonary disease (COPD), also called *chronic obstructive lung disorder*, is the most common. It affects an estimated 30 million Americans and its incidence is rising. It now ranks third among the major causes of death in the United States.

The disorder affects more men than women, probably because until recently, men were more likely to smoke heavily. However, the rate of COPD among women is increasing. Early COPD might not produce symptoms and may cause only minimal disability in many patients, but it tends to worsen with time.

Types of COPD include asthma, chronic bronchitis, emphysema and, more commonly, any combination of these conditions (usually bronchitis and emphysema). Other obstructive disorders include cystic fibrosis and sleep apnea.

COPD affects more men than women. However, the rate among women is increasing.

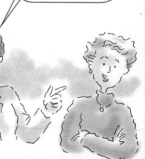

Asthma

Asthma is a chronic inflammatory airway disorder that causes episodic airway obstruction and hyperresponsiveness of the airway to multiple stimuli. It results from bronchospasms, increased mucus secretion, and mucosal edema. Asthma affects as many as 17 million Americans annually. An estimated 6.3 million children have asthma, making it the most common chronic childhood disease. Although reversible, *status asthmaticus*, a prolonged and severe asthma attack that doesn't respond to standard treatment, is life-threatening and can lead to respiratory failure and cardiac arrest. (See *The incidence of asthma*.)

Making things worse

Asthma exacerbations are acute or subacute episodes of worsening shortness of breath, coughing, wheezing, and measurable decreases in expiratory airflow.

Memory jogger

How can you remember the types of chronic obstructive pulmonary disease (COPD)? Simple: Just remember that you really need to "ACE" this one! The types of COPD include:

A — asthma

C — chronic bronchitis

E — emphysema.

What causes it

Many people with asthma, especially children, have intrinsic and extrinsic asthma.

Outside and sensitive

Extrinsic, or *atopic*, asthma begins in childhood. Patients are typically sensitive to specific external (extrinsic) allergens. Extrinsic allergens that can trigger an asthma attack include such elements as pollen, animal dander, house dust or mold, kapok or feather pillows, food additives containing sulfites, and other sensitizing substances. Extrinsic asthma in childhood is commonly accompanied by other hereditary allergies, such as eczema and allergic rhinitis.

A look within

Patients with *intrinsic*, or *nonatopic*, asthma react to internal, nonallergenic factors. Intrinsic factors that can trigger an asthma attack include irritants, emotional stress, fatigue, endocrine changes, temperature variations, humidity variations, exposure to noxious fumes, anxiety, coughing or laughing, and genetic factors. Most episodes occur after a severe respiratory tract infection, especially in adults.

Exercise-induced asthma is a narrowing of the airways that makes it difficult to move air out of the lungs. Symptoms include coughing, wheezing, chest tightness, and prolonged, unexpected shortness of breath after 5 to 20 minutes of exercise. These symptoms are commonly worse in cold, dry air.

I love animals. I wish their dander didn't trigger asthma attacks in some people.

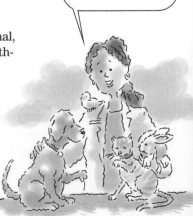

Calling in sick

Many adults acquire an allergic form of asthma or exacerbation of existing asthma from exposure to irritants in the workplace. Chemicals in flour, acid anhydrides, and excreta of dust mites in carpet are a few such agents that trigger asthma.

Genetic messes

Asthma is associated with two genetic influences:
- ability to develop asthma because of an abnormal gene (atopy)
- tendency to develop hyperresponsive airways (without atopy).

A potent mix

Environmental factors interact with inherited factors to cause asthmatic reactions with associated bronchospasms.

How it happens

In asthma, the tracheal and bronchial linings overreact to various stimuli, causing episodic smooth-muscle spasms that severely constrict the airways.

Immunoglobulin (Ig) E antibodies, attached to histamine-containing mast cells and receptors on cell membranes, initiate intrinsic asthma attacks.

When the IgE antibody is exposed to an allergen, such as pollen, the antibody combines with the antigen. On subsequent exposure to the antigen, mast cells degranulate and release mediators. Mast cells in the lung interstitium are stimulated to release histamine and leukotrienes. Histamine attaches to receptor sites in the larger bronchi, where it causes swelling in smooth muscle. Mucous membranes become inflamed, irritated, and swollen. (See *Looking at a bronchiole in asthma*, page 172.)

As a result, expiratory airflow decreases, trapping gas in the airways and causing alveolar hyperinflation. Atelectasis may develop in some lung regions. The increased airway resistance initiates labored breathing. (See *Averting an asthma attack*, page 173.)

Several factors may contribute to bronchoconstriction, including hereditary predisposition; sensitivity to allergens or irritants such as pollutants; viral infections; aspirin, beta-adrenergic blockers, non-steroidal anti-inflammatory agents, and other drugs; tartrazine (a yellow food dye); psychological stress; cold air; and exercise. Asthma can produce status asthmaticus and respiratory failure. (See *Understanding the progression of an asthma attack*, page 174.)

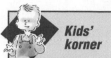

Kids' korner

The incidence of asthma

Asthma can strike at any age but about half of all people with asthma are younger than age 10. In this age-group, asthma affects twice as many boys as girls. About one-third of patients experience asthma onset between ages 10 and 30. In this group, incidence is the same in both genders. Hereditary factors are also important; about one-third of all people with asthma share the disease with at least one immediate family member.

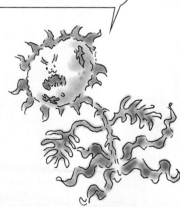

You can't always trust a pretty face. Exposure to my pollen makes mast cells in the lung release histamine. Sorry about that!

Looking at a bronchiole in asthma

Asthma is characterized by bronchospasms, increased mucus secretion, and mucosal edema, all of which contribute to airway narrowing and obstruction. Shown here is a normal bronchiole in cross-section and an obstructed bronchiole, as it appears in asthma.

Normal bronchiole

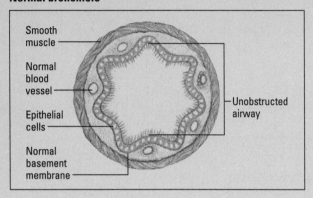

Smooth muscle

Normal blood vessel

Epithelial cells

Normal basement membrane

Unobstructed airway

Obstructed bronchiole

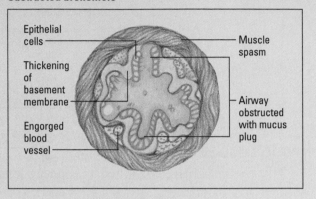

Epithelial cells

Thickening of basement membrane

Engorged blood vessel

Muscle spasm

Airway obstructed with mucus plug

What to look for

An asthma attack can begin slowly or dramatically. Progressive cyanosis, confusion, and lethargy may indicate that the acute asthma attack has progressed to status asthmaticus.

A patient of few words

Typically, the patient reports exposure to a particular allergen followed by a sudden onset of dyspnea, wheezing, and tightness in the chest accompanied by a cough that produces thick, clear or yellow sputum. The patient may complain of feeling suffocated, appear visibly dyspneic, and be able to speak only a few words before pausing to catch his breath.

I'm oxygen deprived. What's your excuse?

Mental status is a sensitive indicator of oxygen deprivation, and the patient may initially be irritable or anxious. As hypoxemia progresses, the patient becomes confused and increasingly lethargic, a sign of impending respiratory failure.

The patient's heart rate is elevated and commonly irregular. Respiratory rate is also well above normal. When the patient begins to tire, his respiratory rate begins to slow, which may be another sign of impending respiratory failure if he's also confused and lethargic.

Averting an asthma attack

This flowchart shows pathophysiologic changes that occur with asthma. Treatments and interventions are introduced to alter the physiologic cascade and stop the asthma attack.

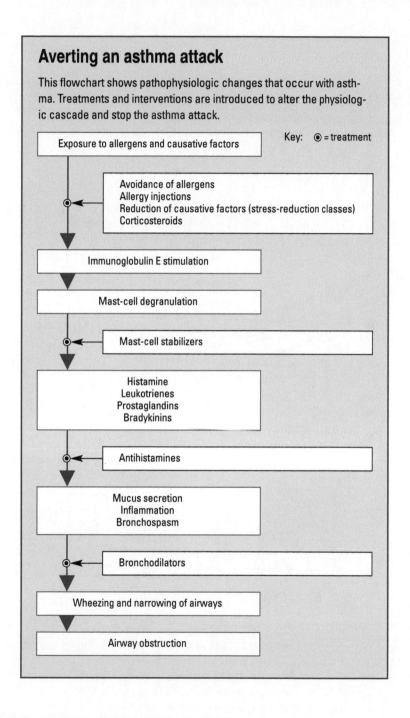

Key: ◉ = treatment

Exposure to allergens and causative factors

Avoidance of allergens
Allergy injections
Reduction of causative factors (stress-reduction classes)
Corticosteroids

Immunoglobulin E stimulation

Mast-cell degranulation

Mast-cell stabilizers

Histamine
Leukotrienes
Prostaglandins
Bradykinins

Antihistamines

Mucus secretion
Inflammation
Bronchospasm

Bronchodilators

Wheezing and narrowing of airways

Airway obstruction

Now I get it!

Understanding the progression of an asthma attack

In asthma, hyperresponsiveness of the airways and bronchospasms occur. These illustrations show the progression of an asthma attack.

Histamine attaches to receptor sites in larger bronchi, which causes swelling of the smooth muscles.

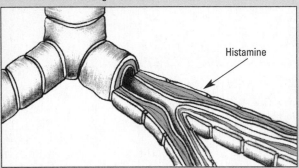

Leukotrienes attach to receptor sites in the smaller bronchi, which causes swelling of smooth muscle there. Leukotrienes also cause prostaglandins to travel to the lungs via the bloodstream, where they enhance the effects of histamine.

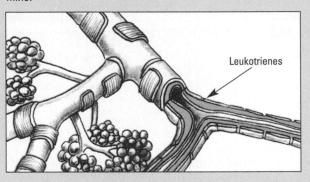

Histamine stimulates the mucous membranes to secrete excessive mucus, further narrowing the bronchial lumen. On inhalation, the narrowed bronchial lumen can still expand slightly; however, on exhalation, the increased intrathoracic pressure closes the bronchial lumen completely.

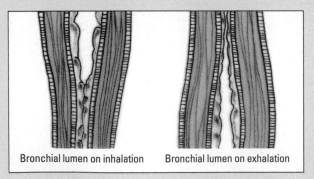

Bronchial lumen on inhalation   Bronchial lumen on exhalation

Mucus fills lung bases, inhibiting alveolar ventilation. Blood is shunted to alveoli in other parts of the lungs but the shunting can't compensate for diminished ventilation.

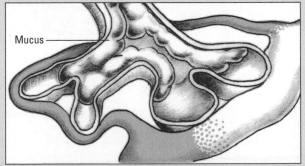

Mucus

Roll out the barrel

On inspection, you may see a barrel chest if the patient has chronic asthma. During an attack, the patient's face may appear pale and diaphoretic and he may use accessory muscles of respiration. The patient generally sits up straight or leans forward slightly. On percussing the chest wall, you may find hyperresonance; palpation may reveal vocal fremitus.

The lungs tell all

When you listen to the lungs, you may hear harsh respirations with inspiratory and expiratory wheezes and, possibly, reduced breath sounds over some areas of the lung. The expiratory phase of respiration is prolonged. Marked wheezing may develop due to increased edema and mucus in the lower airways. Breath sounds and wheezing may suddenly stop because of severe bronchoconstriction and edema. (See *When wheezing stops*.)

What tests tell you

These tests are used to establish an asthma diagnosis:
• *Pulmonary function tests* reveal decreased vital capacity and increased total lung and residual capacities during an acute attack. Peak and expiratory flow rate measurements are less than 60% of baseline.
• *Pulse oximetry* commonly shows that oxygen saturation is less than 90%.
• *Chest X-rays* may show hyperinflation with areas of atelectasis and a flat diaphragm due to increased intrathoracic volume.
• *Arterial blood gas (ABG) analysis* reveals decreasing partial pressure of arterial oxygen (PaO_2) and increasing partial pressure of arterial carbon dioxide ($PaCO_2$).
• An *electrocardiogram (ECG)* shows sinus tachycardia during an attack.
• *Sputum analysis* may indicate increased viscosity, mucus plugs, Curschmann's spirals (casts of airways), Charcot-Leyden crystals, and eosinophils. Cultures may disclose causative organisms if infection is the trigger.
• A *complete blood count* with differential shows an increased eosinophil count secondary to inflammation, and an elevated white blood cell (WBC) and granulocyte count if an acute infection is present.

How it's treated

The best treatment for asthma is prevention. Because patients usually can't avoid precipitating factors completely, several treatments are available to decrease the frequency and severity of asthma attacks.

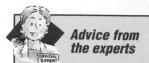

Advice from the experts

When wheezing stops

Even if you no longer hear wheezing in a patient who's having an acute asthma attack, the attack may not be over. When bronchospasm and mucosal swelling become severe, little air moves through the airways; as a result, you won't hear wheezing.

If all other assessment criteria—labored breathing, prolonged expiratory time, and accessory muscle use—point to acute bronchial obstruction, maintain the patient's airway and give oxygen as ordered. The patient may begin to wheeze again when the airways open further.

Prevention

• Asthma attacks may be prevented by identifying and avoiding precipitating factors, such as environmental allergens or irritants.
• When the stimuli can't be removed entirely, desensitization to specific antigens decreases the severity of asthma attacks with future exposure. Desensitization may be more helpful in children than in adults with bronchial asthma.

Drug therapy

Drug therapy is most effective when started soon after the onset of signs and symptoms. ABG measurements help to determine the severity of an asthma attack and the patient's response to treatment, which, for the most part, must be tailored to the patient.
• Bronchodilators, which are usually included in the patient's drug therapy arsenal, decrease bronchoconstriction, reduce bronchial airway edema, and increase pulmonary ventilation. Bronchodilators include rapid-acting epinephrine, methylxanthines (theophylline and aminophylline), and beta$_2$-adrenergic antagonists (albuterol and terbutaline) to decrease bronchoconstriction.
• Anticholinergics are used to increase the effects of bronchodilators. Anticholinergic bronchodilators (such as ipratropium) block acetylcholine, another chemical mediator.
• Corticosteroids (hydrocortisone sodium succinate, prednisone, methylprednisolones, and beclomethasone) are used for their anti-inflammatory and immunosuppressant effects. They decrease bronchoconstriction, reduce bronchial airway edema, and increase pulmonary ventilation.
• Subcutaneous epinephrine counteracts the effects of mediators of an asthma attack.
• Mast-cell stabilizers (cromolyn [Intal] and nedocromil [Tilade]) are useful in patients with atopic asthma who have seasonal disease. Used prophylactically, they block the acute obstructive effects of antigen exposure by inhibiting the degranulation of mast cells. This, in turn, prevents the release of chemical mediators (histamine and leukotrienes) that cause bronchoconstriction and anaphylaxis.
• Antibiotics are prescribed as needed for treatment of infection.

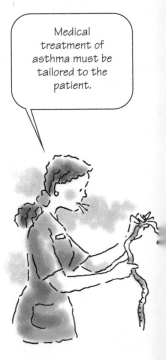

Medical treatment of asthma must be tailored to the patient.

Supportive measures

• Humidified, low-flow oxygen may be used to correct dyspnea, cyanosis, and hypoxemia, and to maintain an oxygen saturation greater than 90%.

• Mechanical ventilation becomes necessary when the patient doesn't respond to initial ventilatory support and drugs, or when respiratory failure develops.
• Relaxation exercises can help to increase circulation and aid in the recovery from an asthma attack.

Comprehensive care: status asthmaticus

Status asthmaticus must be treated promptly to prevent progression to fatal respiratory failure. The patient with increasingly severe asthma that doesn't respond to drug therapy is usually admitted to the intensive care unit for treatment with corticosteroids, epinephrine, sympathomimetic aerosol sprays, and I.V. aminophylline. Such patients require frequent ABG analysis and pulse oximetry to assess respiratory status, especially after ventilator therapy or a change in oxygen concentration. The patient may require endotracheal intubation and mechanical ventilation if his $Paco_2$ increases. (See *How status asthmaticus progresses*, page 178.)

What to do

Effective care for a patient with asthma requires strong assessment skills as well as administration of a variety of medications and therapeutic regimens:
• Start by assessing the severity of asthma. (See *Classifying asthma*, page 179.)
• Administer the prescribed treatments and assess the patient's response.
• Place the patient in high Fowler's position. Encourage pursed-lip and diaphragmatic breathing. Help him to relax.
• Monitor the patient's vital signs. Keep in mind that developing or increasing tachypnea may indicate worsening asthma, and that tachycardia may indicate worsening asthma or drug toxicity.
• Keep in mind that blood pressure readings may reveal pulsus paradoxus, indicating severe asthma. Hypertension may indicate asthma-related hypoxemia.

I get misty

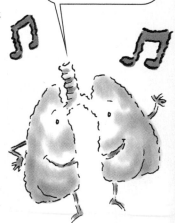

Look at me, I'm as helpless as a kitten in a tree... I get misty (well, actually, humidified).

• Administer prescribed humidified oxygen by nasal cannula at 2 L/minute to ease breathing and increase arterial oxygen saturation (Sao_2). Later, adjust oxygen according to the patient's vital signs and ABG values.
• Anticipate intubation and mechanical ventilation if the patient fails to respond to treatment.

How status asthmaticus progresses

A potentially fatal complication, status asthmaticus arises when impaired gas exchange and heightened airway resistance increase the work of breathing. This flowchart shows the stages of status asthmaticus.

> Obstructed airways hamper gas exchange and increase airway resistance, leading to labored breathing.

> The patient hyperventilates, lowering partial pressure of arterial carbon dioxide ($Paco_2$).

> Respiratory alkalosis and hypoxemia develop.

> Hypoxia and labored breathing tire the patient. His respiratory rate drops to normal.

> $Paco_2$ rises to a higher-than-baseline level (an asthmatic patient's $Paco_2$ is usually low).

> The patient hypoventilates from exhaustion.

> Respiratory acidosis begins as partial pressure of oxygen in arterial blood drops and $Paco_2$ continues to rise.

> Without treatment, the patient experiences acute respiratory failure.

> Hypoxia and cellular death from lack of oxygen and accumulation of carbon dioxide can result.

• Observe the frequency and severity of the patient's cough and note whether it's productive. Next, auscultate his lungs, noting adventitious or absent breath sounds. Maintain adequate oxygenation.

• Treat dehydration with I.V. fluids until the patient can tolerate oral fluids, which help loosen secretions.

Classifying asthma

These lists include current guidelines for classifying asthma severity as mild intermittent, mild persistent, moderate persistent, or severe persistent.

Mild intermittent
• Attacks no more than twice per week
• Nighttime attacks no more than twice per month
• Attacks lasting no longer than a few hours to days
• Attacks of varying severity but without symptoms between attacks

Mild persistent
• Attacks more than twice per week but not every day
• Nighttime attacks more than twice per month
• Attacks that are sometimes severe enough to interrupt regular activities

Moderate persistent
• Daily attacks
• Nighttime attacks more than once per week
• More severe attacks that occur at least twice per week and may last days
• Attacks that require daily use of quick-relief (rescue) medication and necessitate changes in daily activities

Severe persistent
• Continual, severe daily attacks
• Frequent, severe nighttime attacks
• Attacks that require limits on daily activities

• If conservative treatment fails to improve the airway obstruction, anticipate bronchoscopy or bronchial lavage when the area of collapse is a lobe or larger.

Over the long run

• Monitor the patient's respiratory status to detect baseline changes, assess response to treatment, and prevent or detect complications.
• Auscultate the lungs frequently, noting the degree of wheezing and quality of air movement.
• Review ABG levels, pulmonary function test results, and Sao_2 readings.
• If the patient is taking systemic corticosteroids, observe for complications, such as elevated blood glucose levels and friable skin and bruising.
• Minimize cushingoid effects resulting from long-term use of corticosteroids by trying alternate-day dosing or using prescribed inhaled corticosteroids. If the patient is taking corticosteroids by inhaler, watch for signs of candidal infection in the mouth and pharynx, including white patches in the mouth (especially on the patient's tongue or throat), a coated feeling on the tongue, or a sore throat or tongue. Instruct the patient to use an extender device and rinse his mouth after using the inhaler to help prevent these discomforts.
• For patients with moderate to severe chronic disease, consider regular use of an extender device, which may facilitate delivery of inhaled medications.

No place like home

Managing asthma at home

• Teach the patient and his family members to avoid known allergens and irritants.
• Describe prescribed drugs, including their names, dosages, actions, and adverse effects. Be sure to explain special instructions for taking the drugs properly.
• Teach the patient how to use a metered-dose inhaler. If he has difficulty using an inhaler, he may need an extender device to optimize drug delivery and lower the risk of candidal infection with orally inhaled corticosteroids.
• If the patient has moderate to severe asthma, explain how to use a peak-flow meter to measure the degree of airway obstruction. Tell him to keep a record of peak-flow readings and to bring it to medical appointments. Explain the

importance of calling the doctor immediately if the peak flow drops suddenly. (A drop can signal severe respiratory problems.)
• Tell the patient to notify the doctor if he develops a fever higher than 100° F (37.8° C), chest pain, shortness of breath without coughing or exercising, or uncontrollable coughing. An uncontrollable asthma attack requires immediate attention.
• Teach the patient diaphragmatic and pursed-lip breathing, as well as effective coughing techniques.
• Urge the patient to drink at least 3 qt (3 L) of fluid daily to help loosen secretions and maintain hydration.

• Observe the patient's anxiety level. Keep in mind that measures to reduce hypoxemia and breathlessness should relieve anxiety.
• Keep the room temperature comfortable. Use an air conditioner or a fan in hot, humid weather.
• Teach the patient how to use a metered dose inhaler.
• Control exercise-induced asthma by instructing the patient to use a bronchodilator or cromolyn 30 minutes before exercise. Also instruct him to use pursed-lip breathing while exercising. (See *Managing asthma at home.*)

Chronic bronchitis

Chronic bronchitis is a form of COPD. It's marked by excessive production of tracheobronchial mucus that's sufficient to cause a cough for at least 3 months each year for 2 consecutive years. The severity of the disease is linked to the amount of cigarette smoke or other pollutants inhaled, and the duration of the inhalation. A respiratory tract infection typically exacerbates the cough and related symptoms. However, few patients with chronic bronchitis develop significant airway obstruction.

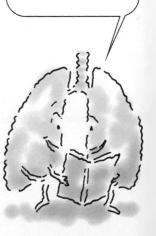

The more you smoke and the longer you inhale, the worse your chronic bronchitis will be.

What causes it

Cigarette smoking is the most common cause of chronic bronchitis. Some studies suggest a genetic predisposition to the disease as well. It's directly correlated to heavy pollution and is more prevalent in people exposed to organic or inorganic dusts and noxious gases. (See *No smoking*.)

How it happens

Chronic bronchitis occurs when irritants are inhaled for a prolonged time. The irritants inflame the tracheobronchial tree, leading to increased mucus production and a narrowed or blocked airway. As the inflammation continues, changes in the cells that line the respiratory tract result in resistance of the small airways and severe ventilation-perfusion ($\dot{V}/\dot{Q}$) imbalance, which decreases arterial oxygenation.

Ch-, ch-, ch-, changes

Chronic bronchitis results in hypertrophy and hyperplasia of the mucous glands, increased goblet cells, ciliary damage, squamous metaplasia of the columnar epithelium, and chronic leukocytic and lymphocytic inflammation of the bronchial walls. (See *Changes in chronic bronchitis*, page 182.)

Hypersecretion of the goblet cells block the free movement of the cilia, which normally sweep dust, irritants, and mucus away from the airways. With mucus and debris accumulating in the airway, the defenses are altered and the patient is prone to respiratory tract infections.

Inflammation, mucus, obstruction — oh, my!

Additional effects include widespread inflammation, airway narrowing, and mucus within the airways. Bronchial walls become inflamed and thickened from edema and accumulation of inflammatory cells, while the effects of smooth-muscle bronchospasm further narrow the lumen. Initially, only large bronchi are involved, but eventually, all airways are affected. Airways become obstructed and closure occurs, especially on expiration. The gas is then trapped in the distal portions of the lungs. Hypoventilation occurs, leading to a $\dot{V}/\dot{Q}$ mismatch and resultant hypoxemia.

Second but not last

Hypoxia and hypercapnia occur secondary to hypoventilation. Pulmonary vascular resistance

Kids' korner

No smoking

While most children experience acute bronchitis at some point, regardless of whether they're exposed to second-hand cigarette smoke, children of parents who smoke are at a higher risk for respiratory tract infections that can lead to chronic bronchitis. Chronic bronchitis during childhood tends to be a symptom of an underlying pulmonary disorder and is a risk factor for developing chronic respiratory problems as an adult.

If the cilia aren't free to sweep dust, irritants, and mucus away from airways, we're all in trouble!

FREE the CILIA NOW!

Changes in chronic bronchitis

In chronic bronchitis, irritants inflame the tracheobronchial tree over time, leading to increased mucus production and a narrowed or blocked airway. As the inflammation continues, goblet and epithelial cells hypertrophy. Because the natural defense mechanisms are blocked, the airways accumulate debris in the respiratory tract. The illustrations below show these changes.

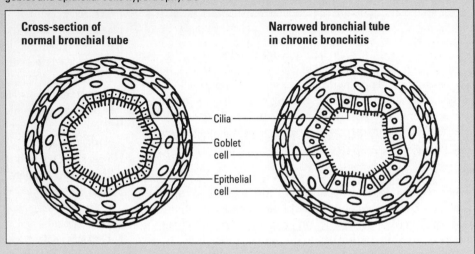

Cross-section of normal bronchial tube

Narrowed bronchial tube in chronic bronchitis

Cilia

Goblet cell

Epithelial cell

(PVR) increases as inflammatory and compensatory vasoconstriction in hypoventilated areas narrows the pulmonary arteries. Increased PVR leads to increased afterload of the right ventricle. With repeated inflammatory episodes, scarring of the airways occurs, and permanent structural changes develop. Respiratory infections can trigger acute exacerbations, and respiratory failure can occur.

Downs and ups

Patients with chronic bronchitis have a diminished respiratory drive. The resulting chronic hypoxia causes the kidneys to produce erythropoietin, which stimulates excessive red blood cell (RBC) production and leads to polycythemia. Although hemoglobin levels are high, the amount of reduced (not fully oxygenated) hemoglobin in contact with oxygen is low; therefore, cyanosis occurs.

What to look for

The patient's history typically reflects a long-time smoker who has frequent upper respiratory tract infections. Usually, the patient seeks treatment for a productive cough and exertional dyspnea. He may describe his cough as initially prevalent in the winter months but gradually becoming a year-round problem with increasingly severe episodes. He also typically reports worsening dyspnea that takes increasingly longer to subside.

C^3 — Cough, cyanosis, compensation

Inspection usually reveals a cough that produces copious gray, white, or yellow sputum due to hypersecretions of goblet cells. The patient may appear cyanotic, and he may use accessory respiratory muscles for breathing due to compensatory attempts to supply the cells with increased oxygen. Vital signs usually include tachypnea due to hypoxia; another typical finding includes substantial weight gain due to edema.

Et tu, feet?

Palpation may disclose pedal edema and neck vein distention due to right-sided heart failure. Auscultation findings include wheezing, prolonged expiratory time due to the body's attempt to keep airways patent, and rhonchi due to air moving through the narrow, mucus-filled passages.

What tests tell you

The following tests may help diagnose chronic bronchitis:
- *Chest X-rays* may show hyperinflation and increased bronchovascular markings.
- *Pulmonary function tests* demonstrate increased residual volume, decreased vital capacity and forced expiratory flow, and normal static compliance and diffusing capacity.
- *ABG analysis* reveals decreased PaO_2 and normal or increased $PaCO_2$.
- *Sputum culture* may reveal many microorganisms and neutrophils.
- *ECG* may reveal atrial arrhythmias, peaked P waves in leads II, III, and aV_F and, occasionally, right ventricular hypertrophy.

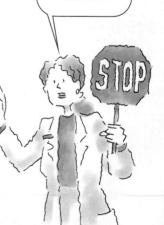

Stop smoking. It's the best way to treat chronic bronchitis.

How it's treated

The most effective treatment for chronic bronchitis is smoking cessation and, to the extent possible, avoidance of air pollutants. Antibiotics can be used to treat recurring infections. Bronchodilators may relieve bronchospasm and facilitate mucus clearance. Adequate fluid intake is essential, and chest physiotherapy may be needed to mobilize secretions. Ultrasonic or mechanical nebulizer treatments may help to loosen and mobilize secretions. Occasionally, a patient responds to corticosteroid therapy.

No place like home

Teaching about chronic bronchitis

• Advise the patient to avoid crowds, as well as people with known infections, and to obtain influenza and *Pneumococcus* immunizations.

• If the patient is receiving home oxygen therapy, explain the treatment rationale. Show him how to operate the equipment.

• Teach the patient and his family how to perform postural drainage and chest percussion. Instruct the patient to maintain each position for 10 minutes before a caregiver performs percussion and the patient coughs. Also teach the patient coughing and deep-breathing techniques to promote good ventilation and to remove secretions.

• Review all medications, including dosages, adverse effects, and reasons the medications have been prescribed. Teach the patient how and when to use an inhaler. Describe adverse reactions and advise him to report such reactions to the doctor immediately.

• Encourage the patient to eat high-calorie, protein-rich meals, and to drink plenty of fluids to prevent dehydration and help loosen secretions.

• If the patient smokes, encourage him to stop. Provide him with smoking-cessation resources or counseling, if necessary.

If another member of the household smokes, explain the risks associated with second-hand smoke, and urge that person to quit or to smoke outdoors.

• Urge the patient to avoid inhaled irritants, such as automobile exhaust fumes, aerosol sprays, and industrial pollutants.

• Warn the patient that exposure to blasts of cold air may precipitate bronchospasm. Suggest that he avoid cold, windy weather, or that he cover his mouth and nose with a scarf or mask if he must go outside.

• If the patient takes methylxanthines such as theophylline, warn him that cigarette or marijuana smoking significantly increases plasma clearance of the medication. Instruct the patient to notify the doctor if he quits smoking; while quitting is, of course, extremely beneficial, patients who do so while taking methylxanthines may experience adverse effects related to higher blood levels of theophylline.

• If appropriate, describe the signs and symptoms of peptic ulcer disease. Instruct the patient to check his stool every day for blood and to notify the doctor if he has persistent nausea, vomiting, heartburn, indigestion, constipation, diarrhea, or bloody stool.

Diuretics may be used to treat edema, and oxygen may be needed to treat hypoxia.

What to do

Use these strategies to manage chronic bronchitis:
• Answer the patient's questions, and encourage him and his family members to express their concerns about the illness. Include the patient and his family members in care decisions. Refer them to other support services as appropriate. (See *Teaching about chronic bronchitis*.)

(Text continues on page 185.)

Asthmatic bronchus

Asthma is a chronic reactive airway disorder that causes episodic airway obstruction. Such obstruction results from bronchospasms, increased mucus secretion, and mucosal edema. It's a type of chronic obstructive pulmonary disease, a group of lung diseases characterized by increased airflow resistance.

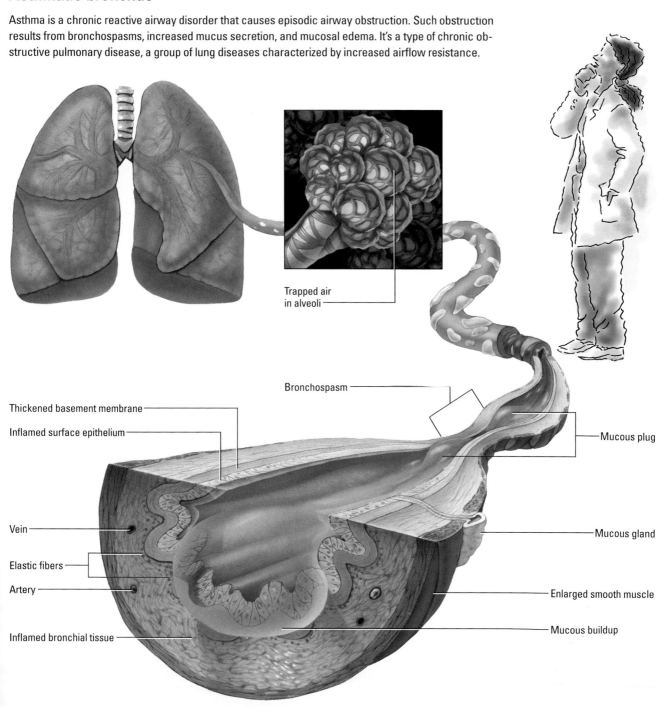

Trapped air
in alveoli

Bronchospasm

Thickened basement membrane

Inflamed surface epithelium

Mucous plug

Vein

Mucous gland

Elastic fibers

Artery

Enlarged smooth muscle

Inflamed bronchial tissue

Mucous buildup

Alveolar changes in ARDS

Acute respiratory distress syndrome (ARDS) is a form of pulmonary edema that can quickly lead to acute respiratory failure. Also known as *shock lung, stiff lung, white lung, wet lung,* or *Da Nang lung,* ARDS may follow direct or indirect injury to the lung. However, diagnosis is difficult and death can occur within 48 hours of onset if ARDS isn't promptly diagnosed and treated.

In phase 1, injury reduces normal blood flow to the lungs. Platelets aggregate and release histamine (H), serotonin (S), and bradykinin (B).

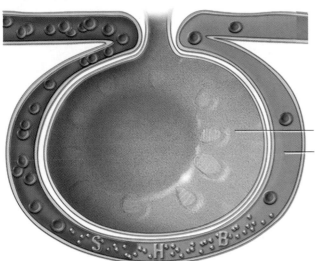

Alveolus

Capillary

In phase 2, those substances—especiall[...] [...]ramine—inflame and damage the alveolocapillary membr[...], [...]creasing capillary permeability. Fluids then shift into the interstitial space.

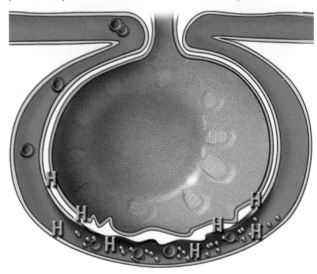

In phase 3, as capillary permeability increases, proteins and fluids leak out, increasing interstitial osmotic pressure and causing pulmonary edema.

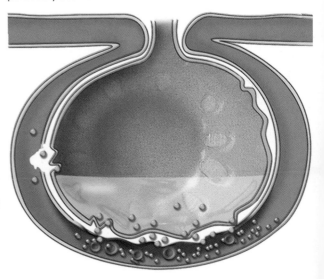

> Injury that occurs with ARDS decreases the ability for blood to reach me.

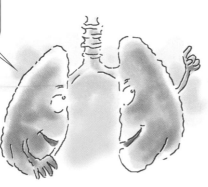

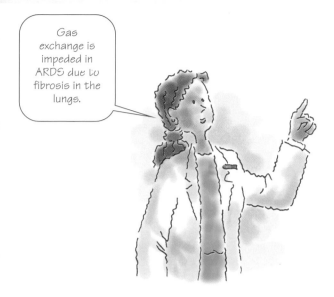

> Gas exchange is impeded in ARDS due to fibrosis in the lungs.

In phase 5, sufficient oxygen (O_2) can't cross the alveolocapillary membrane, but carbon dioxide (CO_2) can and is lost with every exhalation. O_2 and CO_2 levels decrease in the blood.

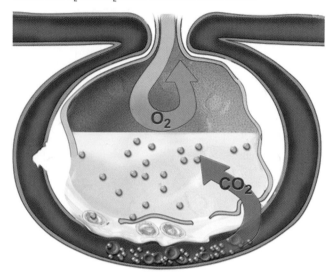

In phase 4, decreased blood flow and fluids in the alveoli damage surfactant and impair the cell's ability to produce more. As a result, alveoli collapse, impeding gas exchange and decreasing lung compliance.

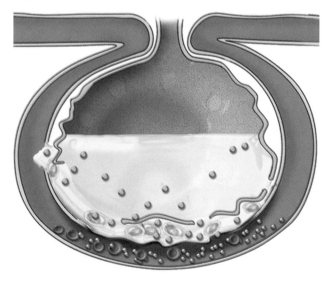

In phase 6, pulmonary edema worsens, inflammation leads to fibrosis, and gas exchange is further impeded.

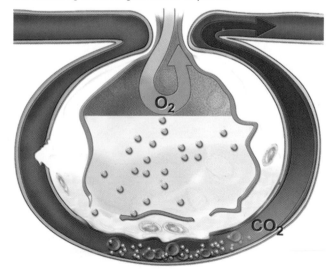

Emphysema

Emphysema, a form of chronic obstructive pulmonary disease, is the abnormal, permanent enlargement of the acini accompanied by destruction of alveolar walls. Obstruction results from tissue changes rather than mucus production, which occurs in asthma and chronic bronchitis. Distinguishing characteristics of emphysema include airflow limitation caused by lack of elastic recoil in the lungs.

Lung changes in emphysema

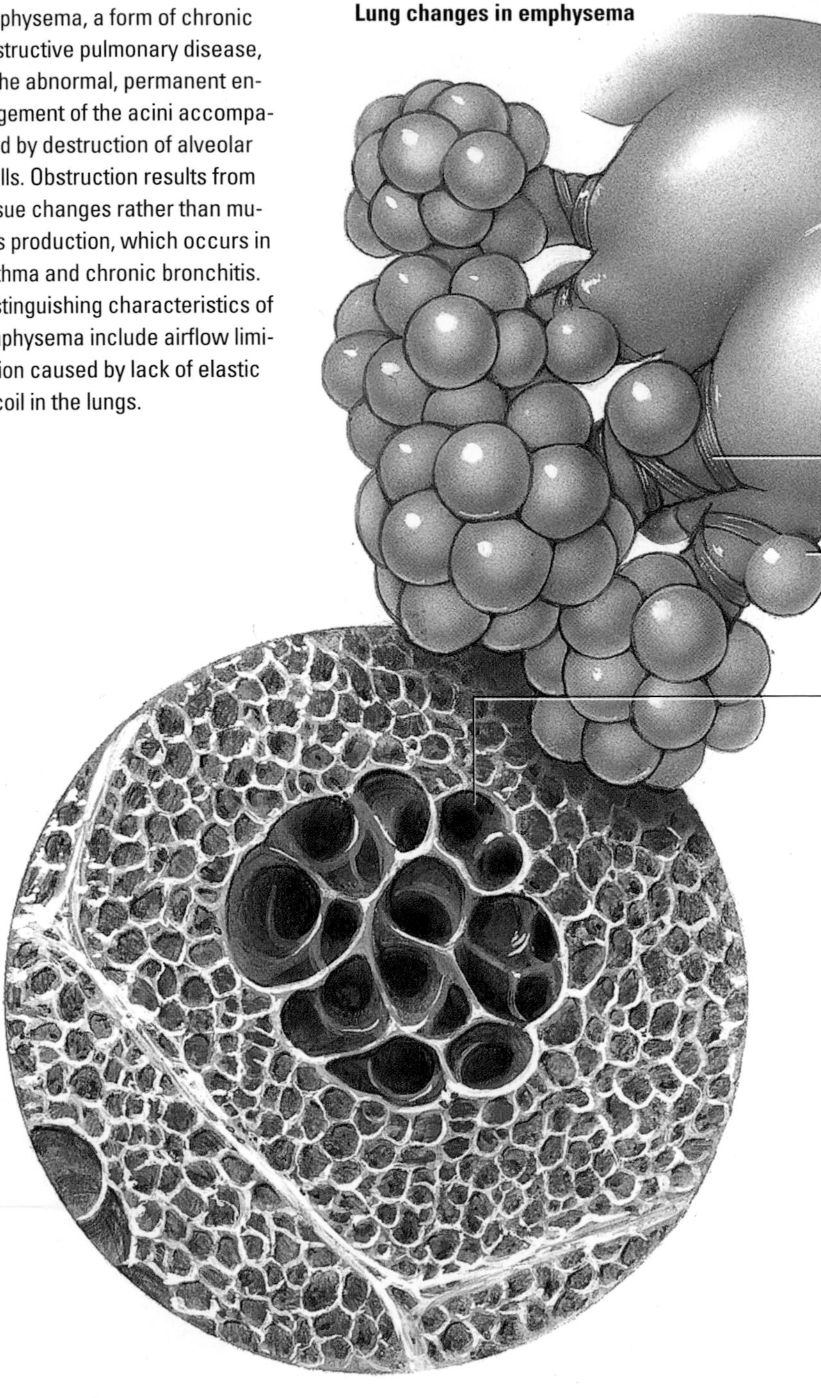

Dilation and destruction of bronchial walls

Smooth muscle

Alveolus

Loss of lung tissue

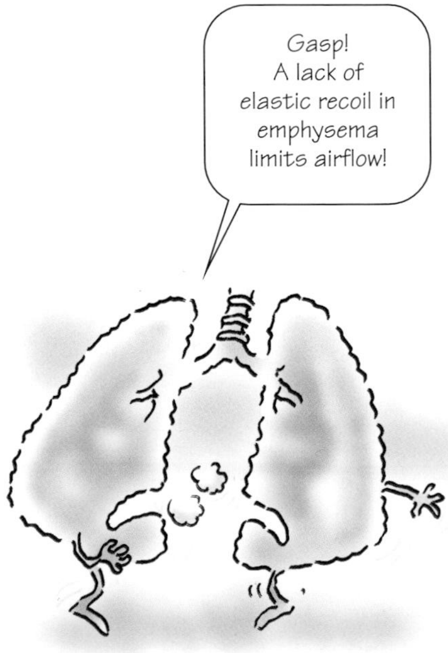

Gasp! A lack of elastic recoil in emphysema limits airflow!

• Assess for changes in baseline respiratory function. Evaluate sputum quality and quantity, restlessness, increased tachypnea, and altered breath sounds. Report changes immediately.

• Perform chest physiotherapy, including postural drainage and chest percussion and vibration for involved lobes, several times daily as needed.

• Weigh the patient three times weekly and assess for edema.

• Provide the patient with a high-calorie, protein-rich diet. Offer small, frequent meals to conserve the patient's energy and prevent fatigue.

• Make sure the patient receives adequate fluids (at least 3 qt [3 L] per day) to loosen secretions.

• Schedule respiratory therapy at least 1 hour before or after meals. Provide oral care after bronchodilator inhalation therapy.

• Encourage daily activity and provide diversional activities as appropriate. To conserve the patient's energy and prevent fatigue, help him to alternate periods of rest and activity.

• Administer medications as ordered, and note the patient's response to them.

Cystic fibrosis

Cystic fibrosis (CF) is a chronic, progressive, inherited disease that affects the exocrine (mucus-secreting) glands. The incidence of CF is highest in people of northern European ancestry, and is the most common fatal genetic disease of white children. The disease is less common in Blacks, Native Americans, and people of Asian ancestry. It occurs with equal frequency in both genders. Although CF is incurable, medical researchers continue to discover better treatments. As a result, life expectancy in people with CF has greatly increased—from age 16 to age 28 or older.

What causes it

CF is transmitted as an autosomal-recessive trait. When both parents are carriers of the recessive gene, they have a 25% chance of transmitting the disease with each pregnancy. More than 100 specific mutations of the gene have been identified.

How it happens

CF increases the viscosity of bronchial, pancreatic, and other mucus gland secretions, obstructing glandular ducts. The accumulation of thick, tenacious secretions in the bronchioles and alveoli

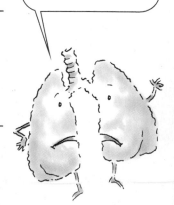

Incidence of CF is highest in people of northern European ancestry and is the most common fatal genetic disease of white children.

causes respiratory changes, eventually leading to severe atelectasis and emphysema.

The disease also causes characteristic GI effects in the intestines, pancreas, and liver. Obstruction of the pancreatic ducts results in a deficiency of several digestive enzymes. This interferes with the digestion of food and the absorption of fat-soluble vitamins (A, D, E, and K). In the pancreas, fibrotic tissue, multiple cysts, thick mucus, and fat replace the acini (small, saclike swellings normally found in this gland), producing signs of pancreatic insufficiency (insufficient insulin production, abnormal glucose tolerance, and glycosuria).

Symptom sources

The immediate causes of symptoms are increased viscosity of bronchial, pancreatic, and other mucous gland secretions and consequent destruction of glandular ducts. CF accounts for almost all cases of pancreatic enzyme deficiency in children. (See *Pediatric symptoms of CF.*)

What to look for

CF can cause bronchiectasis, pneumonia, atelectasis, hemoptysis, dehydration, distal intestinal obstructive syndrome, malnutrition, gastroesophageal reflux, nasal polyps, rectal prolapse, and cor pulmonale. Other, inevitable complications that occur as the disease progresses include hepatic disease, diabetes, pneumothorax, arthritis, pancreatitis, and cholecystitis.

In addition:
• A deficiency of fat-soluble vitamins can lead to clotting problems, retarded bone growth, and delayed sexual development. Males may experience azoospermia; females may experience secondary amenorrhea.
• Hypochloremia and hyponatremia from increased sodium and chloride concentrations in sweat can induce cardiac arrhythmias and potentially fatal shock, especially in hot weather, when sweating is profuse.
• Biliary obstruction and fibrosis may prolong neonatal jaundice. In some patients, cirrhosis and portal hypertension lead to esophageal varices, episodes of hematemesis and, occasionally, hepatomegaly.
• The clinical effects of CF may become apparent soon after birth or may take years to develop. They include major aberrations in sweat gland, respiratory, and GI functions.

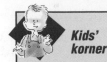
Kids' korner

Pediatric symptoms of CF

Some children display symptoms of cystic fibrosis (CF) at birth, as in a meconium ileus. A meconium ileus occurs because of a missing enzyme; specifically, the enzyme that moistens and makes all body fluids free-flowing. This results in the production of thick, tenacious meconium.

In other children, CF isn't diagnosed until weeks, months, or even years after birth. Some children may have a mild form of the disease, while others have extensive digestive and pulmonary involvement.

Children with CF commonly display a barrel chest, cyanosis, and clubbing of the fingers and toes. They suffer recurring bronchitis and pneumonia, with associated nasal polyps and sinusitis. Death typically results from pneumonia, emphysema, or atelectasis.

Thick and sticky

Tell-tale symptoms reflect obstructive changes in the lungs: wheezy respirations; a dry, nonproductive, paroxysmal cough; dyspnea; and tachypnea. These changes stem from thick, tenacious secretions in the bronchioles and alveoli, and eventually lead to severe atelectasis and emphysema.

Meconium conundrum

The GI effects of CF occur mainly in the intestines, pancreas, and liver. One early symptom is meconium ileus; the neonate with CF doesn't excrete meconium, a dark-green mucilaginous material found in the intestine at birth. He develops symptoms of intestinal obstruction, such as abdominal distention, vomiting, constipation, dehydration, and electrolyte imbalance.

Eventually, obstruction of the pancreatic ducts and resulting deficiency of trypsin, amylase, and lipase prevent the conversion and absorption of fat and protein in the intestinal tract. The undigested food is then excreted in frequent, bulky, foul-smelling, and pale stool with a high fat content.

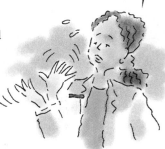

Is it hot In here, or is it me? Sweat gland dysfunction is the most common abnormality in patients with CF.

Common in kids

A common complication in infants and children is rectal prolapse. This stems from malnutrition and wasting of perirectal supporting tissues.

Pancreatic prognosis

While pancreatic insufficiency may occur with CF, about 15% of patients are pancreas-sufficient, having adequate pancreatic exocrine function for normal digestion. These patients have a better prognosis.

What tests tell you

According to the Cystic Fibrosis Foundation, a definitive diagnosis of CF requires all three of these criteria:
• two clearly positive *sweat tests*, using pilocarpine solution (a sweat inducer), and the presence of an obstructive pulmonary disease, confirmed pancreatic insufficiency or failure to thrive, or a family history of CF
• *chest X-rays* that show early signs of lung obstruction
• *stool specimen analysis* that shows the absence of trypsin, suggesting pancreatic insufficiency.

A show of support

The following test results may support the diagnosis:

• *Deoxyribonucleic acid testing* can now locate the delta F 508 mutation (found in about 70% of CF patients. The detection of two pathogenic mutations is diagnostic of CF. This test can also be used for carrier detection and prenatal diagnosis in families with a previously affected child.

• If pulmonary exacerbation exists, *pulmonary function tests* can reveal decreased vital capacity, elevated residual volume due to air entrapments, and decreased forced expiratory volume in 1 second.

• A *liver enzyme test* may reveal hepatic insufficiency.

• A *sputum culture* may reveal organisms that patients typically and chronically colonize, such as *Pseudomonas* and *Staphylococcus*.

• A *serum albumin level test* helps to assess nutritional status.

• *Electrolyte analysis* is used to assess for dehydration.

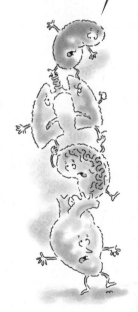

Which CF treatments are appropriate? The answer lies in the organ systems that are involved.

How it's treated

Because CF has no cure, the goal of treatment is to help the patient lead as normal a life as possible. Specific treatments depend on the organ systems involved:

• To combat electrolyte loss through sweat, the patient should generously salt his food and, during hot weather, take salt supplements.

• Oral pancreatic enzymes taken with meals and snacks offset pancreatic enzyme deficiencies. Such supplements improve absorption and digestion and help satisfy hunger without an unreasonable caloric intake. The patient's diet should be high in fat, protein, and calories, and should include vitamin A, D, E, and K supplements.

• To manage pulmonary dysfunction, the patient should undergo chest physiotherapy and nebulization to loosen secretions followed by postural drainage. Breathing exercises should be performed several times per day to help remove lung secretions. The patient shouldn't take antihistamines, which dry mucous membranes, making mucus expectoration difficult.

The alfa aerosol

• *Dornase alfa*, a pulmonary enzyme given by aerosol nebulizer, helps to thin airway mucus, improving lung function and reducing the risk of pulmonary infection.

• A patient with pulmonary infection must loosen and remove mucopurulent secretions by using intermittent nebulizer and pos-

tural drainage to relieve obstruction. Use of a moist tent is controversial because mist particles can become trapped in the esophagus and stomach, never reaching the lungs.
- Broad-spectrum antibiotics are used to control infection.
- Oxygen therapy is used as needed.

New parts and approaches

- Heart-lung transplantation may reduce the effects of the disease.
- Since the discovery of the basic genetic defect of CF, new treatments have been explored. Experimental treatments include drugs such as amiloride and gene therapy. Researchers have targeted the lungs for gene therapy because the most serious pathology occurs there.

What to do

To provide care to the patient with CF:
- Give medications as ordered. Administer pancreatic enzymes with meals and snacks.
- Perform chest physiotherapy, including postural drainage and chest percussion designed for all lobes, several times per day as ordered.
- Administer oxygen therapy as ordered. Check levels of arterial oxygen saturation using pulse oximetry.
- Provide a well-balanced, high-calorie, high-protein diet. Include plenty of fats, which are nutritionally necessary but will be difficult for the patient to digest. Give him enzyme capsules to help combat most of the effects of fat malabsorption. Include vitamin A, D, E, and K supplements if laboratory analysis indicates any deficiencies.
- Make sure the patient receives plenty of liquids to prevent dehydration, especially in warm weather.
- Provide exercise and activity periods to promote health. Encourage the patient to perform breathing exercises to help improve his ventilation.

We're the Vitamin Patrol and we're here to serve and supplement. People with CF need us to combat deficiencies.

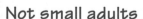

Not small adults

- Provide the young child with play periods, and enlist the help of the physical therapy department. Some pediatric facilities have play therapists and child-life specialists, who provide essential playtime for young patients and help them to deal with their illnesses.

No place like home

Managing CF at home

The following information will assist the patient and his family in managing cystic fibrosis (CF) at home:
• Inform the patient and his family about the disease, and thoroughly explain all treatment measures. Make sure they know about tests that can determine if family members carry the CF gene.
• Teach the patient and his family about all the medications the patient is taking. Explain possible adverse reactions, and urge them to notify the doctor if these reactions occur.
• Teach the patient and his family about aerosol therapy, including intermittent nebulizer treatments before postural drainage. Tell them that these treatments help to loosen secretions and dilate the bronchi.
• Instruct the patient's family in proper methods of chest physiotherapy.
• If the doctor prescribes aerobic exercises, teach the patient how to perform them, and review their importance in maintain-

ing cardiopulmonary and respiratory muscle function and improving activity tolerance.
• Teach the patient and his family about the signs of infection and sudden changes in the patient's condition that should be reported to the doctor. These signs include increased coughing, decreased appetite, sputum that thickens or contains blood, shortness of breath, and chest pain.
• Advise the parents of a child with the disease not to be overly protective. Instead, help them explore ways to enhance their child's quality of life and to foster responsibility and independence from an early age. Stress the importance of good communication; this will enable the child to express his fears and concerns.
• Encourage participation in local organizations, such as the Cystic Fibrosis Foundation, to help meet patient and family needs.

• Provide emotional support to the parents of children with CF. Because it's an inherited disease, the parents may feel enormous guilt. Encourage them to discuss their fears and concerns, and answer their questions as honestly as possible.
• Be flexible with care and visiting hours during hospitalization to allow the child to continue schoolwork and maintain friendships.
• Include the family in all phases of the child's care. If the patient is an adolescent, he may want to perform much of his own treatment protocol. Encourage him to do so. (See *Managing CF at home*.)

Emphysema

Emphysema is another type of COPD. It's the most common cause of death from respiratory disease in the United States. Emphysema affects approximately 2 million Americans and appears to be more prevalent in men than in women. Postmortem findings reveal few adult lungs without some degree of emphysema.

What causes it

In terms of its cause, emphysema has both a genetic and a behavioral component. A genetic deficiency of the enzyme alpha$_1$-antitrypsin (AAT) is responsible for 1% to 3% of all cases of emphysema, and 1 in 3,000 neonates are diagnosed with the disease. Cigarette smoking is thought to cause up to 20% of emphysema cases. Other causative factors are unknown.

How it happens

Primary emphysema has been linked to an inherited deficiency of AAT. This enzyme is a major component of alpha$_1$-globulin and inhibits the activation of several proteolytic enzymes. AAT deficiency is an autosomal-recessive trait that predisposes an individual to develop emphysema; without sufficient AAT, proteolysis (breakdown of proteins) in lung tissues isn't inhibited. In homozygous individuals (those who inherit a trait from both parents), the chance of developing lung disease is as high as 80%; people who smoke have an even greater chance of developing emphysema. Nonsmokers who develop emphysema and those who develop the disease before or during their early 40s are believed to have an AAT deficiency.

Ain't misbehavin' — just noncompliant

In emphysema, recurrent inflammation is associated with the release of proteolytic enzymes from lung cells. The subsequent proteolysis causes irreversible enlargement of the air spaces distal to the terminal bronchioles. Enlargement of air spaces destroys the alveolar walls. This results in a breakdown of elasticity and a loss of fibrous and muscle tissue, thus making the lungs less compliant.

Out of circulation

In normal breathing, the air moves into and out of the lungs to meet metabolic needs. A change in airway size compromises the lung's ability to circulate sufficient air. In patients with emphysema, recurrent pulmonary inflammation damages and eventually destroys the alveolar walls, creating large air spaces.

If we keep this up, we're asking for trouble — shortness of breath, chronic cough... emphysema.

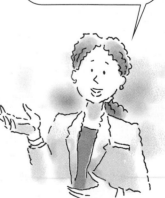

Those who develop emphysema before their mid-40s and are nonsmokers are believed to have an AAT deficiency.

Breakdown and collapse

The alveolar septa (partitions) are initially destroyed, eliminating a portion of the capillary bed and increasing air volume in the acinus. This breakdown leaves the alveoli unable to recoil normally after expanding and results in bronchiolar collapse on expiration. The damaged or destroyed alveolar walls can't support the airways to keep them open.

It's a trap!

The amount of air that can be expired passively diminishes, thus trapping air in the lungs and leading to overdistention. (See *Air trapping in emphysema*.) Hyperinflation of the alveoli produces bullae (air spaces) adjacent to pleura (blebs). Septal destruction also decreases airway calibration. Part of each inspiration is trapped because of increased residual volume and decreased calibration. Septal destruction may affect only the respiratory bronchioles and alveolar ducts, leaving alveolar sacs intact, or it can involve the entire acinus with more random damage that involves the lower lobes of the lungs.

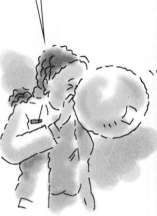

Hyperinflation is bad for the economy, and even worse for the lungs.

It gets complicated

In emphysema, complications may include recurrent respiratory tract infections, cor pulmonale, and respiratory failure. Peptic ulcer disease strikes 20% to 25% of patients with COPD. Additionally, alveolar blebs and bullae may rupture, leading to spontaneous pneumothorax or pneumomediastinum.

What to look for

The patient may report shortness of breath and a chronic cough. His history may reveal a long-term smoking habit, as well as anorexia with resultant weight loss and a general feeling of malaise.

Inspect, palpate, percuss, auscultate

Inspection may reveal a barrel-chested patient who breathes through pursed lips and uses accessory muscles. You may notice peripheral cyanosis, clubbed fingers and toes, and tachypnea. Palpation may reveal decreased tactile fremitus and decreased chest expansion. Percussion may reveal hyperresonance. On auscultation, you may hear decreased breath sounds, crackles and wheezing during inspiration, a prolonged expiratory phase with grunting respirations, and distant heart sounds.

Air trapping in emphysema

After alveolar walls are damaged or destroyed, they can't support the airways and keep them open. The alveolar walls then lose their capability of elastic recoil. Collapse then occurs on expiration.

Normal expiration
Normal expiration, as shown here, involves normal recoil and an open bronchiole.

Impaired expiration
Impaired expiration, as shown here, involves decreased elastic recoil and a narrowed bronchiole.

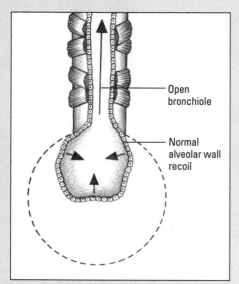

Open bronchiole

Normal alveolar wall recoil

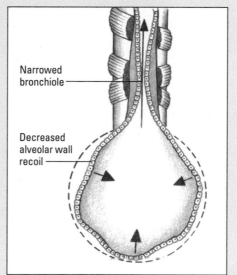

Narrowed bronchiole

Decreased alveolar wall recoil

What tests tell you

- *Chest X-rays* in advanced disease may show a flattened diaphragm, reduced vascular markings at the lung periphery, overaeration of the lungs, a vertical heart, an enlarged anteroposterior chest diameter, and large retrosternal air space.
- *Pulmonary function tests* typically indicate increased residual volume and total lung capacity, reduced diffusing capacity, and increased inspiratory flow.
- *ABG analysis* usually shows reduced Pao_2 and normal $Paco_2$ until late in the disease.
- *ECG* may reveal tall, symmetrical P waves in leads II, III, and aV_F; vertical QRS axis; and signs of right ventricular hypertrophy late in the disease.

• *RBC count* usually demonstrates an increased hemoglobin level late in the disease when the patient has persistent severe hypoxia.

How it's treated

Emphysema management usually includes the use of bronchodilators such as aminophylline to promote mucociliary clearance, antibiotics to treat respiratory tract infection, and immunizations to prevent influenza and pneumococcal pneumonia.

Other treatment measures include adequate hydration and (in selected patients) chest physiotherapy to mobilize secretions. Some patients may require oxygen therapy (at low settings) to correct hypoxia. They may also require transtracheal catheterization to receive oxygen at home. Counseling about the importance of smoking cessation and avoiding smoke and other air pollutants is essential.

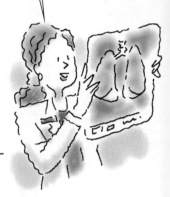

In advanced disease, chest X-rays may show a flattened diaphragm and a large retrosternal airspace, among other things.

What to do

Caring for a patient with emphysema will likely require that you take these measures:
• Provide supportive care and help the patient adjust to lifestyle changes necessitated by a chronic illness.
• Answer the patient's questions about his illness as honestly as possible. Encourage him to express his fears and concerns. Remain with him during periods of extreme stress and anxiety.
• Include the patient and his family members in care-related decisions. Refer the patient to support services, as needed.
• Perform chest physiotherapy, including postural drainage and chest percussion and vibration, several times daily if ordered.
• Provide the patient with a high-calorie, protein-rich diet to promote health and healing. Give small, frequent meals to conserve energy and prevent fatigue.
• Schedule respiratory treatments at least 1 hour before or after meals. Provide oral care after bronchodilator therapy.
• Make sure the patient receives adequate fluids (at least 3 qt [3 L] per day) to loosen secretions.
• Encourage daily activity and provide diversionary activities as appropriate. To conserve energy and prevent fatigue, encourage the patient to alternate periods of rest and activity.
• Administer medications as ordered. Record the patient's response to these medications.
• Watch for complications, such as respiratory tract infections, cor pulmonale, respiratory failure, and peptic ulcer disease. Report complications to the doctor immediately.

Sleep apnea

Sleep apnea is a disruption in breathing during sleep. An episode generally lasts at least 10 seconds and typically occurs more than five times in 1 hour. Sleep apnea affects more men than women; incidence increases with a person's age.

What causes it

Sleep apnea can have a central or neurologic origin, but more commonly it's related to a type of respiratory obstruction. The soft palate or tongue may obstruct the upper airway. Factors that contribute to sleep apnea include obesity, a large uvula, a neck that is shorter than normal, or enlarged tonsils or adenoids. (See *Pickwickian syndrome*, page 196.)

How it happens

Skeletal muscles relax during sleep. This relaxation displaces the tongue and other anatomic structures of the head and neck.

The displacement can result in obstruction of the upper airway even though the chest wall continues to move. Absence of breathing causes an increase in arterial carbon dioxide levels and lowers the pH level. These changes stimulate the nervous system and the sleeping person responds after 10 or more seconds of apnea. This arousal episode serves to correct the obstruction and breathing resumes. The cycle repeats itself as often as every 5 minutes during sleep, affecting the patient's ability to get a restful night of sleep.

Sleep apnea affects more men than women. That's a good thing for me — I barely get enough sleep as it is!

What to look for

In obstructive sleep apnea, snoring, excessive daytime sleepiness, intellectual impairment, memory loss, and cardiorespiratory symptoms may be noted. In central sleep apnea, the patient will likely complain of sleeping poorly, a morning headache, or daytime fatigue. Many of these symptoms are related to the patient's inability to sleep soundly due to frequent waking patterns.

Pickwickian syndrome

Defined as a group of symptoms that primarily affect patients with extreme obesity, Pickwickian syndrome takes its name from a character in Dickens' novel *The Pickwick Papers,* who seemed to have many traits of this disease.

The major health problem associated with this disease is sleep apnea caused by excessive fatty tissue surrounding the chest muscles. This fat strains the heart, lungs, and diaphragm, and contributes to breathing difficulties.

Symptoms
Symptoms of Pickwickian syndrome include:
• excessive sleepiness during the day
• shortness of breath
• disturbed sleep at night
• flushed face or a bluish tint to the face
• elevated blood pressure
• enlarged liver
• elevated red blood cell count
• sleep apnea.

Diagnostic tests
Tests to help diagnose Pickwickian syndrome include:
• echocardiogram to determine heart enlargement or pulmonary hypertension
• sleep latency tests to assess the degree of sleepiness during the day
• magnetic resonance imaging and computed tomography scans, or upper airway studies to detect heart enlargement.

Treatment
Pickwickian syndrome is reversible. Weight loss and exercise are the main treatment strategies. Typical methods for managing sleep apnea should be employed in patients with this syndrome.

What tests tell you

Polysomnography is the most common test used to diagnosis sleep apnea. This test is performed during an overnight sleep study, generally conducted in a sleep lab environment. An overnight sleep study has the benefit of allowing the patient to experience all stages of sleep. The patient wears monitoring devices and is observed during sleep. The equipment used assesses the depth of sleep, stage of sleep, respiratory effort required, oxygen saturation, and muscle movement.

How it's treated

Mild cases of sleep apnea may be resolved by weight loss or a change in sleeping position. Devices that prevent obstruction by the tongue or neck structures can be used to eliminate displacement of these structures and prevent sleep apnea. Severe cases commonly require surgical intervention.

Making the cut?

Nonsurgical intervention usually involves the use of a bilevel positive airway pressure (BiPAP) system. This ventilation system serves to hold the airways open during sleep. A nasal continuous positive airway pressure (CPAP) system continuously delivers positive airway pressure.

Surgical intervention may involve an adenoidectomy (removal of the adenoids), a uvulectomy (removal of the uvula), or reconstruction of the entire oropharynx. Laser or traditional surgery may be used. The final resort may be the creation of a tracheostomy.

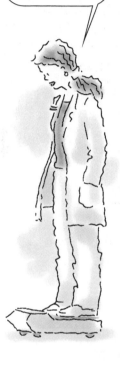

Lose a little weight, get more sleep. In mild sleep apnea cases, weight loss might be the answer.

What to do

Providing care to a patient with sleep apnea may require a range of interventions. Nurses are advised to:
• Educate the patient and his family about the disorder and its possible causes.
• Perform an assessment and collect a health history to determine contributing causes for the condition.
• Using the health history, assess the patient's sleep patterns, including his degree of fatigue during the day due to interrupted sleep patterns and interference in his ability to function.
• Encourage a smoking cessation program if the patient smokes.
• Encourage a weight loss program for the obese patient.
• Provide information and teaching on the use of a BiPAP or CPAP device.
• To ensure optimal function, make sure the nasal or full-face mask that's used with the BiPAP or CPAP device fits properly.
• Provide preoperative and postoperative teaching for patients and their significant others if a tracheostomy or surgical intervention is necessary.

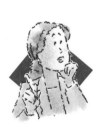

Quick quiz

1. Intrinsic (nonatopic) asthma can be caused by:
    A.   animal dander.
    B.   pollen.
    C.   mold or household dust.
    D.   anxiety.

Answer: D. Patients with intrinsic asthma react to internal, non-allergic factors such as anxiety.

2. The most common cause of chronic bronchitis is:
    A.   heart failure.
    B.   cigarette smoke.
    C.   reaction to antibiotic therapy.
    D.   dehydration.

Answer: B. Cigarette smoke is the leading cause of chronic bronchitis. The severity of the disease is linked to the amount of cigarette smoke or other pollutants inhaled.

3.   Increased bronchial, pancreatic, and other mucus gland secretions, as well as obstructed glandular ducts are caused by:
   A.   chronic bronchitis.
   B.   emphysema.
   C.   cystic fibrosis.
   D.   asthma.

Answer: C. Cystic fibrosis is a chronic, progressive, inherited disease affecting the mucus secreting glands of the body.

4.   In sleep apnea, the absence of breathing leads to:
   A.   decreased arterial CO_2 and lower pH levels.
   B.   increased arterial CO_2 and lower pH levels.
   C.   increased arterial CO_2 and higher pH levels.
   D.   decreased arterial CO_2 and higher pH levels.

Answer: B. Absence of breathing leads to an increase in arterial CO_2 and lowers the pH level. These changes stimulate the nervous system and, after 10 or more seconds of apnea, the sleeping person responds by breathing until the next episode occurs.

Scoring

☆☆☆   If you answered all four items correctly, splendid. There's no obstruction in your understanding of obstructive disorders!

☆☆   If you answered three items correctly, good job. Your obstructive disorders knowledge is close to maximum saturation!

☆   If you answered fewer than three items correctly, don't sweat it. Review the chapter and you'll be breathing easy in no time!

7

Restrictive disorders

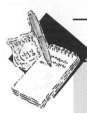

Just the facts

In this chapter, you'll learn:

♦ common restrictive disorders and their potential causes

♦ ways to recognize a restrictive disorder affecting the respiratory tract

♦ diagnostic tests used to confirm a restrictive disorder

♦ treatments for a variety of restrictive respiratory conditions.

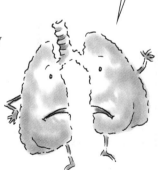

Lung capacity decreases in restrictive disorders. I don't like the sound of that!

Understanding restrictive disorders

Restrictive disorders affect the interstitium of the lungs (alveoli, blood vessels and surrounding supporting tissues). In restrictive disorders, a decrease in the lung capacity results from the inability of the lungs to expand and relax at the rate and completeness the diaphragm and intercostal muscles demand. With restrictive pulmonary disease, thickening of the lung tissues can occur and will result in a decrease in arterial oxygen levels.

Restrictive disorders reduce vital capacity and the functional residual capacity, but airflow remains normal. Conditions such as pulmonary fibrosis damage the lung tissue and result in loss of elasticity. Often the onset of these disorders is slow and insidious and dyspnea is the most common symptom.

Acute respiratory distress syndrome

Acute respiratory distress syndrome (ARDS) is a type of pulmonary edema not related to heart failure. It's also known as *shock*, *white lung*, *wet lung*, or *Da Nang lung*. ARDS may follow direct or indirect lung injury and can quickly lead to acute respiratory failure.

The three hallmark features of ARDS are:

 bilateral patchy infiltrates on chest X-ray

 no signs or symptoms of heart failure

 no improvement in partial pressure of arterial oxygen (PaO_2) despite increasing oxygen delivery.

The prognosis for the patient with ARDS varies depending on the cause and the patient's age and health status before developing the syndrome. (See *ARDS in children.*)

What causes it

Some of the most common predisposing factors for ARDS are:
- sepsis
- lung injury from trauma such as airway contusion
- other trauma-related factors, such as fat emboli, shock, and multiple blood transfusions (trauma or non-trauma-related)
- shock (trauma- or non-trauma-related)
- disseminated intravascular coagulation
- pancreatitis
- massive blood transfusions
- burns
- cardiopulmonary bypass
- drug overdose
- aspiration of stomach contents
- pneumonitis
- near drowning
- pneumonia
- inhalation of noxious gases (such as ammonia or chlorine).

How it happens

In ARDS, the tissues lining the alveoli and the pulmonary capillaries are injured directly, by aspiration of gastric contents or inhalation of noxious gases, or indirectly, by chemical mediators released into the bloodstream in response to systemic disease. (See *Understanding ARDS.*)

Inflammation — it's such a follower

The injured tissues release cytokines and other molecules that cause inflammation as white blood cells collect at the site and swelling occurs. The tissues become more permeable to fluid and

Kids' korner

ARDS in children

Acute respiratory distress syndrome (ARDS) is a significant cause of mortality in children. Children at risk for ARDS include those with infections that cause fluid accumulation in the lungs. Children with any type of lung infection should receive prompt treatment to avoid this serious condition.

Welcome to the injury site. Please make room for the cytokines, and those other inflammation-causing molecules. (Boy, it's getting crowded in here!)

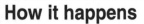

Now I get it!

Understanding ARDS

Here's how acute respiratory distress syndrome (ARDS) progresses:

☝ Injury reduces normal blood flow to the lungs. Platelets aggregate and release histamine (H), serotonin (S), and bradykinin (B).

✌ The released substances inflame and damage the alveolar capillary membrane, increasing capillary permeability. Fluids then shift into the interstitial space.

🤟 Capillary permeability increases and proteins and fluids leak out, increasing interstitial osmotic pressure and causing pulmonary edema.

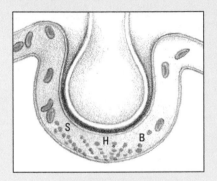

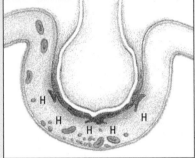

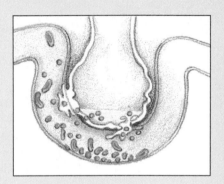

🖐 Decreased blood flow and fluids in the alveoli damage surfactant and impair the cell's ability to produce more. The alveoli then collapse, thus impairing gas exchange.

🖐 Oxygenation is impaired but carbon dioxide (CO_2) easily crosses the alveolar capillary membrane, and is expired. Blood oxygen (O_2) and CO_2 levels are low.

🖐 Pulmonary edema worsens and inflammation leads to fibrosis. Gas exchange is further impeded.

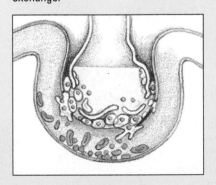

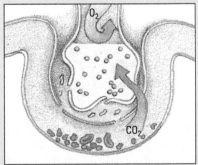

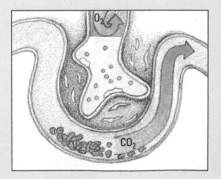

proteins, and the hydrostatic pressure gradient between the alveoli and the capillaries is reversed.

Sorry! Gas exchange closed due to illness

Proteins and fluid begin to move from the capillaries into the alveoli, which impairs gas exchange in those alveoli. As the process continues, the alveoli collapse (atelectasis), and gas exchange becomes impossible.

Ventilation prevention

The fluid that accumulates in the interstitial spaces, alveolar spaces, and small airways causes the lungs to stiffen, preventing air from moving into the lungs (ventilation).

Shunt stunts

As alveoli fill with fluid or collapse, the capillaries surrounding the alveoli fail to absorb oxygen. The body responds by shunting blood away from these alveoli, a process called *right-to-left shunting*.

Responses to the big buildup — how distressing!

As fluid builds up in the alveoli, the patient develops thick, frothy sputum and marked hypoxemia with increasing respiratory distress. As pulmonary edema worsens, inflammation leads to fibrosis, further impeding gas exchange.

Off-line alkaline

Tachypnea due to respiratory distress causes alkalosis as carbon dioxide (CO_2) levels decrease. The body tries to compensate and restore the normal blood pH range through metabolic acidosis. The lack of oxygen also forces the body into anaerobic metabolism, which adds to the acidosis. Unless gas exchange is restored and this process is reversed, acidosis worsens until all organ systems are affected and, subsequently, fail.

What to look for

ARDS occurs in four stages, each with these typical signs and symptoms:

 Stage I develops hours to days after the initial injury in response to decreasing oxygen levels in the blood. This stage involves dyspnea, especially on exertion. Respiratory and heart rates are normal to high. Auscultation may reveal diminished breath sounds, particularly when the patient is tachypneic.

Stage II symptoms are sometimes incorrectly attributed to trauma. This stage is marked by increased respiratory distress. The respiratory rate is high and the patient may use accessory muscles to breathe. He may appear restless, apprehensive, and mentally sluggish or agitated. He may have a dry cough or frothy sputum. The heart rate is elevated and the skin is cool and clammy. Lung auscultation may reveal basilar crackles.

Stage III involves obvious respiratory distress with tachypnea, use of accessory breathing muscles, and decreased mental acuity. The patient exhibits tachycardia with arrhythmias (usually premature ventricular contractions) and labile blood pressure. The skin is pale and cyanotic. Auscultation may disclose diminished breath sounds, basilar crackles, and rhonchi. This stage generally requires endotracheal (ET) intubation and mechanical ventilation.

Stage IV is characterized by decreasing respiratory and heart rates. The patient's mental status nears loss of consciousness. The skin is cool and cyanotic. Breath sounds are severely diminished to absent.

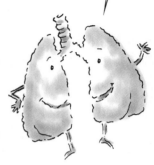

If all the world's a stage, can I choose stage I?

What tests tell you

These test results are used to diagnose ARDS:
• *Arterial blood gas (ABG) analysis* initially shows decreased Pao_2 despite oxygen supplementation. Because of tachypnea, partial pressure of arterial carbon dioxide ($Paco_2$) is also decreased, causing an increase in blood pH (respiratory alkalosis). As ARDS worsens, $Paco_2$ increases and pH decreases as the patient becomes acidotic. This imbalance is worsened by metabolic acidosis caused by a lack of oxygen, which, in turn, forces the body to switch to anaerobic metabolism.
• Initially, *chest X-rays* may be normal. Basilar infiltrates begin to appear in about 24 hours. In later stages, lung fields have a ground-glass appearance and, eventually, as fluid fills the alveoli, white patches appear. Ultimately, in later stages of ARDS, these patches may cover both lung fields in their entirety.
• *Pulmonary artery (PA) catheterization* may be used to identify the cause of pulmonary edema through pulmonary artery wedge pressure (PAWP) measurement. PAWP is 18 mm Hg or lower than normal in patients with ARDS.
• A *differential diagnosis* is essential to rule out cardiogenic pulmonary edema, pulmonary vasculitis, and diffuse pulmonary hemorrhage. Tests used to determine the causative agent can include sputum analysis, blood cultures, toxicology tests, and serum amylase levels (to rule out pancreatitis).

How it's treated

The goal of therapy is to correct the original cause of ARDS, if possible, and to provide enough oxygen to allow normal body processes to continue until the lungs begin to heal.
• Antibiotics and steroids may be administered to fight infection and minimize inflammation.
• Diuretics may be needed to reduce interstitial and pulmonary edema. In later stages of ARDS, however, vasopressors are usually prescribed to maintain blood pressure and blood supply to critical tissues.
• Respiratory support is most important. Humidified oxygen delivered through a tight-fitting mask and continuous positive airway pressure may be adequate. ET intubation and mechanical ventilation are commonly required. Positive end-expiratory pressure (PEEP) may prevent alveolar collapse. High-frequency jet ventilation is sometimes used. Suctioning, as necessary, removes accumulated secretions from the tracheobronchial tree.
• Prone positioning may improve the patient's oxygenation.

More meds

Additional medications are generally required when intubation and mechanical ventilation are instituted. Sedatives, including opioids and, sometimes, neuromuscular-blocking agents, minimize restlessness and allow ventilation.

Memory jogger

How can you remember the key treatments for acute respiratory distress syndrome (ARDS)? Simple: Just remember its abbreviation! The main treatments for ARDS include:

A — antibiotics

R — respiratory support

D — diuretics

S — situate (place the patient in a prone position).

What to do

ARDS requires careful monitoring and supportive care. When your patient isn't intubated, watch carefully for signs of respiratory failure, which can happen quickly and, when it does occur, necessitates intubation and mechanical ventilation. In addition, follow these measures:
• Assess the patient's respiratory status at least every 2 hours; more often if indicated. Note respiratory rate, rhythm, and depth. Report dyspnea and accessory muscle use. Be alert for inspiratory retractions.
• Administer oxygen as ordered. Monitor fraction of inspired oxygen levels.
• Auscultate lungs bilaterally for adventitious or diminished breath sounds. Inspect the color and character of sputum; clear, frothy sputum indicates pulmonary edema. To maintain PEEP, suction only as needed.
• Check ventilator settings often. Assess oxygen saturation continuously by pulse oximetry or mixed venous oxygen saturation

($S\bar{v}O_2$) by PA catheter. Monitor serial ABG levels; document and report changes in arterial oxygen saturation (SaO_2) as well as metabolic and respiratory acidosis and PaO_2 changes.

• Monitor vital signs. Institute continuous cardiac monitoring and observe for arrhythmias that may result from hypoxemia, acid-base disturbances, or electrolyte imbalance.

• Monitor the patient's level of consciousness, noting confusion or mental sluggishness.

• Be alert for signs of treatment-induced complications, including arrhythmias, disseminated intravascular coagulation, GI bleeding, infection, malnutrition, paralytic ileus, pneumothorax, pulmonary fibrosis, renal failure, thrombocytopenia, and tracheal stenosis.

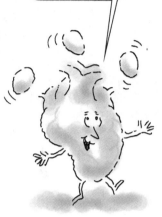

Monitor me all you want. If I were arrhythmic, could I do this? I don't think so!

I wanna be sedated...

• Give sedatives as ordered to reduce restlessness. Administer sedatives and analgesics at regular intervals if the patient on mechanical ventilation is receiving neuromuscular blocking agents.

• Provide routine eye care and instill artificial tears to prevent corneal drying and abrasion from the loss of the blink reflex in mechanically ventilated patients receiving neuromuscular blocking agents.

• Administer anti-infective agents as ordered if the underlying cause is sepsis or infection.

• Place the patient in a comfortable position that maximizes air exchange, such as semi-Fowler's or high Fowler's position. A continuous rotation bed or prone positioning may be needed.

• Allow for periods of rest to prevent fatigue and reduce oxygen demand.

• If your patient has a PA catheter in place, know the desired PAWP level and check readings as indicated. Watch for decreasing $S\bar{v}O_2$. Because PEEP may reduce cardiac output, check for hypotension, tachycardia, and decreased urine output.

• Evaluate the patient's serum electrolyte levels frequently, as ordered. Monitor urine output hourly to ensure adequate renal function. Measure intake and output. Weigh the patient daily.

• Record caloric intake. Administer tube feedings and parenteral nutrition, as ordered.

• Perform passive range-of-motion exercises to maintain joint mobility. Provide meticulous skin care to prevent breakdown.

Acute respiratory failure

When the lungs can't sufficiently maintain arterial oxygenation or eliminate CO_2, acute respiratory failure results. Unchecked and untreated, this condition can lead to decreased oxygenation of the body tissues and metabolic acidosis.

In patients with essentially normal lung tissue, respiratory failure usually produces hypercapnia (an above-normal amount of CO_2 in the arterial blood) and hypoxemia (a deficiency of oxygen in the arterial blood).

In patients with chronic obstructive pulmonary disease (COPD), however, respiratory failure is signaled only by an acute drop in ABG levels and clinical deterioration. The reason? Patients with COPD consistently have high $Paco_2$ levels and low Pao_2 levels, but are able to compensate and maintain a normal, or near-normal, pH level.

What causes it

Conditions that cause alveolar hypoventilation, ventilation-perfusion ($\dot{V}/\dot{Q}$) mismatch, or right-to-left shunting can lead to respiratory failure. These conditions include:
• COPD
• bronchitis
• pneumonia
• bronchospasm
• ventilatory failure
• pneumothorax
• atelectasis
• cor pulmonale
• pulmonary edema
• pulmonary emboli
• central nervous system (CNS) disease
• CNS depression due to head trauma, or misuse of opioids, sedatives, or tranquilizers.

How it happens

In patients with acute respiratory failure, gas exchange is diminished by any combination of the following factors:
• alveolar hypoventilation
• $\dot{V}/\dot{Q}$ mismatch
• intrapulmonary shunting.

Imbalances associated with respiratory failure include hypervolemia, hypovolemia, hypokalemia, hyperkalemia, respiratory acidosis, respiratory alkalosis, and metabolic acidosis. Let's look at each one individually. (See *What happens in acute respiratory failure.*)

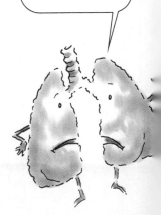

Hypervolemia?
Hypokalemia?
Acidosis? Uh-oh!
I think gas exchange is becoming unbalanced.

Now I get it!

What happens in acute respiratory failure

Three major malfunctions account for impaired gas exchange and subsequent acute respiratory failure: alveolar hypoventilation, ventilation-perfusion ($\dot{V}/\dot{Q}$) mismatch, and intrapulmonary (right-to-left) shunting.

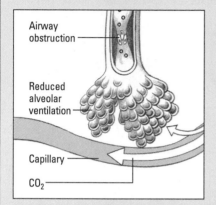

Airway obstruction

Reduced alveolar ventilation

Capillary

CO_2

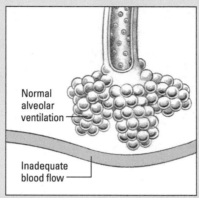

Normal alveolar ventilation

Inadequate blood flow

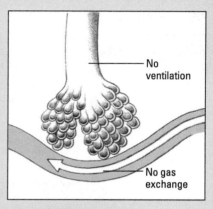

No ventilation

No gas exchange

Alveolar hypoventilation

In alveolar hypoventilation (shown above as the result of airway obstruction), the amount of oxygen brought to the alveoli is diminished. This causes a drop in the partial pressure of arterial oxygen and an increase in alveolar carbon dioxide (CO_2). The accumulation of CO_2 in the alveoli prevents diffusion of adequate amounts of CO_2 from the capillaries, which increases the partial pressure of arterial CO_2.

$\dot{V}/\dot{Q}$ mismatch

$\dot{V}/\dot{Q}$ mismatch, the leading cause of hypoxemia, occurs when insufficient ventilation exists with a normal flow of blood or when, as shown above, normal ventilation exists with an insufficient flow of blood. Partial pressure of arterial oxygen is low, but partial pressure of arterial carbon dioxide is normal because of normal ventilation in some parts of the lung.

Intrapulmonary shunting

As shown above, intrapulmonary shunting occurs when blood passes from the right side of the heart to the left side without being oxygenated.

Hypervolemia

Prolonged respiratory treatments, such as nebulizer use, can lead to inhalation and absorption of water vapor. Excessive fluid absorption may also result from increased lung capillary pressure or permeability, which typically occurs in ARDS. The excessive fluid absorption may precipitate pulmonary edema.

Causes of respiratory failure

Problems with the brain, lungs, muscles and nerves, or pulmonary circulation can impair gas exchange and cause respiratory failure. Here's a list of conditions that can cause respiratory failure:

Brain
- Anesthesia
- Cerebral hemorrhage
- Cerebral tumor
- Drug overdose
- Head trauma
- Skull fracture

Lungs
- Acute respiratory distress syndrome
- Asthma
- Chronic obstructive pulmonary disease
- Cystic fibrosis
- Flail chest
- Massive bilateral pneumonia
- Sleep apnea
- Tracheal obstruction

Muscles and nerves
- Amyotrophic lateral sclerosis
- Guillain-Barré syndrome
- Multiple sclerosis
- Muscular dystrophy
- Myasthenia gravis
- Polio
- Spinal cord trauma

Pulmonary circulation
- Heart failure
- Pulmonary edema
- Pulmonary embolism

Hypovolemia

Because the lungs remove water daily through exhalation, an increased respiratory rate can promote excessive loss of water. Excessive loss can also occur with fever or any other condition that increases the metabolic rate and, thus, the respiratory rate. (See *Causes of respiratory failure*.)

Hyperkalemia

In acidosis, excess hydrogen ions move into the cell. Potassium ions then move out of the cell and into the blood to balance the positive charges between the two fluid compartments. Hyperkalemia may result.

Hypokalemia

If a patient begins to hyperventilate and alkalosis results, hydrogen ions will move out of the cells, and potassium ions will move from the blood into the cells. That shift can cause hypokalemia.

Respiratory acidosis

Respiratory acidosis, which is due to hypoventilation, results from the inability of the lungs to eliminate sufficient quantities of CO_2. The excess CO_2 combines with water to form carbonic acid. Increased carbonic acid levels result in decreased pH, which contributes to respiratory acidosis.

Respiratory alkalosis

Respiratory alkalosis develops from an excessively rapid respiratory rate, or hyperventilation, and causes excessive CO_2 elimination. Loss of CO_2 decreases the blood's acid-forming potential and results in respiratory alkalosis.

Metabolic acidosis

Conditions that cause hypoxia cause cells to use anaerobic metabolism. That metabolism creates an increase in the production of lactic acid, which can lead to metabolic acidosis.

What to look for

Hypoxemia and hypercapnia, which are characteristic of acute respiratory failure, stimulate strong compensatory responses from all body systems, especially the respiratory, cardiovascular, and CNS.

Leading with the lungs

When the body senses hypoxemia or hypercapnia, the respiratory center responds by increasing respiratory depth and, subsequently, respiratory rate. Signs of labored breathing — flared nostrils, pursed-lip exhalation, and the use of accessory breathing muscles, among others — may signify respiratory failure.

As respiratory failure worsens, muscle retractions between the ribs, above the clavicle, and above the sternum may also occur. The patient is dyspneic and may become cyanotic. Auscultation of the chest reveals diminished or absent breath sounds over the affected area. You may also hear wheezes, crackles, or rhonchi. Respiratory arrest may occur.

The heart heats up

The sympathetic nervous system usually compensates by increasing the heart rate and constricting blood vessels in an effort to improve cardiac output. The patient's skin may become cool, pale, and clammy. Eventually, as myocardial oxygenation diminishes, cardiac output, blood pressure, and heart rate drop. Arrhythmias develop, and cardiac arrest may occur.

S.O.S. from the CNS

Even a slight disruption in oxygen supply and CO_2 elimination can affect brain function and behavior. Hypoxia initially causes anxiety and restlessness, which can progress to marked confusion, agitation, and lethargy. Headache, the primary indicator of hypercapnia, occurs as cerebral vessels dilate in an effort to increase the brain's blood supply. If the CO_2 level continues to rise, the patient is at risk for seizures and coma. (See *Recognizing worsening respiratory failure.*)

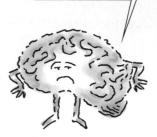

Please don't mess with the CNS! One tiny disruption can wreak havoc with my function and behavior.

What tests tell you

The following tests can help diagnose respiratory failure and guide its treatment:
• *ABG analysis* changes indicate respiratory failure. Always compare ABG results with your patient's baseline values. For a patient with previously normal lungs, the pH is usually less than 7.35, the Pao_2 less than 50 mm Hg, and the $Paco_2$ greater than 50 mm Hg. In a patient with COPD, an acute drop in the Pao_2 level of 10 mm Hg or more indicates respiratory failure. *Keep in mind that patients with chronic COPD have a chronically low Pao_2, increased $Paco_2$, increased bicarbonate levels, and normal pH.*
• *Chest X-rays* may identify an underlying pulmonary condition.
• *Electrocardiogram (ECG)* changes may reveal arrhythmias.
• Changes in *serum potassium levels* may be related to acid-base balance.

How it's treated

The underlying cause of acute respiratory failure must be addressed and the oxygen and CO_2 levels improved.

Saturate with oxygen

Oxygen is given in controlled concentrations, commonly using a Venturi mask. The goal of oxygen therapy is to prevent oxygen toxicity by administering the lowest dose of oxygen for the shortest period of time, while achieving an oxygen saturation of at least 90% or a Pao_2 level of at least 60 mm Hg.

Intubate and ventilate

Intubation and mechanical ventilation are indicated if conservative treatment fails to raise oxygen saturation above 90%. The patient may also be intubated and ventilated if acidemia continues, if he becomes exhausted, or if respiratory arrest occurs. Intubation provides a patent airway. Mechanical ventilation decreases the

---

Recognizing worsening respiratory failure

The following assessment findings are commonly seen in patients with worsening respiratory failure:
• arrhythmias
• bradycardia
• cyanosis
• diminished or absent breath sounds over affected area (as well as wheezes, crackles, or rhonchi)
• dyspnea
• hypotension
• muscle retractions.

work of breathing, ventilates the lungs, and improves oxygenation.

PEEP therapy may be ordered during mechanical ventilation to improve gas exchange. PEEP maintains positive pressure at the end of expiration, thus preventing the airways and the alveoli from collapsing between breaths.

Open those airways

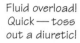
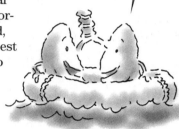

Fluid overload! Quick — toss out a diuretic!

Bronchodilators, especially inhalants, are used to open the airways. If the patient can't inhale effectively or is on a mechanical ventilator, he may receive a bronchodilator via a nebulizer. A corticosteroid, theophylline, and an antibiotic may also be ordered, as well as chest physiotherapy (including postural drainage, chest percussion, and chest vibration). Suctioning may be required to clear the airways. I.V. fluids may be ordered to correct dehydration and help thin secretions. A diuretic may be used if the patient is experiencing fluid overload.

What to do

To care effectively for a patient with respiratory failure, follow these guidelines:
• Assess respiratory status; monitor rate, depth, and character of respirations, checking breath sounds for abnormalities.
• Monitor vital signs frequently.
• Monitor the patient's neurologic status; it may become depressed as respiratory failure worsens.
• Ongoing respiratory assessment should include accessory muscle use, changes in breath sounds, ABG analysis, secretion production and clearance, and respiratory rate, depth, and pattern. Notify the doctor if interventions don't improve the patient's condition.
• Monitor fluid status by maintaining accurate fluid intake and output records. Obtain daily weights.
• Evaluate serum electrolyte levels for abnormalities that can occur with acid-base imbalances.
• Evaluate ECG results for arrhythmias.
• Monitor oxygen saturation values with a pulse oximeter.
• Monitor ABG levels to assess ventilation.

Maintain and administer

• Intervene as needed to correct underlying respiratory problems and associated alterations in acid-base status.
• Keep a handheld resuscitation bag at the bedside.
• Maintain patent I.V. access as ordered for medication and I.V. fluid administration.

- Administer oxygen as ordered to help maintain adequate oxygenation and to restore the normal respiratory rate.
- Use caution when administering oxygen to a patient with COPD. Increased oxygen levels can depress the breathing stimulus.
- Make sure the ventilator settings are at the ordered parameters.
- Perform chest physiotherapy and postural drainage as needed to promote adequate ventilation.
- If the patient is retaining CO_2, encourage slow, deep breaths with pursed lips. Urge him to cough up secretions. If he can't mobilize secretions, use suction when necessary. (See *Teaching about respiratory failure.*)
- Unless the patient is retaining fluid or has heart failure, increase his fluid intake to 2 qt (2 L)/day, to help liquefy secretions.

A little TLC

- Reposition the immobilized patient every 1 to 2 hours.
- Position the patient for optimum lung expansion. Sit the conscious patient upright as tolerated in a supported, forward-leaning position to promote diaphragm movement. Supply an over-the-bed table and pillows for support.
- If the patient isn't on a ventilator, avoid giving him a narcotic or other CNS depressant because either may further suppress respirations.

Serve and protect

- Limit carbohydrate intake and increase protein intake because carbohydrate metabolism causes more CO_2 production than protein metabolism.
- Calm and reassure the patient while giving care. Anxiety can raise oxygen demands.
- Pace care activities to maximize the patient's energy level and to provide needed rest. Limit his need to respond verbally; talking may cause shortness of breath.
- Implement safety measures as needed to protect the patient. Reorient the confused patient.

Don't be a stranger

- Stress the importance of returning for routine follow-up appointments with the doctor.
- Explain how to recognize signs and symptoms of overexertion, fluid retention, and heart failure. These may include a weight gain of 2 to 3 lb (0.9 to 1.4 kg) per day, edema of the feet or ankles, nausea, loss of appetite, or abdominal tenderness.
- Help the patient develop the knowledge and skills he needs to perform pulmonary hygiene. Encourage adequate hydration to

No place like home

Teaching about respiratory failure

Make sure to cover these points with your patient, and then evaluate what he's learned:
- basics of the condition and its treatments
- proper pulmonary hygiene and coughing techniques
- need for proper rest
- need to quit smoking, if applicable
- prescribed medications
- warning signs and symptoms and adverse reactions to medications—and when to report them
- importance of follow-up appointments
- diet restrictions, if appropriate.

thin secretions—but instruct the patient to notify the doctor of any signs of fluid retention or heart failure.
• Chart all instructions given and care provided.

Asbestosis

Asbestosis is characterized by diffuse interstitial pulmonary fibrosis resulting from prolonged exposure to airborne asbestos particles. Asbestosis may develop many years (about 15 to 20) after regular exposure to asbestos has ended.

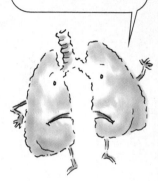

Asbestos exposure causes pleural plaques and mesotheliomas of the pleura and peritoneum. Gulp!

What causes it

Sources of asbestos exposure include asbestos mining and milling, the construction industry (in which asbestos is used in a prefabricated form), and the fireproofing and textile industries. Asbestos is also used in the production of paints, plastics, and brake and clutch linings. Asbestos-related diseases develop in families of asbestos workers as a result of exposure to fibrous dust shaken off workers' clothing at home. Such diseases develop in the general public as a result of exposure to fibrous dust or waste piles from nearby asbestos plants.

How it happens

Asbestosis is a form of pneumoconiosis. It follows prolonged inhalation of respirable asbestos fibers (about 50 microns long and 0.5 microns wide). Asbestos exposure causes pleural plaques and mesotheliomas of the pleura and peritoneum. A potent cocarcinogen, asbestos heightens a cigarette smoker's risk for lung cancer. In fact, an asbestos worker who smokes is 90 times more likely to develop lung cancer than a smoker who never worked with asbestos.

Asbestosis may progress to pulmonary fibrosis with respiratory failure and cardiovascular complications, including pulmonary hypertension and cor pulmonale.

Now you have another reason not to smoke—especially if you work with asbestos!

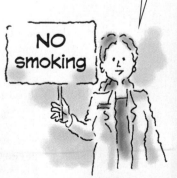

What to look for

The patient with asbestosis typically relates a history of occupational, family, or neighborhood exposure to asbestos fibers. The average exposure time is about 10 years. He may report exertional dyspnea. With extensive fibrosis, he may report dyspnea even at rest. In advanced disease, the patient may complain of a dry cough (may be productive in smokers), chest pain (often pleuritic), and recurrent respiratory tract infections.

Inspect and auscultate

Inspection findings may include tachypnea and clubbing of the fingers. With auscultation, you may hear characteristic dry crackles in the lung bases.

What tests tell you

The following tests may help diagnose asbestosis or the extent of respiratory involvement:

• *Chest X-rays* may show fine, irregular, and linear diffuse infiltrates. If the patient has extensive fibrosis, X-rays may disclose lungs with a honeycomb or ground-glass appearance. Films may also show pleural thickening and pleural calcification, bilateral obliteration of costophrenic angles and, in later disease stages, an enlarged heart with a classic "shaggy" border.

• *Pulmonary function tests* may suggest decreased vital capacity, forced vital capacity (FVC), and total lung capacity; decreased or normal forced expiratory volume in 1 second (FEV_1); a normal ratio of FEV_1 to FVC; and reduced diffusing capacity for carbon monoxide when fibrosis destroys alveolar walls and thickens the alveolocapillary membrane.

• *ABG analysis* may reveal decreased PaO_2 and CO_2 from hyperventilation.

How it's treated

Chest physiotherapy techniques, such as controlled coughing and postural drainage with chest percussion and vibration, may be implemented to relieve respiratory signs and symptoms and, in advanced disease, manage hypoxia and cor pulmonale.

A spray a day

Aerosol therapy, inhaled mucolytics, and increased fluid intake (at least 3 qt [3 L] daily) can also help to relieve respiratory symptoms. Hypoxia requires oxygen administration by cannula or mask (up to 2 L/minute) or by mechanical ventilation if the patient's arterial oxygen level can't be maintained above 40 mm Hg.

Core treatment for cor

Diuretic agents, digoxin preparations, and salt restriction may be necessary for patients with cor pulmonale. Respiratory tract infections require prompt antibiotic therapy.

What to do

When caring for a patient with asbestosis, consider these interventions:
• Provide supportive care and help the patient adjust to lifestyle changes necessitated by chronic illness.
• Be alert for changes in baseline respiratory function. Also watch for changes in sputum quality and quantity, restlessness, increased tachypnea, and changes in breath sounds. Report these immediately.
• Perform chest physiotherapy, including postural drainage and chest percussion and vibration for involved lobes, several times daily.
• Weigh the patient three times weekly.
• Provide high-calorie, high-protein foods. Offer small, frequent meals to conserve the patient's energy and prevent fatigue.
• Make sure the patient receives adequate fluids to loosen secretions.
• Schedule respiratory therapy at least 1 hour before or after meals. Provide mouth care after inhalation bronchodilator therapy.
• Encourage daily activity and provide diversions as appropriate. Help conserve the patient's energy and prevent fatigue by alternating rest and activity.
• Administer medication as ordered and note the patient's response.
• Watch for complications, such as pulmonary hypertension and cor pulmonale.

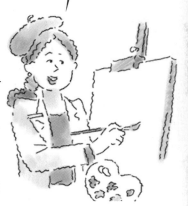

Provide diversions for the patient with asbestosis.

Atelectasis

Atelectasis (collapsed or airless condition of all or part of the lung) may be chronic or acute, and commonly occurs to some degree in patients undergoing abdominal or thoracic surgery. The prognosis depends on prompt removal of the airway obstruction, relief of hypoxia, and reexpansion of the collapsed lobules or lung.

What causes it

Atelectasis may result from:
• bronchial occlusion by mucus plugs (a common problem in heavy smokers or people with COPD, bronchiectasis, or cystic fibrosis)

- occlusion by foreign bodies
- bronchogenic carcinoma
- inflammatory lung disease
- oxygen toxicity
- pulmonary edema
- any condition that inhibits full lung expansion or makes deep breathing painful, such as abdominal surgical incisions, rib fractures, tight dressings, and obesity
- prolonged immobility
- mechanical ventilation using constant, small tidal volumes without intermittent deep breaths
- CNS depression (as in drug overdose), which eliminates periodic sighing.

How it happens

In atelectasis, incomplete expansion of lobules (clusters of alveoli) or lung segments leads to partial or complete lung collapse. Because parts of the lung are unavailable for gas exchange, unoxygenated blood passes through these areas unchanged, resulting in hypoxemia.

What to look for

Your assessment findings will vary with the cause and degree of hypoxia, and may include:
- dyspnea (possibly mild and subsiding without treatment if atelectasis involves only a small area of the lung, or severe if massive collapse occurs)
- cyanosis, decreased breath sounds
- anxiety, diaphoresis
- dull sound on percussion if a large portion of the lung is collapsed
- hypoxemia, tachycardia
- substernal or intercostal retraction
- compensatory hyperinflation of unaffected areas of the lung
- mediastinal shift to the affected side.

What tests tell you

The following tests aid in diagnosing atelectasis:
- *Chest X-ray* shows characteristic horizontal lines in the lower lung zones. Dense shadows accompany segmental or lobar collapse, and are commonly associated with hyperinflation of neighboring lung zones during widespread atelectasis. However, exten-

sive areas of "micro-atelectasis" may exist in the absence of any abnormalities on the patient's chest X-ray.
• *Bronchoscopy* may be performed when the cause of atelectasis is unknown. This is done to rule out an obstructing neoplasm or a foreign body.

How it's treated

Atelectasis is treated with incentive spirometry, chest percussion, postural drainage, and frequent coughing and deep-breathing exercises. If these measures fail, bronchoscopy may help remove secretions. Humidity and bronchodilators can improve mucociliary clearance and dilate airways, and are sometimes used with a nebulizer. Atelectasis secondary to an obstructing neoplasm may require surgery or radiation therapy.

What to do

To keep the patient's airways clear and to relieve hypoxia, follow these guidelines:
• To prevent atelectasis after surgery, encourage the patient to cough, turn, and breathe deeply every 1 to 2 hours, as ordered. Teach the patient to splint his incision when coughing. Reposition the postoperative patient gently and frequently, and help him walk as soon as possible. Administer adequate analgesics to control pain.
• During mechanical ventilation, tidal volume should be maintained at 10 to 15 ml/kg of the patient's body weight to ensure adequate lung expansion. Use the sigh mechanism on the ventilator, if appropriate, to intermittently increase tidal volume at the rate of three to four sighs per hour.
• Humidify inspired air and encourage adequate fluid intake to mobilize secretions. Loosen and clear secretions with postural drainage and chest percussion.
• Assess breath sounds and ventilatory status frequently, and report any changes.
• Evaluate the patient. Secretions should be clear and the patient should show no signs of hypoxia.

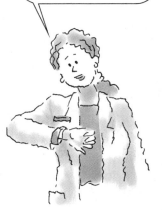

It's been 2 hours. It's time to cough, turn, and breathe. Doctor's orders to prevent atelectasis.

Bronchopulmonary dysplasia

Bronchopulmonary dysplasia (BPD) is a chronic pulmonary disorder that occurs in severely ill neonates who have received high concentrations of oxygen for long periods of time, and prolonged assistance from mechanical ventilation.

What causes it

BPD is caused by prolonged exposure to oxygen, leading to oxygen toxicity. In 90% of BPD cases, the neonates are born prematurely; many of these neonates develop respiratory distress syndrome (RDS) related to lung immaturity. Other potential causes include lung injury from mechanical ventilation, neonatal pulmonary hypertension, damage to the lungs from high-pressure oxygen therapy, surfactant deficiency, inflammation caused by oxygen exposure, ligation of a patent ductus arteriosus, genetic predisposition, bacteria, and viruses. BPD usually develops in neonates within 4 weeks of birth.

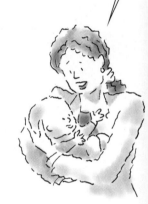

It's not your fault, little one. You were born early, and your alveoli haven't had time to mature.

How it happens

The alveoli are the air sacs of the lungs. In BPD, alveoli are poorly developed, generally due to premature birth. Alveoli development occurs between 36 weeks' gestation and 18 months after birth. In a healthy neonate, normal alveoli maturation occurs by the 6th month after birth. However, in the premature neonate, the alveoli haven't had time to mature and are, therefore, incapable of normal function.

Surfactant is also thought to play a role in BPD. Surfactant typically lines the alveoli but, in premature birth, this lining hasn't developed fully. As a result, the neonate will experience decreased lung compliance and increased airway resistance, and will require oxygen therapy and mechanical ventilation.

What to look for

The following signs and symptoms may be noted with BPD:
- tachycardia
- tachypnea
- chest retraction
- retraction of the ribs
- cough
- paradoxical respirations (movement of the chest and abdomen in opposite directions with each breath)
- wheezing
- abnormal posture
- respiratory distress
- episodic cyanosis
- symptoms of a respiratory infection (irritability, fever, nasal congestion, cough, change in breathing patterns).

What tests tell you

These tests can help diagnose BPD and guide its treatment:
- *Chest X-ray* reveals pulmonary changes such as bronchiolar metaplasia and interstitial fibrosis.
- *ABG analysis* reveals hypoxemia.

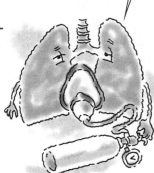

I think I need a ventilator. I'm feeling a bit deflated.

How it's treated

Treatment usually focuses on ventilator support, which delivers pressure to the lungs to keep the tissue inflated and provide necessary oxygen. As the neonate's oxygenation improves, oxygen concentrations and pressures are slowly reduced. When the neonate is successfully weaned from the ventilator, oxygen therapy via a mask or nasal cannula is commonly required for several weeks to months.

Nutritional support is another important area of treatment for BPD. Neonates are generally fed I.V. or through a gastric tube. Caloric needs increase with the added energy demand required for breathing. Fluids may be restricted and diuretics may be added to the medication regimen to prevent fluid overload. Surfactant therapy may be initiated.

Corticosteroids may be added to the treatment regimen to reduce swelling. Bronchodilators may be included in the treatment regimen to open the airway and ease airflow. Antibiotics may be required if infection is diagnosed or suspected. All attempts should be made to limit the neonate's exposure to infection, including limiting the number of visitors, particularly children.

What to do

Follow these guidelines when providing care to a neonate with BPD:
- Maintain adequate oxygenation through the use of oxygen therapy and positive pressure ventilation.
- Assess breath sounds and ventilatory status frequently and report any changes.
- Monitor pH, partial pressure of CO_2, and partial pressure of oxygen carefully.
- Assess oxygenation via pulse oximetry and ABG analysis.
- Establish an indwelling arterial line early in the acute management phase of this condition.
- Decrease oxygen concentrations and pressure as tolerated by the neonate to prevent prolonged oxygen toxicity.

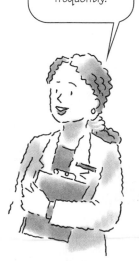

When dealing with BPD, assess the neonate's breath sounds frequently.

• Collaborate with the dietitian to provide additional calories and nutritional support for the neonate.
• Administer medications (bronchodilators, corticosteroids, antibiotics) as prescribed.
• Provide information and support to the neonate's parents and other family members.

Idiopathic pulmonary fibrosis

Idiopathic pulmonary fibrosis (IPF) is a chronic and typically fatal interstitial pulmonary disease. About 50% of patients with its diagnosis die within 5 years. Once thought to be a rare condition, it's now more common. The incidence of IPF is slightly higher in men than in women, and in smokers than in nonsmokers. It occurs most commonly in people ages 50 to 70, and rarely appears before age 40 or after age 80. IPF is one of several types of interstitial lung diseases, all of which should be ruled out before a diagnosis of IPF is confirmed.

What causes it

IPF is the result of a cascade of events that involve inflammatory, immune, and fibrotic changes in the lungs. Despite many studies and hypotheses, the stimulus that begins the progression remains unknown. Viral and genetic causes have been considered, but there's currently no solid evidence to support either theory.

How it happens

Despite no clear cause for IPF, it *is* clear that chronic inflammation plays an important role. Inflammation sets into motion the injury, as well as the fibrosis that ultimately distorts and impairs the structure and function of the alveolo-capillary gas exchange surface. Lung biopsy reveals swollen alveolar walls with chronic inflammatory cellular infiltrate composed of mononuclear cells and polymorphonuclear leukocytes. Intra-alveolar inflammatory cells can be found in early stages of the disease. As the disease progresses, excessive collagen and fibroblasts fill the interstitium. In advanced stages, the alveolar walls are destroyed and replaced by honeycombing cysts.

What to look for

The usual presenting symptoms of IPF are dyspnea and a dry, hacking, commonly paroxysmal cough. Most people have had

Calm yourself, Watson. A clear cause for IPF may be eluding us, but as for injury and fibrosis, inflammation is clearly a prime suspect!

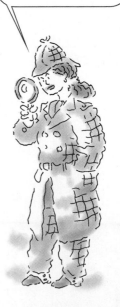

these symptoms for several months or years before seeking medical attention. Auscultation typically reveals expiratory crackles, especially in the bases of the lungs. Bronchial breath sounds become audible later, when airway consolidation develops. Rapid, shallow breathing occurs, especially with exercise.

Clubbing of the fingertips has been noted in more than 40% of patients with IPF. Late in the disease, cyanosis and pulmonary hypertension commonly occur. As the disease progresses, profound hypoxemia and severe, debilitating dyspnea are noted.

What tests tell you

Diagnosis begins with a thorough patient history to exclude more common causes of interstitial lung disease. Of particular interest are environmental and occupational exposures (to agents including coal dust, asbestos, silica, and beryllium), connective tissue disorders (including scleroderma and rheumatoid arthritis), and exposure to drugs such as amiodarone, tocainide, and crack cocaine. The following tests aid in the diagnosis of IPF:

• *Lung biopsy* is the gold standard for diagnosing IPF. Biopsies may be performed through a thoracoscope or a bronchoscope. Histologic features of the biopsy tissue vary, depending on the stage of the disease.

• *Chest X-rays* may show four distinct patterns: interstitial, reticulonodular, ground-glass, or honeycomb. Although X-rays don't help confirm the presence of an abnormality, and correlate poorly with the histologic findings and pulmonary function tests, they may be used to track the progression of the disease.

• *High-resolution computed tomography scans* provide superior views of the four patterns seen on X-ray films, and are routinely used to confirm an IPF diagnosis.

• *Pulmonary function tests* show reductions in vital capacity and total lung capacity, and demonstrates impaired diffusing capacity for carbon monoxide. Simple spirometry may not show an abnormality.

• *ABG analysis* and *pulse oximetry readings* reveal hypoxemia. Hypoxemia progressively worsens as the disease progresses. Oxygenation will also decline with exercise.

• *Bronchoscopy* accesses bronchioalveolar lavage fluid, which exhibits increases in the number and percentage of polymorphonuclear leukocytes and alveolar macrophages. Lymphocytes may be low, normal, or elevated.

How it's treated

Oxygen therapy can't change the pathology of IPF but it can prevent the problems related to dyspnea and tissue hypoxia in the early stages of the disease. Initially, the patient may require little or no supplemental oxygen while at rest; he will, however, need more as the disease progresses, and during episodes of exertion.

Drug therapy is largely unsuccessful and controversial. This is due to the lack of controlled studies to evaluate treatment modalities, the poor understanding of the factors that may influence the patient's response to treatment, and the difficulty diagnosing the disease in its early stages. IPF is extremely variable, which makes evaluation of a consistent response to treatment difficult. Lung transplantation may be successful for younger, otherwise healthy individuals.

What to do

Care of a patient with IPF will likely include the following interventions:
• Explain all diagnostic tests to the patient, who may experience anxiety and frustration about the many tests required to establish the diagnosis.
• Monitor oxygenation at rest and on exertion. Oxygen flow rates will likely be prescribed for the level of activity at which the patient is performing. A higher oxygen flow rate will be ordered for use during exertion, to maintain adequate oxygenation.
• As IPF progresses, the patient's oxygen requirements will increase. A non-rebreathing mask may be required to supply high oxygen percentages. Eventually, maintaining adequate oxygenation may become impossible despite maximum oxygen flow rates.
• Most patients will require oxygen therapy at home. (See *At home with IPF.*)
• Encourage the patient to be as active as possible.
• Monitor the patient for adverse reactions to drug therapy.
• Teach the patient about prescribed medications, especially adverse effects. Also teach the patient and his family members infection prevention techniques.
• Encourage good nutritional habits. Small frequent meals with high nutritional value may be necessary if dyspnea interferes with eating.
• Provide emotional support for the patient and family members as they deal with the patient's increasing disability, dyspnea, and probable death.

No place like home

At home with IPF

Follow these guidelines when discharging a patient with idiopathic pulmonary fibrosis (IPF):
• Make appropriate referrals to discharge planners, respiratory care practitioners, and home equipment vendors to ensure continuity of care when the patient goes home.
• Tell the patient or caregiver to arrange the bed and necessary equipment for daily functioning in an area that doesn't require the patient to climb stairs frequently, if at all.
• Encourage the patient to use breathing exercises and relaxation and energy conservation techniques. Explain that all of these strategies will help him to manage severe dyspnea.

RDS of the neonate

Respiratory distress syndrome (RDS) of the neonate, also known as *hyaline membrane disease*, is the most common cause of neonatal death; in the United States alone, it kills about 40,000 neonates every year. The syndrome occurs most exclusively in neonates born before 37 weeks' gestation; it occurs in about 60% of those born before 28 weeks' gestation.

RDS of the neonate is marked by widespread alveolar collapse. Occurring mainly in premature neonates and in sudden infant death syndrome, it strikes apparently healthy neonates. It's most common in neonates of mothers who have diabetes, and in those delivered by cesarean birth; however, it may also occur suddenly after antepartum hemorrhage.

In RDS of the neonate, premature neonates develop a widespread alveolar collapse due to surfactant deficiency. If untreated, the syndrome causes death within 72 hours after birth in up to 14% of neonates weighing less than 5.5 lb (2,500 g). Aggressive management and mechanical ventilation can improve the prognosis, although some surviving neonates are left with BPD. Mild cases of the syndrome subside after about 3 days.

What causes it

Common causes of RDS include:
- surfactant deficiency
- structural lung immaturity.

How it happens

Surfactant, a lipoprotein present in alveoli and respiratory bronchioles, helps to lower surface tension, maintain alveolar patency, and prevent alveolar collapse, particularly at the end of expiration. Although the neonatal airways are developed by 27 weeks' gestation, the intercostal muscles are weak and the alveoli and capillary blood supply is immature. Surfactant deficiency causes a higher surface tension. The alveoli aren't able to maintain patency and begin to collapse.

Collapse, hypoxia, injury

With alveolar collapse, ventilation is decreased and hypoxia develops. The resulting pulmonary injury and inflammatory reaction lead to edema and swelling of the interstitial space, thus impeding gas exchange between the capillaries and the functional alveoli.

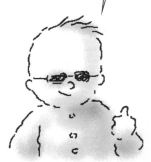

Thanks to the surfactant, now I'm breathing easy!

The inflammation also stimulates production of hyaline membranes composed of white fibrin, which accumulate in the alveoli. These deposits further reduce gas exchange in the lung. They also decrease lung compliance, resulting in an increase in the work of breathing.

Decreases, increases, shunts

Decreased alveolar ventilation results in a decreased ventilation-perfusion ratio and pulmonary arteriolar vasoconstriction. The pulmonary vasoconstriction can result in increased right cardiac volume and pressure, causing blood to be shunted from the right atrium through a patent foramen ovale to the left atrium. Increased pulmonary resistance also results in deoxygenated blood passing through the ductus arteriosus, totally bypassing the lungs, and causing a right-to-left shunt. The shunt further increases hypoxia.

Because of immature lungs and an already increased metabolic rate, the neonate must expend more energy to ventilate collapsed alveoli. This further increases oxygen demand and contributes to cyanosis. The neonate attempts to compensate with rapid, shallow breathing, causing an initial respiratory alkalosis as CO_2 is expelled. The increased effort at lung expansion causes respirations to slow and respiratory acidosis to occur, leading to respiratory failure.

What to look for

Suspect RDS of the neonate in a patient with a history that includes preterm birth (before 28 weeks' gestation), cesarean delivery, maternal history of diabetes, or antepartal hemorrhage. Signs and symptoms of RDS may include:

- rapid, shallow respirations due to hypoxia
- intercostal, subcostal, or sternal retractions due to hypoxia
- nasal flaring due to hypoxia
- audible expiratory grunting (a natural compensatory mechanism that produces PEEP to prevent further alveolar collapse)
- hypotension due to cardiac failure
- peripheral edema due to cardiac failure
- oliguria due to vasoconstriction of the kidneys.

It gets worse...

In severe cases, these signs and symptoms may also occur:
- apnea due to respiratory failure
- bradycardia due to cardiac failure

• cyanosis from hypoxemia, right-to-left shunting through the foramen ovale, or right-to-left shunting through the atelectatic lung areas
• pallor due to decreased circulation
• frothy sputum due to pulmonary edema and atelectasis
• low body temperature, resulting from an immature nervous system and inadequate subcutaneous fat
• diminished air entry and crackles on auscultation due to atelectasis.

... And complicated

Possible complications of RDS include:
• respiratory failure
• cardiac failure
• BPD.

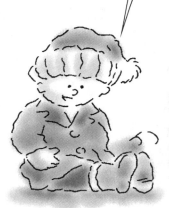

Low body temperature may be a sign of RDS of the neonate.

What tests tell you

• *Chest X-rays* may be normal for the first 6 to 12 hours in 50% of patients, although later films show a fine reticulonodular pattern and dark streaks, indicating air-filled, dilated bronchioles.
• *ABG analysis* reveals a diminished Pao_2 level; a normal, decreased, or increased $Paco_2$ level; and a reduced pH, indicating a combination of respiratory and metabolic acidosis.
• *Lecithin-sphingomyelin ratio* helps to assess prenatal lung development in neonates at risk for this syndrome; this test is usually ordered if a cesarean delivery will be performed before 36 weeks' gestation.

How it's treated

Correcting RDS of the neonate typically involves:
• warm, humidified, oxygen-enriched gases administered by oxygen hood or, if such treatment fails, by mechanical ventilation to promote adequate oxygenation and reverse hypoxia
• administration of surfactant by an ET tube to prevent atelectasis
• mechanical ventilation with PEEP or continuous positive airway pressure (CPAP) administered by nasal prongs (which forces the alveoli to remain open on expiration and promotes increased surface area for exchange of oxygen and CO_2)
• high-frequency oscillation ventilation if the neonate can't maintain adequate gas exchange. This form of ventilation provides satisfactory minute volume (total air breathed in 1 minute) with lower airway pressures

• a radiant warmer or an Isolette to help maintain thermoregulation and reduce metabolic demands
• I.V. fluids to promote adequate hydration and maintain circulation with capillary refill of less than 2 seconds (and maintain fluid and electrolyte balance)
• sodium bicarbonate to control acidosis
• tube feedings or total parenteral nutrition
• prophylactic antibiotics for underlying infections
• diuretics to reduce pulmonary edema
• corticosteroids possibly administered to the mother to stimulate surfactant production in a fetus at high risk for preterm birth
• delayed delivery of a neonate (if premature labor) in an effort to prevent RDS.

What to do

Neonates with RDS require continual assessment and monitoring in a neonatal ICU. Follow these measures:
• Closely monitor blood gases as well as fluid intake and output. If the neonate has an umbilical catheter (arterial or venous), check for arterial hypotension or abnormal central venous pressure. Watch for complications, such as infection, thrombosis, and decreased circulation to the legs. If the neonate has a transcutaneous oxygen monitor, change the site of the lead placement every 2 to 4 hours to avoid burning the skin.
• Weigh the neonate once or twice daily. To evaluate his progress, assess skin color, rate and depth of respirations, severity of retractions, nostril flaring, frequency of expiratory grunting, frothing at the lips, and restlessness.

Prescribing PEEP

• Regularly assess the effectiveness of oxygen or ventilator therapy. Evaluate every change in fraction of inspired oxygen and PEEP or CPAP by monitoring SaO_2 or ABG levels. Be sure to adjust PEEP or CPAP as indicated, based on findings.
• When the neonate is on mechanical ventilation, watch carefully for signs of barotrauma (increase in respiratory distress and subcutaneous emphysema) and accidental disconnection from the ventilator. Check ventilator settings frequently. Be alert for signs of complications of PEEP or CPAP therapy, such as decreased cardiac output, pneumothorax, and pneumomediastinum. Mechanical ventilation increases the risk of infection in premature neonates, so preventive measures are essential. (Mechanical ventilation in neonates is usually done in a pressure-limited mode rather than the volume-limited mode used in adults.)

• As needed, arrange for follow-up care with a neonatal ophthalmologist to check for retinal damage. Premature neonates in an oxygen-rich environment are at increased risk for developing retinopathy of prematurity.

• Teach the parents about their neonate's condition and, if possible, let them participate in his care to encourage normal parent-neonate bonding. Advise parents that full recovery may take up to 12 months. When the prognosis is poor, prepare the parents for the neonate's impending death, and offer emotional support.

• Help reduce RDS mortality by detecting respiratory distress early. Recognize intercostal retractions and grunting, especially in a premature neonate, as signs of RDS; make sure the neonate receives immediate treatment.

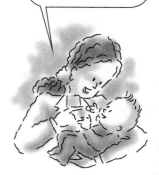

Detecting respiratory distress early will help reduce RDS mortality. Something everyone wants!

Sarcoidosis

Sarcoidosis is a multisystemic, granulomatous disorder that characteristically produces lymphadenopathy, pulmonary infiltration, and skeletal, liver, eye, or skin lesions. It occurs most commonly in adults ages 20 to 40. In the United States, sarcoidosis occurs predominantly among blacks and affects twice as many women as men.

The disease can eventually lead to pulmonary fibrosis, with resultant pulmonary hypertension and cor pulmonale. Even so, acute sarcoidosis usually resolves within 2 years. Chronic, progressive sarcoidosis, which is uncommon, is associated with pulmonary fibrosis and progressive pulmonary disability.

What causes it

The cause of sarcoidosis is unknown, but several possibilities exist. The disease may result from a hypersensitivity response — possibly from T-cell imbalance — to such agents as atypical mycobacteria, fungi, and pine pollen. The incidence is slightly higher within families, suggesting a genetic predisposition. Inhalation of chemicals, such as zirconium and beryllium, may also trigger the disease.

How it happens

Although the exact mechanism of the disease is unknown, research suggests a T-cell problem and, more specifically, a lymphokine production problem. In other granulomatous diseases such as tuberculosis, granuloma formation occurs from inadequate pathogen clearance by macrophages. These macrophages require the help of T cells that secrete lymphokines which, in turn, activate less effective macrophages to become aggressive phagocytes. Lack of lymphokine secretion by T cells may help explain granuloma formation in sarcoidosis.

What to look for

The patient with sarcoidosis may report pain in the wrists, ankles, and elbows; general fatigue and a feeling of malaise; and unexplained weight loss. He may also complain of breathlessness and shortness of breath on exertion, and may have a nonproductive cough and substernal pain.

I spy with my little eye...

On inspection, you may observe erythema nodosum, subcutaneous skin nodules with maculopapular eruptions, and punched-out lesions on the fingers and toes. You may also note weakness and cranial or peripheral nerve palsies. When you inspect the nose, you may see extensive nasal mucosal lesions. Inspection of the eyes commonly reveals anterior uveitis. Glaucoma and blindness occasionally occur in advanced disease.

Palpate and auscultate

You may be able to palpate bilateral hilar and right paratracheal lymphadenopathy and splenomegaly, and you may hear such arrhythmias as premature beats on auscultation.

What tests tell you

• A positive *Kveim-Siltzbach skin test* points to sarcoidosis. In this test, the patient receives an skin intradermal injection of an antigen prepared from human sarcoidal spleen or lymph nodes from patients with sarcoidosis. If he has active sarcoidosis, granuloma develops at the injection site in 2 to 6 weeks. When coupled with a biopsy at the injection site that shows discrete epithelioid cell granuloma, the test confirms the diagnosis.

Diagnostic support group

Several other tests are used to support the diagnosis:
• *Chest X-rays* demonstrate bilateral hilar and right paratracheal adenopathy, with or without diffuse interstitial infiltrates. Occasionally, they show large nodular lesions in lung parenchyma.
• *Lymph node, skin,* or *lung biopsy* discloses noncaseating granulomas with negative cultures for mycobacteria and fungi.

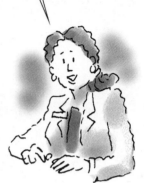

The patient with sarcoidosis might have such symptoms as malaise, weight loss, breathlessness, and substernal pain.

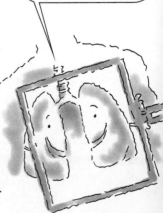

X-rays show bilateral hilar and right paratracheal adenopathy. I hope they don't find any diffuse interstitial infiltrates.

• *Pulmonary function tests* indicate decreased total lung capacity and compliance, and reduced diffusing capacity.
• *ABG analysis* shows a decreased PaO_2.
• *Tuberculin skin tests*, *fungal serologies*, *sputum cultures* (for mycobacteria and fungi), and *biopsy cultures* are negative and help rule out infection.

How it's treated

Asymptomatic sarcoidosis requires no treatment. However, sarcoidosis that causes ocular, respiratory, CNS, cardiac, or systemic symptoms (such as fever and weight loss) requires treatment with systemic or topical corticosteroids. The same is true of sarcoidosis that produces hypercalcemia or destructive skin lesions. Such therapy usually continues for 1 to 2 years, but some patients may need lifelong therapy. A patient with hypercalcemia also requires a low-calcium diet and protection from direct exposure to sunlight. If the patient has a significant response to the tuberculin skin tests, showing tuberculosis reactivation, he needs isoniazid therapy.

What to do

Care of a patient with sarcoidosis will likely include the following interventions:
• Watch for and report any complications. Also note any abnormal laboratory results (showing anemia, for example) that could alter patient care.
• If the patient has arthralgia, administer analgesics as ordered. Record signs of progressive muscle weakness.
• Provide a nutritious, high-calorie diet and plenty of fluids. If the patient has hypercalcemia, speak to the dietitian about a low-calcium diet. Weigh the patient regularly to detect weight loss.
• Monitor the patient's respiratory function. Check chest X-rays for the extent of lung involvement, and note and record any increase in or first-time bloody sputum. If the patient has pulmonary hypertension or end-stage cor pulmonale, monitor ABG levels, watch for arrhythmias, and administer oxygen as needed.
• Listen to the patient's fears and concerns, and remain with him during periods of extreme stress and anxiety. Encourage him to identify actions and care measures that help make him more comfortable and relaxed. Then try to perform these measures, and encourage the patient to do so as well.
• Whenever possible, include the patient in care decisions, and include family members in all phases of the patient's care. (See *Going home with sarcoidosis*.)

No place like home

Going home with sarcoidosis

The following guidelines provide information to consider when preparing a patient with sarcoidosis for discharge:
• Stress the need for compliance with the prescribed steroid therapy. Emphasize the importance of not skipping doses.
• Instruct the patient to take steroids with food.
• Make sure the patient understands the need for regular, careful follow-up examinations and treatment.
• Encourage the patient to wear medical identification jewelry to identify himself as a corticosteroid user.
• Discuss the patient's increased vulnerability to infection, and review ways to minimize exposure to illness.
• Refer the patient with failing vision to community support and resource groups, including the American Foundation for the Blind, if necessary.

Silicosis

Silicosis is the most common form of pneumoconiosis. Those who work around silica dust, such as foundry workers, boiler scalers, and stone cutters, have the highest incidence of the disease. (See *Berylliosis: Another type of pneumoconiosis.*) Silica in its pure form is found in the manufacture of ceramics (flint) and building materials (sandstone). It occurs in mixed form in the production of construction materials (cement). It's also found in powder form (silica flour) in paints, porcelain, scouring soaps, and wood fillers, and in the mining of gold, lead, zinc, and iron.

What causes it

Silicosis is caused by the inhalation of silica dust due to:
• manufacture of ceramics and building materials
• use of the mixed or powder form
• mining of gold, lead, zinc, and iron.

Sand blasters, tunnel workers, and others exposed to high concentrations of respirable silica may develop acute silicosis after 1 to 3 years. Those exposed to lower concentrations of free silica can develop accelerated silicosis, usually after about 10 years of exposure.

How it happens

In silicosis, small particles of mineral dust are inhaled and deposited in the respiratory bronchioles, alveolar ducts, and alveoli. The surfaces of these particles generate silicon-based radicals that lead to the production of hydroxy, hydrogen peroxide, and other oxygen radicals that damage cell membranes and inactivate cell proteins.

Don't eat my dust!

Alveolar macrophages ingest the particles of mineral dust, become activated, and release cytokines, such as tumor necrosis factor and others that attract other inflammatory cells. The inflammation damages resident cells and the extracellular matrix. Fibroblasts are stimulated to produce collagen, resulting in fibrosis.

Berylliosis: Another type of pneumoconiosis

Berylliosis—a type of pneumoconiosis—is a systemic granulomatous disease that mainly affects the lungs. It's an occupational disease that commonly affects workers in beryllium alloy, ceramics, foundry, grinder, cathode ray tube, gas mantle, missile, and nuclear reactor industries.

Berylliosis occurs in two forms: acute nonspecific pneumonitis and chronic noncaseating granulomatous disease with interstitial fibrosis, which can cause death from respiratory failure and cor pulmonale. In about 10% of patients with acute berylliosis, chronic disease develops 10 to 15 years after exposure.

Symptoms	Diagnostic tests	Treatment
Symptoms of berylliosis include: • an itchy rash • a beryllium ulcer • swelling and ulceration of the nasal mucosa • septal perforation • tracheitis • bronchitis (dry cough) • chest tightness • substernal pain • tachycardia • worsening dyspnea.	Tests that may help diagnose berylliosis or the extent of respiratory involvement include: • chest X-rays detect pulmonary edema • pulmonary function studies demonstrate decreased vital capacity as fibrosis stiffens the lungs • ABG analysis findings indicate diminished partial pressure of arterial oxygen (Pao_2) and CO_2 • a positive beryllium patch test establishes a patient's hypersensitivity to beryllium but doesn't confirm the diagnosis • tissue biopsy and spectrographic analysis, if positive, support, but don't confirm, the diagnosis • urinalysis may identify beryllium excreted in urine, indicating exposure to the metal.	• A beryllium ulcer requires excision or curettage. • If the patient has hypoxia, he may need oxygen delivered by nasal cannula or mask (usually 1 to 2 L/minute). • If the patient has severe respiratory failure, he may need mechanical ventilation if the Pao_2 falls below 40 mm Hg. • The patient with acute berylliosis usually receives corticosteroid therapy in an attempt to alter the disease's progression; maintenance therapy may be lifelong for chronic cases. • Respiratory symptoms may respond to bronchodilators, increased fluid intake (at least 3 qt [3 L] daily), and chest physiotherapy. • Diuretic agents, digoxin preparations, and sodium restriction may help the patient with cor pulmonale.

What to look for

The patient will have a history of long-term industrial exposure to silica dust. He may complain of dyspnea on exertion, which he's likely to attribute to "being out of shape" or "slowing down." If the disease has progressed to the chronic and complicated stage, the patient may report a dry cough, especially in the morning.

When you inspect the patient, you may note decreased chest expansion and tachypnea. If he has advanced disease, he may also act lethargic and look confused. You may percuss areas of increased and decreased resonance. On auscultation, you may hear fine to medium crackles, diminished breath sounds, and an intensified ventricular gallop on inspiration—a hallmark of cor pulmonale.

What tests tell you

The following tests may help diagnose silicosis or the extent of respiratory involvement:
- *Chest X-rays* in simple silicosis show small, discrete, nodular lesions distributed throughout both lung fields, although they typically concentrate in the upper lung zones. The lung nodes may appear enlarged and may show eggshell calcification. In complicated silicosis, X-rays show one or more conglomerate masses of dense tissue.
- *Pulmonary function tests* demonstrate reduced FVC in complicated silicosis. If the patient has obstructive disease (emphysematous silicosis areas), FEV_1 is reduced. A patient with complicated silicosis also has reduced FEV_1 but has a normal or high ratio of FEV_1 to FVC. When fibrosis destroys alveolar walls and obliterates pulmonary capillaries, or when it thickens the alveolocapillary membrane, the diffusing capacity for carbon monoxide falls below normal. Both restrictive and obstructive disease reduce maximal voluntary ventilation.
- *ABG analysis* reveals a normal PaO_2 in simple silicosis that may drop significantly below normal in late stages or complicated disease. The patient has normal $PaCO_2$ in the early stages of the disease but hyperventilation may cause it to drop below normal. If restrictive lung disease develops—particularly if the patient is hypoxic and has severe alveolar ventilatory impairment—$PaCO_2$ may increase above normal.

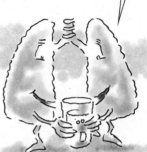

Increased fluid intake helps relieve respiratory signs and symptoms. Sloncha! Salud! Cheers!

How it's treated

The goal in treating silicosis is to relieve respiratory symptoms, manage hypoxia and cor pulmonale, and prevent respiratory tract infections and irritations. Treatment includes careful observation for the development of tuberculosis.

Drink up!

Daily bronchodilation aerosols and increased fluid intake (at least 3 qt [3 L] daily) relieve respiratory signs and symptoms. Steam inhalation and chest physiotherapy (such as controlled coughing and segmental bronchial drainage) with chest percussion and vibration help clear secretions.

In severe cases, the patient may need oxygen by cannula, mask, or mechanical ventilation (if he can't maintain arterial oxygenation). Respiratory tract infection warrants prompt antibiotic administration.

What to do

When caring for a patient with silicosis, consider these interventions:

• Assess for changes in baseline respiratory function, including changes in sputum quality and quantity, restlessness, increased tachypnea, and changes in breath sounds. Report any changes to the doctor immediately.

• Perform chest physiotherapy, including postural drainage and chest percussion and vibration designed for involved lobes, several times each day.

• Provide the patient with a high-calorie, high-protein diet, preferably in small, frequent meals.

• Schedule respiratory therapy at least 1 hour before or after meals. Provide oral care after bronchodilator therapy.

• Make sure the patient receives enough fluids to loosen secretions.

• Encourage daily activity and provide the patient with diversional activities as appropriate. To conserve his energy, alternate periods of rest and activity.

• Administer medication as ordered. Monitor the patient for desired response and for adverse reactions.

• Watch for complications, such as pulmonary fibrosis, right ventricular hypertrophy, and cor pulmonale.

• Help the patient adjust to the lifestyle changes associated with a chronic illness. Answer his questions, and encourage him to express his concerns about his illness.

• Stay with him during periods of extreme stress and anxiety, and include the patient and family members in care decisions whenever possible.

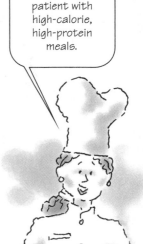

Provide the patient with high-calorie, high-protein meals.

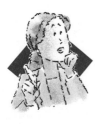

Quick quiz

1. In stage I of ARDS, what symptoms are commonly assessed?
   A. Use of accessory muscles to breath and observed restlessness
   B. Dyspnea, diminished breath sounds, and normal to elevated respiratory rates
   C. Tachycardia with arrhythmias and a labile blood pressure
   D. Decreasing heart rate and respiratory rates and cyanosis

Answer: B. Stage I of ARDS involves dyspnea, especially on exertion. Respiratory and heart rates are generally normal to high.

2.   When assessing a patient with atelectasis, you would expect to observe:
    A.   bradycardia.
    B.   hypertension.
    C.   high-pitched sound on percussion.
    D.   dyspnea, depending on the degree of lung involvement.

Answer: D. Dyspnea may be mild and subside without treatment if atelectasis involves only a small area of the lung, or severe if a massive collapse occurs.

3.   Of the following patients, the one most likely to develop idiopathic pulmonary fibrosis is:
    A.   a 2-year-old child with a history of frequent respiratory infection.
    B.   a 35-year-old female with a history of pneumonia twice in 1 year.
    C.   a 52-year-old man with a history of smoking.
    D.   an 84-year-old man with a history of working in a fertilizer factory.

Answer: C. IPF occurs slightly more commonly in men than women, and in smokers more than in nonsmokers. It occurs most commonly in people ages 50 to 70 and rarely appears before age 40 or after age 80.

4.   The greatest risk factor for developing bronchopulmonary dysplasia is:
    A.   premature birth.
    B.   maternal smoking.
    C.   familial history of asthma.
    D.   respiratory rate of 55 breaths per minute.

Answer: A. In approximately 90% of BPD cases, the neonates are born prematurely.

Scoring

☆☆☆ If you answered all four items correctly, bravo! Your knowledge of restrictive disorders knows no bounds.

☆☆ If you answered three items correctly, wow! You're close to an unrestricted understanding of restrictive disorders.

☆ If you answered fewer than three items correctly, don't get deflated! Take a deep breath and read the chapter again.

Vascular lung disorders

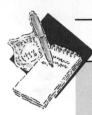

Just the facts

In this chapter, you'll learn:

♦ several vascular lung disorders and their potential causes

♦ the pathophysiology of vascular lung disorders

♦ ways to recognize and diagnose vascular lung disorders

♦ treatments for a variety of vascular lung disorders.

Understanding vascular lung disorders

Vascular lung disorders affect the vascular structures of the lungs. Normal pulmonary vasculature is a low-pressure, low-resistance system. It includes pulmonary arteries, pulmonary veins, pulmonary capillaries, pulmonary lymphatics, and broncial circulation.

Conditions that affect any of these vascular components can result in a vascular lung disorder and compromised respiratory function.

Cor pulmonale

Cor pulmonale is a condition in which hypertrophy (an increase in the size of an organ that's not related to tumor growth) and dilation of the right ventricle develop secondary to disease affecting the structure or function of the lungs or their vasculature. This condition is also known as *right ventricular hypertrophy*.

Cor pulmonale can occur at the end stage of various chronic disorders of the lungs, pulmonary vessels, chest wall, and respiratory control center. This condition doesn't stem from congenital disorders or conditions affecting the left side of the heart.

It says here that vascular lung disorders affect the vascular structures of the lungs. This can compromise respiratory function.

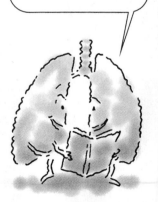

What causes it

About 85% of patients with cor pulmonale also have chronic obstructive pulmonary disease (COPD) and about 25% of patients with bronchial COPD eventually develop cor pulmonale. The disorder is most common in smokers and in middle-aged and elderly males, but the incidence of cor pulmonale is rising in the female population. Prognosis for patients with cor pulmonale is poor because it occurs late in the course of the individual's underlying condition, and with other irreversible diseases. (See *Cor pulmonale in children.*)

So much in common

Common causes of cor pulmonale include:
• disorders that affect the pulmonary parenchyma
• COPD
• bronchial asthma
• primary pulmonary hypertension
• vasculitis
• pulmonary emboli
• external vascular obstruction resulting from a tumor or an aneurysm
• kyphoscoliosis (excessive curvature of the spine)
• pectus excavatum (funnel chest)
• muscular dystrophy
• poliomyelitis
• obesity (Pickwickian syndrome)
• living at high altitudes (chronic mountain sickness).

How it happens

In cor pulmonale, pulmonary hypertension increases the heart's workload. To compensate, the right ventricle increases in size (hypertrophies) to force blood through the lungs. As long as the heart can compensate for the increased pulmonary vascular resistance, signs and symptoms reflect only the underlying disorder.

Increased afterload causes severe right ventricular enlargement in patients with cor pulmonale. An occluded vessel impairs the heart's ability to generate enough pressure. Pulmonary hypertension results from the increased blood flow needed to oxygenate the tissues.

In the red

In response to hypoxemia, the bone marrow produces more red blood cells (RBCs), causing polycythemia. The blood's viscosity increases, which further aggravates pulmonary hyper-

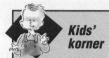

Kids' korner

Cor pulmonale in children

In children, cor pulmonale can be a complication of cystic fibrosis or of hemosiderosis, upper airway obstruction, scleroderma, extensive bronchiectasis, neuromuscular diseases that affect respiratory muscles, or abnormalities of the respiratory control area.

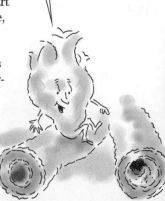

An occluded vessel sure does make it hard to generate enough pressure. I can't work under these conditions!

tension, causing an increase in the right ventricle's workload, and subsequent heart failure. (See *Understanding cor pulmonale*.)

Obstruction and constriction

In chronic obstructive disease, increased airway obstruction further compromises airflow. The resulting hypoxia and hypercapnia can have vasodilatory effects on systemic arterioles (minute arterial branches with distal ends that lead to capillaries). Hypoxia then increases pulmonary vasoconstriction. The liver becomes palpable and tender because it's enlarged and displaced in a downward position near the diaphragm.

All systems — not go

Compensatory mechanisms begin to fail and larger amounts of blood remain in the right ventricle at the end of diastole (the period of the cardiac cycle when the muscle fibers lengthen, the heart dilates, and the cavities fill with blood). The presence of this "extra" blood causes ventricular dilation. Increasing intrathoracic pressures impede venous return and increase jugular vein pressure. Peripheral edema can occur and right ventricular hypertrophy increases progressively. The main pulmonary arteries enlarge, pulmonary hypertension increases, and heart failure occurs.

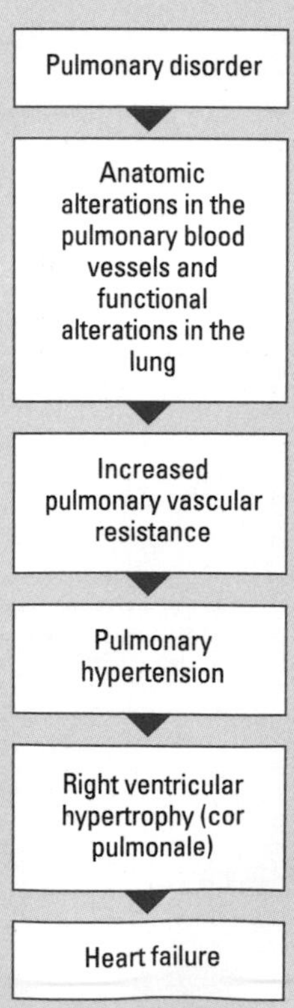

What to look for

Symptoms of cor pulmonale can change based on the stage of the condition. A patient in the early stages may have the following symptoms:
- chronic, productive cough resulting from attempts to clear secretions from the lungs
- exertional dyspnea due to hypoxia
- wheezing respirations from a narrowed airway
- fatigue and weakness due to hypoxemia.

Progressive but not progress

Patients with progressive cor pulmonale may have the following symptoms:
- dyspnea at rest due to hypoxemia
- tachypnea due to a response to decreased oxygenation to the tissues
- orthopnea (difficulty breathing if not in an upright position) due to pulmonary edema
- dependent edema due to right-sided heart failure
- distended neck veins due to pulmonary hypertension
- decreased cardiac output
- enlarged, tender liver related to polycythemia (excessive RBCs) and decreased cardiac output

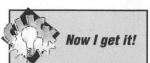

Now I get it!

Understanding cor pulmonale

Although pulmonary restrictive disorders (such as fibrosis or obesity), obstructive disorders (such as bronchitis), and primary vascular disorders (such as recurrent pulmonary emboli) may cause cor pulmonale, these disorders share a common pathway, as shown below.

Pulmonary disorder

↓

Anatomic alterations in the pulmonary blood vessels and functional alterations in the lung

↓

Increased pulmonary vascular resistance

↓

Pulmonary hypertension

↓

Right ventricular hypertrophy (cor pulmonale)

↓

Heart failure

- distention of the jugular vein caused by pressure over the liver from right-sided heart failure
- right upper quadrant discomfort due to liver involvement
- tachycardia due to decreased cardiac output and increased hypoxia
- weakened pulses due to decreased cardiac output.

What tests tell you

Several tests are available to assist in diagnosing cor pulmonale:
- *Pulmonary artery pressure measurements* show increased right ventricular and pulmonary artery pressures, stemming from increased pulmonary vascular resistance. Right ventricular systolic and pulmonary artery systolic pressure will exceed 30 mm Hg; pulmonary artery diastolic pressure will exceed 15 mm Hg.
- An *echocardiogram* or an *angiogram* can demonstrate right ventricular enlargement. An echocardiogram can help to estimate pulmonary artery pressure, while also ruling out structural and congenital lesions.
- *Chest X-rays* show large, central pulmonary arteries. Right ventricular enlargement is indicated by enlargement of the right side of the heart's silhouette on an anterior chest film.
- *Arterial blood gas (ABG) analysis* shows decreased partial pressure of arterial oxygen (PaO_2). It's commonly less then 70 mm Hg and usually no more then 90 mm Hg with the patient on room air.
- An *electrocardiogram (ECG)* commonly demonstrates arrhythmias, such as premature atrial and ventricular contractions, and atrial fibrillation during severe hypoxia. It may also show right bundle-branch block, right axis deviation, prominent P waves and inverted T waves in right precordial leads, and right ventricular hypertrophy.
- *Pulmonary function test* findings are consistent with the underlying pulmonary disease. Hematocrit is generally greater than 50%.

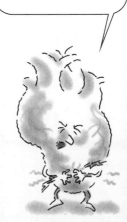

Cor pulmonale is a lot of pressure — increased pressures on the right, decreased PaO_2, and now, arrhythmias.

How it's treated

Treatment of cor pulmonale is aimed at reducing hypoxia, increasing the patient's exercise tolerance and, when possible, correcting the underlying condition. In addition to bed rest, treatment may include:
- cardiac glycoside (digoxin) to strengthen cardiac contractions
- antibiotics when respiratory infection is present

Now I get it!

Polycythemia and phlebotomy

In response to hypoxemia, the bone marrow produces more red blood cells (RBCs), causing polycythemia.

Polycythemia

Physical findings of polycythemia include:
- ruddy, cyanotic skin
- emphysema and hypoxemia without hepatosplenomegaly or hypertension
- clubbing of the fingers (if the underlying disease is cardiac).

Phlebotomy

Phlebotomy may be required to rapidly reduce high RBC levels quickly. The frequency of phlebotomy and the amount of blood removed each time (typically, 350 to 500 ml) will be determined by the patient's condition.

Follow these guidelines to ensure that the procedure is carried out effectively, while keeping the patient as comfortable as possible:
- Explain the procedure to the patient.

- Before starting the phlebotomy procedure, check the patient's blood pressure, heart rate, and respiratory rate.
- Keep the patient in a supine position during the procedure to prevent syncope or vertigo.
- If the patient develops tachycardia or clamminess, or complains of vertigo, stop the procedure immediately and notify the physician.
- Immediately after the phlebotomy procedure, check the patient's blood pressure and heart rate.
- Encourage the patient to drink at least 24 oz (720 ml) of fluid after the procedure, or replace slowly through an I.V. source.
- Because iron is lost during phlebotomy, monitor the patient and lab studies for signs of iron deficiency, including pallor, weight loss, weakness, and glossitis.
- Monitor serum iron, total iron-binding capacity, and ferritin levels to assess the adequacy of the patient's iron stores.

- culture and sensitivity of a sputum specimen, to assist in selecting the appropriate antibiotic for the infection
- administration of potent pulmonary artery vasodilators (such as diazoxide, nitroprusside, hydralazine, angiotensin-converting enzyme inhibitors, calcium channel blockers, and prostaglandins) in primary pulmonary hypertension
- delivery of oxygen by mask or cannula in concentrations ranging from 24% to 40%, depending on the PaO_2 levels (see *COPD and oxygen therapy*)
- in acute cases, possible mechanical ventilation
- low-salt diet, restricted fluid intake, and administration of diuretics, such as furosemide, to reduce edema
- possible phlebotomy to reduce the elevated RBC count caused by polycythemia (see *Polycythemia and phlebotomy*)
- anticoagulants in small doses to reduce the risk of thromboembolism
- tracheostomy for the patient with an upper airway obstruction
- steroid therapy in patients with vasculitis or an acute exacerbation of COPD.

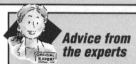

Advice from the experts

COPD and oxygen therapy

Generally, patients with underlying chronic obstructive pulmonary disease (COPD) shouldn't receive high concentrations of oxygen because of possible subsequent respiratory depression. Excessive oxygen therapy may eliminate the hypoxic respiratory drive, causing carbon dioxide narcosis.

At home with cor pulmonale

When preparing a patient with cor pulmonale for discharge, follow these guidelines:
• Make sure the patient understands the importance of maintaining a low-salt diet, weighing himself daily, and watching for and reporting edema.
• Teach the patient to assess for edema by pressing the skin over the shin with one finger, holding it for 1 or 2 seconds, and then checking for a finger impression (indicative of edema).
• Instruct the patient to allow for frequent rest periods and to perform breathing exercises regularly.
• If the patient needs supplemental oxygen therapy at home, refer him to an agency that can help him obtain the necessary equipment.
• If the patient has been placed on anticoagulant therapy, emphasize the need to watch for

bleeding and signs of bleeding (epistaxis, hematuria, bruising) and to report these signs to the doctor.
• Encourage the patient to return for periodic laboratory tests to monitor partial thromboplastin time, fibrinogen level, platelet count, hematocrit, hemoglobin levels, and prothrombin time.
• Because pulmonary infection commonly worsens chronic obstructive pulmonary disease and cor pulmonale, stress the importance of reporting early signs of infection. Instruct the patient to avoid crowds, as well as people with pulmonary infections.
• Advise the patient to avoid nonprescribed medications such as sedatives, which may depress the ventilatory drive.

What to do

Therapy for cor pulmonale aims at reducing hypoxemia and pulmonary vasoconstriction, increasing exercise tolerance and correcting the underlying condition when possible. The following interventions will serve as a guide when caring for a patient with cor pulmonale:
• Plan diet carefully with the patient and the staff dietitian. The patient may lack energy and tire easily when eating, so small, frequent meals are preferred over three large meals per day.
• Prevent fluid retention by limiting the patient's fluid intake to 1 to 2 qt (1 to 2 L) per day and providing a low-sodium diet.
• Monitor serum potassium levels closely if the patient is receiving diuretics. Low serum potassium levels can increase the risk of arrhythmias associated with cardiac glycosides.
• Watch the patient for signs of digoxin toxicity. Such signs include anorexia, nausea, vomiting, and yellow halos around visual images.

• Monitor for cardiac arrhythmias. Teach the patient to check his radial pulse before taking digoxin or any cardiac glycoside. The patient should be instructed to notify the doctor if a change in pulse rate is detected.
• Reposition the bedridden patient frequently to prevent atelectasis.
• Provide meticulous respiratory care, including oxygen therapy. Teach COPD patients to perform pursed-lip breathing exercises.
• Periodically measure ABG levels and watch for signs of respiratory failure, such as a change in pulse rate; deep, labored respirations; and increased fatigue on exertion. (See *At home with cor pulmonale.*)

Pulmonary edema

Pulmonary edema is a common complication of cardiac disorders. It's marked by an accumulation of fluid in extravascular spaces of the lung. The disorder can occur as a chronic condition or it can develop quickly and become rapidly fatal.

What causes it

Pulmonary edema usually results from left-sided heart failure caused by arteriosclerotic, cardiomyopathic, hypertensive, or valvular heart disease.

Factors that may predispose a patient to pulmonary edema include:
• barbiturate or opiate poisoning
• heart failure
• I.V. fluids infused in excessive volumes or at an overly rapid rate
• impaired pulmonary lymphatic drainage (from Hodgkin's disease or obliterative lymphangitis after radiation)
• inhalation of irritating gases
• mitral stenosis and left atrial myxoma (which impair left atrial emptying)
• pneumonia
• pulmonary venoocclusive disease.

How it happens

Normally, pulmonary capillary hydrostatic pressure, capillary oncotic pressure, capillary permeability, and lymphatic drainage are in balance. When this balance is disrupted or the lymphatic drainage system is obstructed, fluid infiltrates the lung and pul-

Now I get it!

Understanding pulmonary edema

In pulmonary edema, diminished function of the left ventricle causes blood to back up into pulmonary veins and capillaries. The increasing capillary hydrostatic pressure pushes fluid into the interstitial spaces and alveoli. These illustrations show a normal alveolus (left) and an alveolus affected by pulmonary edema (right).

Normal alveolus

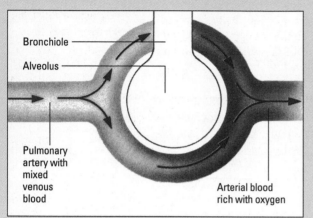

Alveolus in pulmonary edema

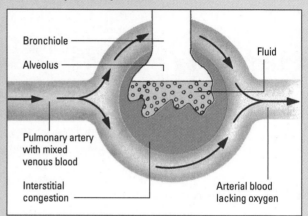

monary edema results. If pulmonary capillary hydrostatic pressure increases, the compromised left ventricle requires increased filling pressures to maintain adequate cardiac output. These pressures are transmitted to the left atrium, the pulmonary veins, and the pulmonary capillary bed, forcing fluids and solutes from the intravascular compartment into the interstitium of the lungs. The interstitium overloads with fluid, which floods the peripheral alveoli and impairs gas exchange.

Got no pull

If colloid osmotic pressure decreases, the hydrostatic force that regulates intravascular fluids (the natural pulling force) is lost because there's no opposition. Fluid flows freely into the interstitium and alveoli, impairing gas exchange and leading to pulmonary edema. (See *Understanding pulmonary edema.*)

Today's weather — expect interstitial flooding...

A blockage of the lymph vessels can result from compression that comes from edema or tumor fibrotic tissue, and increased

> Pulmonary edema is marked by an accumulation of fluid in my extravascular spaces. Geez, Louise — get me outta here!

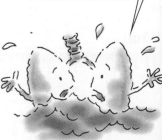

systemic venous pressure. Hydrostatic pressure in the large pulmonary veins increases, the pulmonary lymphatic system can't drain correctly into the pulmonary veins, and excess fluid moves into the interstitial space. Pulmonary edema then results from fluid accumulation.

...and leaking plasma proteins

Capillary injury, such as occurs in acute respiratory distress syndrome or with inhalation of toxic gases, increases capillary permeability. The injury causes plasma proteins and water to leak out of the capillaries and move into the interstitium, increasing the interstitial oncotic pressure, which is normally low. As the level of interstitial oncotic pressure approaches that of capillary oncotic pressure, the water begins to move out of the capillaries and into the lungs, resulting in pulmonary edema.

What to look for

The patient's health history may include a predisposing factor for pulmonary edema. The patient typically complains of a persistent cough. He may report getting a cold and being dyspneic on exertion. He may experience paroxysmal nocturnal dyspnea and orthopnea.

Take a look-see

On inspection, you may note restlessness and anxiety. With severe pulmonary edema the patient's breathing may be visibly labored and rapid. His cough may sound intense and produce frothy, bloody sputum. In advanced stages the patient's level of consciousness decreases.

Distention, clams, and crackles

Typical palpation findings include neck vein distention. In acute pulmonary edema, the skin feels sweaty, cold, and clammy. Auscultation may reveal crepitant crackles and a diastolic (S_3) gallop. In severe pulmonary edema, you may hear wheezing as the alveoli and bronchioles fill with fluid. The crackles become more diffuse. (See *Act quickly with pulmonary edema*.)

What's more

Additional findings include worsening tachycardia, decreasing blood pressure, thready pulse, and decreased cardiac output. In advanced pulmonary edema, breath sounds diminish.

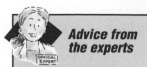

Advice from the experts

Act quickly with pulmonary edema

If you detect inspiratory crackles, dry cough, or dyspnea, notify the doctor immediately. Results from chest X-rays may not be available until 24 hours after you have assessed the patient. Don't wait for the X-ray results if you suspect pulmonary edema because the symptoms will worsen and may eventually progress to respiratory or metabolic acidosis, with subsequent cardiac or respiratory arrest.

Listen to your patient! Persistent cough? Dyspnea on exertion? His history can provide important clues.

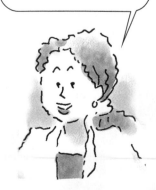

What tests tell you

Clinical features of pulmonary edema help to establish a working diagnosis. Diagnostic tests provide the following information:
• *ABG analysis* usually shows hypoxia with variable partial pressures of arterial carbon dioxide, depending on the patient's degree of fatigue. ABG results may also reveal metabolic acidosis.
• *Chest X-rays* show diffuse haziness of the lung fields and, usually, cardiomegaly and pleural effusion.
• *Pulse oximetry* may reveal decreasing levels of arterial oxygen saturation.
• *Pulmonary artery catheterization* is used to identify left-sided heart failure (indicated by elevated pulmonary artery wedge pressures [PAWP]). These findings help to rule out acute respiratory distress syndrome, in which wedge pressure usually remains normal.
• An *ECG* may disclose evidence of previous or current myocardial infarction.

How it's treated

Treatment of pulmonary edema aims to reduce extravascular fluid, improve gas exchange and myocardial function and, if possible, correct underlying disease.

Ventilate, dilate, and mobilize

High concentrations of oxygen can be administered by cannula or mask. (Typically, the patient with pulmonary edema doesn't tolerate a mask.) If the patient's arterial oxygen levels remain too low, assisted ventilation can improve oxygen delivery to the tissues and usually improves acid-base balance. A bronchodilator, such as aminophylline, may decrease bronchospasm and enhance myocardial contractility. Diuretics, such as furosemide, ethacrynic acid, and bumetanide, increase urination, which helps to mobilize extravascular fluid.

Be positive

Treatment of myocardial dysfunction includes positive inotropic agents, such as digoxin and amrinone, to enhance contractility. Pressor agents may be given to enhance contractility and to promote vasoconstriction in peripheral vessels.

Got rhythm

Antiarrhythmics may also be given, particularly in arrhythmias related to decreased cardiac output. Occasionally, arterial vasodila-

> I got rhythm, I got music, I got antiarrhythmics, who could ask for anything more?

tors such as nitroprusside can decrease peripheral vascular resistance, preload, and afterload.

Back in the flow

Morphine may reduce anxiety and dyspnea and dilate the systemic venous bed, promoting blood flow from pulmonary circulation to the periphery. However, using morphine in the patient with respiratory distress can also compromise respirations. Have resuscitation equipment available in case the patient stops breathing.

Rotation ups and downs

Other treatments include rotating tourniquets and phlebotomy, both of which reduce preload. However, phlebotomy also removes hemoglobin, which may worsen the patient's hypoxemia. (See *Pulmonary edema interventions*, page 246.)

What to do

When caring for a patient with pulmonary edema, consider these interventions:
• Help the patient relax to promote oxygenation, control bronchospasm, and enhance myocardial contractility.
• Reassure the patient, who's likely to be frightened by his inability to breathe normally. Provide emotional support to family members as well.
• Place the patient in high Fowler's position to enhance lung expansion.
• Administer oxygen as ordered.
• Assess the patient's condition frequently and document his responses to treatment. Monitor ABG and pulse oximetry values, oral and I.V. fluid intake, urine output and, in the patient with a pulmonary artery catheter, pulmonary end-diastolic and PAWPs. Check the cardiac monitor often and report changes immediately.
• Watch for complications of such treatments as electrolyte depletion, oxygen therapy, and mechanical ventilation.
• Monitor vital signs every 15 to 30 minutes while administering nitroprusside in dextrose 5% in water by I.V. drip. During use, protect the solution from light by wrapping the bottle or bag with aluminum foil. Discard unused nitroprusside solution after 4 hours. Watch for arrhythmias in patients receiving digoxin, and for marked respiratory depression in those receiving morphine.
• Carefully record the time morphine is given and the amount administered. (See *At home with pulmonary edema*.)

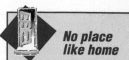

No place like home

At home with pulmonary edema

When preparing a patient with pulmonary edema for discharge, follow these guidelines:
• Urge the patient to follow the prescribed medication regimen.
• Explain all procedures to the patient and family members.
• Describe the early signs of fluid overload and the importance of reporting them.
• Explain the reasons for sodium restrictions. List high-sodium foods and drugs.
• Review all prescribed medications with the patient.
• If the patient takes digoxin, teach him to monitor his pulse rate and stress the need to report signs of toxicity. Encourage consumption of potassium-rich foods.
• If the patient takes a vasodilator, teach him the signs of hypotension and emphasize the need to avoid alcohol.
• Discuss ways to conserve physical energy.

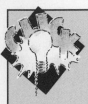

Now I get it!

Pulmonary edema interventions

To care for a patient with suspected pulmonary edema, obtain the patient history, assist with diagnostic tests, and assess respiratory, mental, and cardiovascular status. The flowchart below outlines likely signs and symptoms and appropriate interventions for each of these assessments. Continue to observe the patient with unremarkable symptoms for possible changes that might indicate disease progression.

Respiratory status	Mental status	Cardiovascular status
Signs and symptoms include orthopnea, dyspnea, cough, frothy sputum, crackles, and wheezing.	Signs and symptoms include restlessness, anxiety, shortness of breath, and confusion.	Signs and symptoms include hypotension; cold, clammy skin; irregular pulse; and S_3 heart sound.
Notify the doctor and administer oxygen, place the patient in an upright position with legs dangling, monitor arterial blood gas levels, administer bronchodilators as ordered, and auscultate for breath sounds frequently.	Notify the doctor and provide emotional support. Remain with the patient and explain all procedures.	Notify the doctor and administer cardiopulmonary treatment as ordered, including digoxin, diuretics, and aminophylline. Apply rotating tourniquets as ordered.

Administer I.V. morphine as ordered.

Monitor vital signs, intake and output, and serum electrolyte levels. Document findings.

Acute phase resolves.	Condition deteriorates.

Prepare patient for transfer to intensive care unit.

Pulmonary embolism

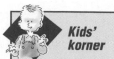

A pulmonary embolism is an obstruction of the pulmonary arterial bed by a dislodged thrombus or a foreign substance. Pulmonary infarction, or lung tissue death from a pulmonary embolus, is sometimes mild and may not produce symptoms. However, when a massive embolism involves more than 50% obstruction of pulmonary artery circulation, it can be rapidly fatal.

What causes it

Pulmonary embolism usually results from dislodged thrombi that originate in the leg veins. Other, less common, sources of thrombi include pelvic veins, renal veins, hepatic veins, the right side of the heart, and the arms. (See *At risk for pulmonary embolism*, page 248.)

How it happens

Trauma, clot dissolution, sudden muscle spasm, intravascular pressure changes, or a change in peripheral blood flow can cause the thrombus to loosen or fragment. Then the thrombus—now called an *embolus*—floats to the heart's right side and enters the lung through the pulmonary artery. There, the embolus may dissolve, continue to fragment or grow. (See *Pulmonary emboli in children.*)

Collapse, atelectasis, death

If the embolus occludes the pulmonary artery, alveoli collapse and atelectasis develops. If the embolus enlarges, it may occlude most or all of the pulmonary vessels, causing death.

Rare but serious

Although rare, the emboli can contain air, fat, amniotic fluid, tumor cells, or talc from drugs intended for oral administration that are injected I.V. by addicts. Pulmonary embolism may lead to pulmonary infarction, especially in patients with chronic heart or pulmonary disease.

What to look for

Total occlusion of the main pulmonary artery is rapidly fatal; smaller or fragmented emboli produce symptoms that vary with

---

Kids' korner

Pulmonary emboli in children

Suspect pulmonary embolism when chest pain and dyspnea develop in a child with a recent history of:
• surgery
• major trauma
• a long period of immobility.

Pulmonary emboli are treated as a medical emergency. To immediately treat the dyspnea, elevate the child's head and administer oxygen through a mask or nasal cannula.

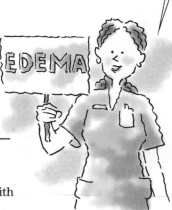

Look out for leg edema! It could be a sign of pulmonary embolism.

Now I get it!

At risk for pulmonary embolism

Many disorders and treatments heighten the risk of pulmonary embolism. At particular risk are surgical patients. For example, the anesthetic used during surgery can injure lung vessels, and surgery itself or prolonged bed rest can promote venous stasis, which compounds the risk. Below are lists of predisposing disorders and other conditions that increase the risk of pulmonary embolism.

Predisposing disorders
- Lung disorders, especially chronic types
- Cardiac disorders
- Infection
- Diabetes mellitus
- History of thromboembolism, thrombophlebitis, or vascular insufficiency
- Sickle cell disease
- Autoimmune hemolytic anemia
- Polycythemia
- Osteomyelitis
- Long-bone fracture
- Manipulation or disconnection of central lines

Venous stasis
- Prolonged bed rest or immobilization
- Obesity
- Age 40 and older
- Burns
- Recent childbirth
- Orthopedic casts

Venous injury
- Surgery, particularly of the legs, pelvis, abdomen, or thorax
- Leg or pelvic fractures or other injuries
- I.V. drug abuse
- I.V. therapy

Increased blood coagulability
- Cancer
- Use of high-dose estrogen oral contraceptives or hormone replacement

the size, number, and location of the emboli. Dyspnea is usually the first symptom of pulmonary embolism and may be accompanied by anginal or pleuritic chest pain. Other clinical features include tachycardia, productive cough (sputum may be blood-tinged), and low-grade fever.

Splinting, edema, and crackles — oh my!

Less common signs include massive hemoptysis, splinting of the chest, and leg edema. A large embolus may produce cyanosis, syncope, and distended jugular veins. Signs of shock (such as weak, rapid pulse and hypotension) and signs of hypoxia (such as restlessness) may also occur. Cardiac auscultation occasionally reveals a right ventricular S_3 audible at the lower sternum, and increased intensity of a pulmonary component of S_2. Crackles and a pleural friction rub may be heard at the infarction site.

(Text continues on page 249.)

Types of pneumonia

Pneumonia is an acute infection of the lung parenchyma that commonly impairs gas exchange. The prognosis is generally good for people who have normal lungs and adequate host defenses before the onset of pneumonia. Pneumonia is typically classified according to location: *bronchopneumonia* involves the distal airways and alveoli; *lobular pneumonia,* part of a lobe; *lobar pneumonia,* an entire lobe.

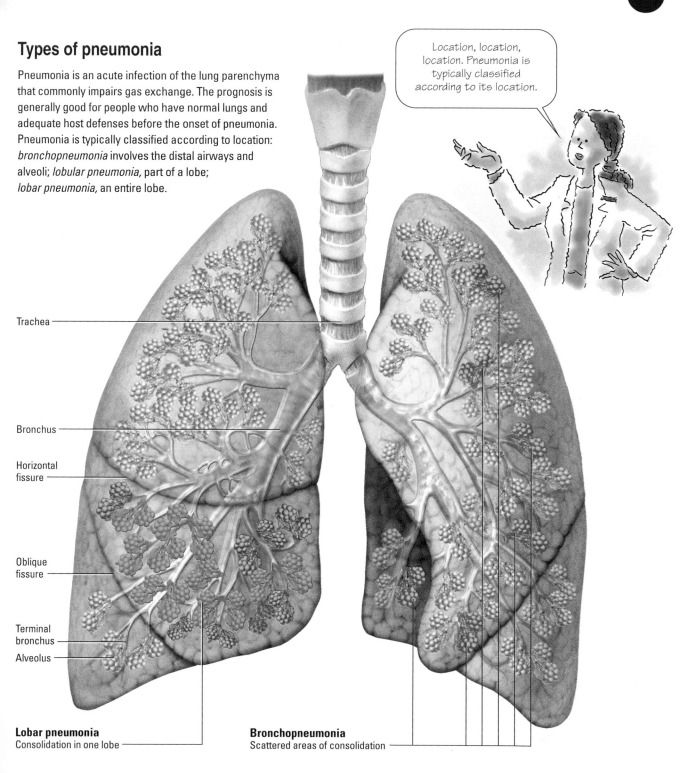

Location, location, location. Pneumonia is typically classified according to its location.

Trachea

Bronchus

Horizontal fissure

Oblique fissure

Terminal bronchus

Alveolus

Lobar pneumonia
Consolidation in one lobe

Bronchopneumonia
Scattered areas of consolidation

How pulmonary edema develops

Pulmonary edema is an accumulation of fluid in the extravascular spaces of the lungs. It's a common complication of cardiac disorders and may occur as a chronic condition or may develop quickly and rapidly become fatal.

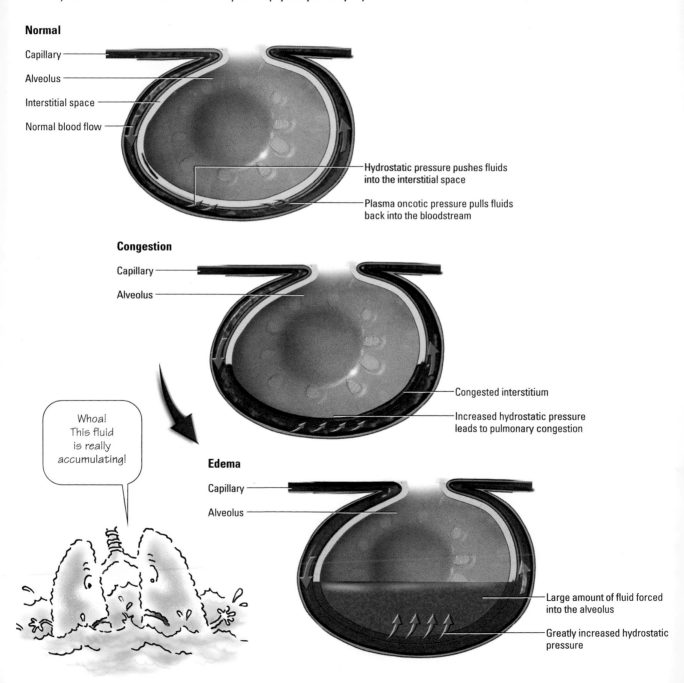

Normal

Capillary

Alveolus

Interstitial space

Normal blood flow

Hydrostatic pressure pushes fluids into the interstitial space

Plasma oncotic pressure pulls fluids back into the bloodstream

Congestion

Capillary

Alveolus

Congested interstitium

Increased hydrostatic pressure leads to pulmonary congestion

Whoa! This fluid is really accumulating!

Edema

Capillary

Alveolus

Large amount of fluid forced into the alveolus

Greatly increased hydrostatic pressure

Tumor infiltration in lung cancer

Lung cancer has long been the most common cause of cancer death in men, and since 1987, it's been the most common cause of cancer death in women. Lung cancer usually develops in the wall or epithelium of the bronchial tree. Its most common types are epidermoid (squamous cell), adenocarcinoma, small cell (oat cell), and large cell (anaplastic).

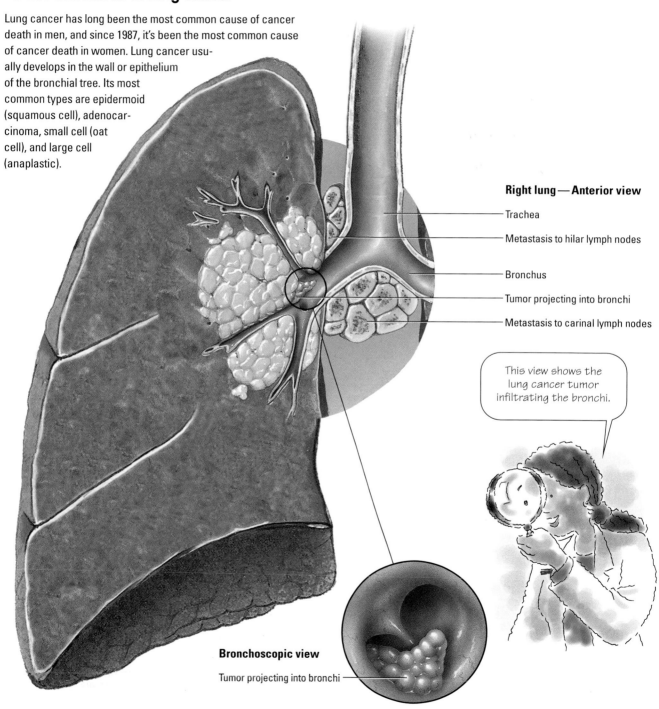

Right lung — Anterior view

- Trachea
- Metastasis to hilar lymph nodes
- Bronchus
- Tumor projecting into bronchi
- Metastasis to carinal lymph nodes

This view shows the lung cancer tumor infiltrating the bronchi.

Bronchoscopic view

Tumor projecting into bronchi

Sites of pulmonary emboli

Pulmonary embolism is a complication in hospitalized patients. It occurs when there's an obstruction of the pulmonary arterial bed by a dislodged thrombus, heart valve vegetation, or foreign substance.

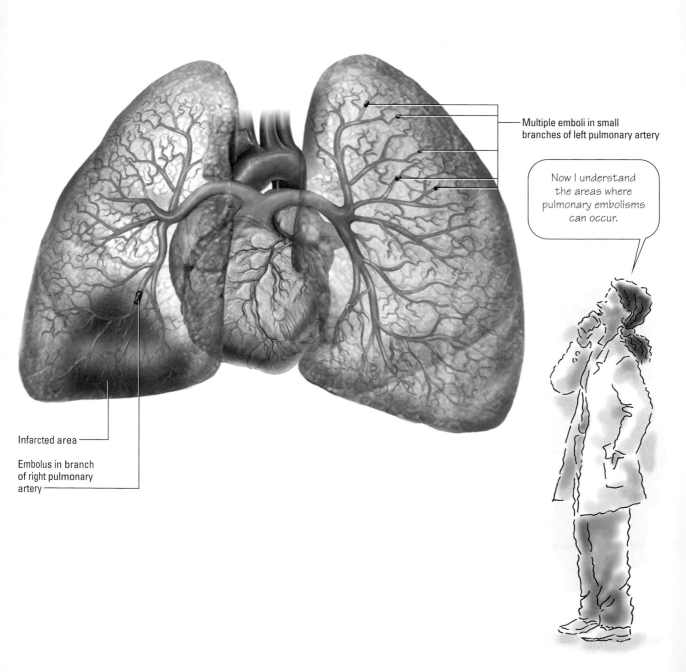

Multiple emboli in small branches of left pulmonary artery

Now I understand the areas where pulmonary embolisms can occur.

Infarcted area

Embolus in branch of right pulmonary artery

What tests tell you

The patient history should reveal predisposing conditions for pulmonary embolism, including deep vein thrombosis (DVT). A triad of factors leading to DVT formation includes stasis, endothelial injury, and hypercoagulability. Risk factors for DVT include long car or plane trips, extended periods of immobility (after surgery, serious illness, or injury), cancer, pregnancy, hypercoagulability, use of certain drug therapies (such as the estrogen preparations in some hormone replacement regimens, hormonal contraceptives, and dehydration), and previous DVTs.

These tests support the diagnosis of pulmonary embolism:
• *Chest X-rays* help to rule out other pulmonary diseases. In addition, they shows areas of atelectasis, diaphragm elevation and pleural effusion, prominence of the pulmonary artery and focal oligemia of blood vessels and, occasionally, the characteristic wedge-shaped infiltrate suggestive of pulmonary infarction.
• *Lung scans* show perfusion defects in areas beyond occluded vessels; however, it doesn't rule out microemboli.
• *Pulmonary angiography* is the most definitive test, but requires a skilled angiographer and radiologic equipment; it also poses some risk to the patient. The decision to use pulmonary angiography depends on the degree of uncertainty about the diagnosis and the need to avoid unnecessary anticoagulant therapy in a high-risk patient.
• *ECG* findings are inconclusive but help distinguish pulmonary embolism from myocardial infarction. In extensive embolism, the ECG may show right axis deviation; right bundle-branch block; tall, peaked P waves; depressed ST segments and inverted T waves (indicative of right-sided heart strain); and supraventricular tachyarrhythmias. A pattern that's sometimes observed is S_1, Q_3, and T_3 (S wave in lead I, Q wave in lead III, and inverted T wave in lead III).
• *Auscultation* occasionally reveals a right ventricular S_3 gallop and increased intensity of a pulmonary component of S_2. Also, crackles and a pleural rub may be heard at the embolism site.
• *ABG analysis* reveals a decrease in PaO_2 and in partial pressure of arterial carbon dioxide. These findings are characteristic but aren't always present in patients with pulmonary embolism.

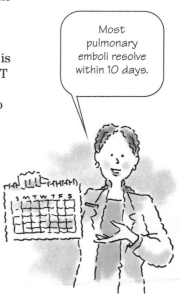

Most pulmonary emboli resolve within 10 days.

How it's treated

Treatment aims to prevent recurrence and maintain adequate cardiovascular and pulmonary function as the obstruction resolves. Because most emboli resolve within 10 days, treatment consists of oxygen therapy as needed and anticoagulation with heparin to inhibit new thrombus formation. (See *Anticoagulation therapy cautions.*)

Massive and shocking

Patients with massive pulmonary embolism and shock may require thrombolytic therapy with tissue plasminogen activator or streptokinase to enhance fibrinolysis of the pulmonary emboli and remaining thrombi. Hypotension related to pulmonary emboli may be treated with vasopressors. To treat septic emboli, you must evaluate the source of the infection.

Seek the septic source

Treatment of septic emboli requires antibiotic therapy as well as evaluation of the source of infection, particularly in cases of endocarditis. Anticoagulants aren't used to treat septic emboli.

Surgery: reservations only

Surgery to interrupt the inferior vena cava is reserved for patients for whom anticoagulants are contraindicated (for example, because of age, recent surgery, or blood dyscrasia) and for those who have had recurrent emboli during anticoagulant therapy. It should be performed only when pulmonary embolism is confirmed by angiography.

Surgery consists of vena caval ligation, plication, or insertion of an umbrella filter for blood returning to the heart and lungs. A combination of low-dose heparin and dihydroergotamine (Migranal) may be administered to prevent postoperative venous thromboembolism.

What to do

- Give oxygen by nasal cannula or mask.
- Check ABG levels if new emboli develop or dyspnea worsens.
- Be prepared to provide equipment for endotracheal intubation and assisted ventilation if breathing is severely compromised. If necessary, prepare to transfer the patient to an intensive care unit, per facility policy.
- Administer heparin as ordered through I.V. push or continuous drip.
- Monitor coagulation studies daily and after changes in heparin dosage. Maintain adequate hydration to avoid the risk of hypercoagulability.
- After the patient is stable, encourage him to move about often and assist with isometric and range-of-motion exercises. Monitor the temperature and color of the patient's feet to check for veno-

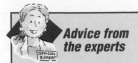

Advice from the experts

Anticoagulation therapy cautions

Make sure to advise the patient taking anticoagulants to:
- watch for signs of bleeding, such as bloody stool, petechiae, nose bleeds (epistaxis), blood in the urine, and large ecchymoses
- take medications exactly as ordered and avoid taking any additional medications (even for headaches or colds)
- avoid changing medication doses unless first approved by the doctor
- shave using an electric razor to prevent excessive bleeding from a cut
- use a soft toothbrush to prevent bleeding of the gums.

stasis. Never vigorously massage the patient's legs. Walk the patient as soon as possible after surgery to prevent venostasis.
• Report frequent pleuritic chest pain so that analgesics can be prescribed.
• Evaluate the patient. His vital signs should be within normal limits and he should show no signs of bleeding after anticoagulant therapy.

Pulmonary hypertension

Pulmonary hypertension refers to chronically elevated pulmonary artery pressure (PAP), with systolic pressure over 30 mm Hg, and a mean PAP over 18 mm Hg. Primary or idiopathic pulmonary hypertension is characterized by increased PAP and increased pulmonary vascular resistance, both without an obvious cause.

Secondary pulmonary hypertension results from existing cardiac or pulmonary disease, or both. The prognosis in secondary hypertension depends on the severity of the underlying disorder. (See *Causes of secondary pulmonary hypertension*, page 252.)

What causes it

Primary, or idiopathic, pulmonary hypertension has no known cause. Yet, the known tendency for the disease to occur within families points to a hereditary defect. It also occurs more commonly in those with collagen disease and is thought to result from altered immune mechanisms. Primary pulmonary hypertension is most common in women between ages 20 and 40, and is usually fatal within 3 to 4 years. Mortality is highest in pregnant women.

Spread the blame

Secondary pulmonary hypertension may result from existing cardiac disease, including:
• left-sided heart failure
• ventricular septal defect
• patent ductus arteriosus.
 Pulmonary causes include:
• COPD
• vasoconstriction of the arterial bed due to hypoxemia and acidosis.

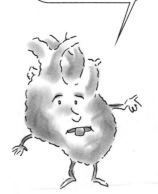

Secondary pulmonary hypertension results from existing cardiac or pulmonary disease — or both.

Now I get it!

Causes of secondary pulmonary hypertension

Secondary pulmonary hypertension can stem from alveolar hypoventilation, vascular obstruction, or primary cardiac disease.

Alveolar hypoventilation

Alveolar hypoventilation can result from diseases that cause alveolar destruction, such as chronic obstructive pulmonary disease (the most common cause in the United States), sarcoidosis, diffuse interstitial pneumonia, malignant metastases, and scleroderma. It may also stem from obesity or kyphoscoliosis, which don't damage lung tissue but prevent the chest wall from expanding sufficiently to let air into the alveoli.

Either way, the resulting decreased ventilation increases pulmonary vascular resistance. Hypoxemia resulting from this ventilation-perfusion mismatch also causes vasoconstriction, further increasing vascular resistance. The result is pulmonary hypertension.

Vascular obstruction

Vascular obstruction can arise from pulmonary embolism or vasculitis. It can also result from disorders that cause obstructions of small or large pulmonary veins, such as left atrial myxoma, idiopathic venoocclusive disease, fibrosing mediastinitis, and mediastinal neoplasm.

Primary cardiac disease

Primary cardiac disease can be congenital or acquired. Congenital defects that cause left-to-right shunting include patent ductus arteriosus, and atrial or ventricular septal defects. This shunting into the pulmonary artery reroutes blood through the lungs (twice), causing pulmonary hypertension.

Acquired cardiac diseases, such as rheumatic valvular disease and mitral stenosis, result in left ventricular failure that diminishes the flow of oxygenated blood from the lungs. This increases pulmonary vascular resistance and right ventricular pressure.

How it happens

In primary pulmonary hypertension, the smooth muscle in the pulmonary artery wall hypertrophies for no apparent reason, narrowing the small pulmonary artery (arteriole) or obliterating it completely. In addition, fibrous lesions also form around the vessels, impairing distensibility and increasing vascular resistance. Pressures in the left ventricle, which receives blood from the lungs, remain normal. However, the increased pressures generated in the lungs are transmitted to the right ventricle, which supplies the pulmonary artery. Eventually, the right ventricle fails (cor pulmonale). Although oxygenation isn't severely affected initially, hypoxia and cyanosis eventually occur, and death results from cor pulmonale.

It's all your fault.

Hey, let's face it. Both of us could be the culprits.

About those alveoli

Alveolar hypoventilation can result from diseases caused by alveolar destruction, or from disorders that prevent the chest wall from expanding sufficiently to allow air into the alveoli. The resulting decreased ventilation increases pulmonary vascular resistance. Hypoxemia resulting from this ventilation-perfusion mismatch also causes vasoconstriction, further increasing vascular resistance and resulting in pulmonary hypertension.

Valves, ventricles, and vascular obstruction

Coronary artery disease or mitral valvular disease causing increased left ventricular filling pressures can result in secondary pulmonary hypertension. A ventricular septal defect and patent ductus arteriosus cause secondary pulmonary hypertension by increasing blood flow through the pulmonary circulation through left-to-right shunting. Pulmonary emboli and chronic destruction of alveolar walls, as seen in emphysema, cause secondary pulmonary hypertension by obliterating or obstructing the pulmonary vascular bed.

Secondary pulmonary hypertension can also occur by vasoconstriction of the vascular bed, which can occur with conditions such as hypoxemia, acidosis, or both. Conditions resulting in vascular obstruction can also cause pulmonary hypertension because blood is prevented from flowing appropriately through the vessels.

Secondary pulmonary hypertension can be reversed if the hypertension is resolved. If hypertension persists, hypertrophy occurs in the medial smooth muscle layer of the arterioles. The larger arteries stiffen, and hypertension progresses. Pulmonary pressures begin to approach systemic blood pressure levels, causing right ventricular hypertrophy and, eventually, cor pulmonale. Death may occur 10 to 15 years after diagnosis.

Cardiac primer

Primary cardiac diseases may be congenital or acquired. Congenital defects cause a left-to-right shunting, rerouting blood through the lungs twice and causing pulmonary hypertension. Acquired cardiac diseases, such as rheumatic valvular disease and mitral stenosis, result in left-sided heart failure that diminishes the flow of oxygenated blood from the lungs. This diminished flow increases pulmonary vascular resistance and right ventricular pressure.

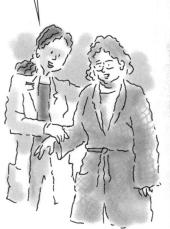

It's important to start moving after surgery. A little walking goes a long way toward preventing venostasis.

What to look for

Patients with pulmonary hypertension typically report increasing dyspnea on exertion, as well as weakness, syncope, and fatigue.

Look, touch, and listen

Look for the signs of pulmonary hypertension, including:
- tachycardia
- tachypnea with mild exertion
- decreased blood pressure
- changes in mental status, from restlessness to agitation or confusion
- signs of right-sided heart failure, such as ascites and jugular vein distention
- an easily palpable right ventricular lift and a reduced carotid pulse
- possible peripheral edema
- decreased diaphragmatic excursion and respiration
- point of maximal impulse displaced beyond the midclavicular line
- systolic ejection murmur; a widely split S_2 and an S_3 or S_4 sound; or decreased breath sounds and loud, turbulent sounds heard on auscultation.

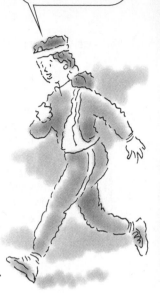

Feeling any dyspnea or weakness? They could be signs of pulmonary hypertension.

What tests tell you

- *ABG analysis* reveals hypoxemia.
- *ECG* changes consistent with right ventricular hypertrophy include right axis deviation and tall or peaked P waves in inferior leads.
- *Pulmonary artery catheterization* reveals increased PAP, with systolic pressure above 30 mm Hg. It may also show increased PAWP if the underlying cause is left atrial myxoma, mitral stenosis, or left-sided heart failure; otherwise, PAWP is normal.
- *Pulmonary angiography* is used to detect filling defects in pulmonary vasculature.
- *Pulmonary function tests* may show decreased flow rates and increased residual volume in underlying obstructive disease. In underlying restrictive disease, they may show reduced total lung capacity.
- *Radionuclide imaging* reveals abnormal right and left ventricular function.
- *Echocardiography* allows assessment of ventricular wall motion and may show valvular dysfunction. It's also used to identify right ventricular enlargement, abnormal septal configuration, and reduced left ventricular cavity size.

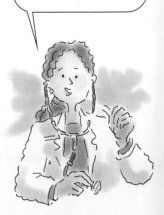

Listen for signs of pulmonary hypertension such as decreased breath sounds.

• *Perfusion lung scanning* may yield normal findings or may reveal multiple patchy and diffuse filling defects not consistent with pulmonary embolism.

How it's treated

Treatment measures for pulmonary hypertension commonly include:
• oxygen therapy to correct hypoxemia
• fluid restriction to decrease preload and minimize the workload of the right ventricle
• possible heart-lung transplantation in severe cases with irreversible changes.

Diverse drugs

Your patient may receive:
• inotropic medications, such as digoxin, to increase cardiac output
• diuretics to decrease intravascular volume and venous return
• calcium channel blockers and other vasodilators (possibly including continuous vasodilator infusion therapy) to reduce myocardial workload and oxygen consumption
• bronchodilators to relax smooth muscles and increase airway patency
• beta-adrenergic blockers to reduce cardiac workload and improve oxygenation
• anticoagulant therapy, if indicated by concurrent hypercoagulability.

What to do

• Assess cardiopulmonary status. Auscultate heart and breath sounds, being alert for S_3 heart sounds, murmurs, or crackles that indicate heart failure. Monitor vital signs, oxygen saturation, and heart rhythm.
• Assess hemodynamic status, including PAP and PAWP, every 2 hours or more often, depending on the patient's condition, and report any changes.
• Monitor intake and output closely and obtain daily weights. Institute fluid restriction as ordered.
• Administer medications as ordered to promote adequate heart and lung function. Assess for potential adverse reactions, such as postural hypotension, from diuretics and beta-adrenergic blockers.
• Administer supplemental oxygen as ordered, and organize care to allow for rest periods. (See *At home with pulmonary hypertension.*)

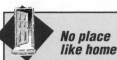

No place like home

At home with pulmonary hypertension

When preparing a patient with pulmonary hypertension for discharge, follow these guidelines:
• Teach the patient to report to the doctor such symptoms as increasing shortness of breath, swelling, increasing weight gain, and increasing fatigue.
• Fully explain the medication regimen.
• If the patient smokes, explain the risks and encourage him to stop.
• If necessary, review dietary restrictions with the patient and provide information and recipes for a low-sodium diet.
• Teach the patient taking a potassium-wasting diuretic about foods that are high in potassium.
• Warn the patient not to overexert himself; suggest frequent rest periods between activities.
• If the patient needs special equipment for home use, contact the social service department for assistance.

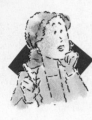

Quick quiz

1. Polycythemia commonly occurs with cor pulmonale in response to:

    A.   hypertension.
    B.   dehydration.
    C.   hypercarbia.
    D.   hypoxemia.

Answer: D. Increased RBC production is a compensatory response to hypoxemia and commonly occurs with cor pulmonale.

2. Typically, the first symptom of a pulmonary embolism is:

    A.   hypothermia.
    B.   bradycardia.
    C.   dyspnea.
    D.   green-tinged sputum.

Answer: C. Dyspnea is usually the first symptom of pulmonary embolism, and may be accompanied by anginal or pleuritic chest pain.

3. Which of the following statements regarding idiopathic pulmonary hypertension is false?

    A.   It's characterized by increased PAP and increases pulmonary vascular resistance.
    B.   It results from existing cardiac or pulmonary disease, or both.
    C.   It occurs more commonly in individuals with collagen disease.
    D.   Mortality is highest in pregnant women.

Answer: B. Secondary pulmonary hypertension results from existing cardiac or pulmonary disease, or both. The prognosis for patients with secondary hypertension depends on the severity of the underlying disorder.

Scoring

☆☆☆ If you answered all three items correctly, zowee! You have a vast vascular disorders knowledge.

☆☆ If you answered two items correctly, great work! Your vascular understanding is expanding.

☆ If you answered fewer than two items correctly, don't expire! Review the chapter and keep on pumping!

Traumatic injuries

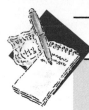

Just the facts

In this chapter, you'll learn:

♦ characteristics of several traumatic respiratory injuries and their potential causes

♦ ways to recognize and diagnose a traumatic injury affecting the respiratory system

♦ treatments for various traumatic respiratory injuries.

Understanding traumatic injuries

Traumatic respiratory injuries are often life-threatening, and have been a contributing factor to more than 25% of trauma-related deaths. They include blunt chest injury, inhalation injury, penetrating chest injury, and pneumothorax.

Blunt chest injury

Chest trauma is usually categorized as penetrating or blunt. Many of these injuries are blunt chest injuries, which result from sudden compression or positive pressure caused by direct impact to an organ and the surrounding tissues.

Blunt chest injuries include myocardial contusion and rib and sternal fractures. The fractures may be simple, multiple, displaced, or jagged, and may cause potentially fatal complications, such as hemothorax, pneumothorax, and hemorrhagic shock. A patient with a blunt chest injury may develop flail chest.

> Most blunt chest injuries result from car accidents.

What causes it

Most blunt chest injuries result from motor vehicle accidents. Such injury occurs from the impact of the chest hitting the steering wheel. Other common causes include falls, sports injuries, and blast injuries.

How it happens

Blunt chest trauma can cause extensive injury to the lungs, chest wall, pleural space, and vessels of the body. Blunt injuries are commonly associated with greater mortality rates than penetrating chest injuries.

Flail chest

Multiple rib fractures may lead to a condition called *flail chest*. With flail chest, a portion of the chest wall "caves" in, causing a loss of chest wall integrity that prevents adequate lung inflation. Bruised skin, extreme pain caused by rib fracture and disfigurement, paradoxical chest movements, and rapid, shallow respirations are all signs and symptoms of flail chest.

Tachycardia, hypotension, respiratory acidosis, and cyanosis can also occur with flail chest. Paradoxical breathing patterns are described as collapse of the injured chest wall and expansion of the uninjured chest wall during inhalation. During exhalation, the injured chest wall moves out and the uninjured chest wall moves in. (See *Flail chest: Paradoxical breathing*.)

Flail chest can also cause tension pneumothorax, a condition in which air enters the chest but can't be ejected during exhalation; life-threatening thoracic pressure build-up causes lung collapse and subsequent mediastinal shift. The cardinal signs and symptoms of tension pneumothorax include tracheal deviation (away from the affected side), cyanosis, severe dyspnea, absent breath sounds (on the affected side), agitation, jugular vein distention, and shock.

Hemothorax

When a rib lacerates lung tissue or an intercostal artery, hemothorax occurs, causing blood to collect in the pleural cavity, compressing the lung and limiting respiratory capacity. It can also result from rupture of large or small pulmonary vessels. Massive hemothorax is the most common cause of shock following chest trauma. Although slight bleeding occurs even with mild pneumothorax, such bleeding resolves very quickly, usually without changing the patient's condition.

Pulmonary contusion

Blunt trauma injuring the lung tissue can cause a pulmonary contusion and potentially lead to respiratory failure. Pulmonary con-

Now I get it!

Flail chest: Paradoxical breathing

A patient with a blunt chest injury may develop flail chest, which results in paradoxical breathing, as described here.

Inhalation
- Injured chest wall collapses in.
- Uninjured chest wall moves out.

Exhalation
- Injured chest wall moves out.
- Uninjured chest wall moves in.

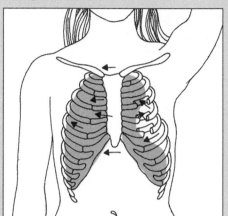

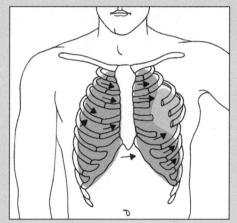

tusions are the most common chest injury seen in the United States and are commonly related to vehicular accidents.

Common symptoms noted with this condition include dyspnea, restlessness, hemoptysis, tachycardia, crackles, decreased lung compliance, atelectasis, arterial blood gas (ABG) analysis results indicating hypoxemia and hypercarbia, and a chest X-ray revealing local or diffuse patchy, poorly delineated densities or irregular infiltrates. Treatment options for pulmonary contusions include intubation and mechanical ventilation, hemodynamic monitoring and, possibly, thoracotomy if massive hemorrhage is suspected.

Other complications

Myocardial contusions produce electrocardiogram (ECG) abnormalities. Laceration or rupture of the aorta is nearly always immediately fatal. In rare cases, aortic laceration may develop 24 hours after blunt injury, so patient observation is critical.

Aortic laceration may develop up to 24 hours after blunt chest injury, so patient observation is critical!

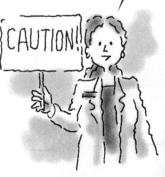

CAUTION!

Diaphragmatic rupture (usually on the left side) causes severe respiratory distress. Unless treated early, abdominal viscera may herniate through the rupture into the thorax, compromising both circulation and the vital capacity of the lungs.

Other complications of blunt chest trauma include cardiac tamponade, pulmonary artery tears, large myocardial tears (which can be rapidly fatal), small myocardial tears (which can cause pericardial effusion), ventricular rupture, and bronchial, tracheal, or esophageal tears or rupture.

What to look for

A history of trauma with dyspnea, chest pain, and other typical symptoms suggest a blunt chest injury. When assessing the patient, percussion over the lung will reveal dullness in hemothorax and tympany in tension pneumothorax. Auscultation may reveal a change in position of the loudest heart sound in tension pneumothorax or muffled heart sounds in cardiac tamponade. Blunt chest injuries commonly cause severe pain, which is notable during respirations. The patient can typically locate the site of the pain with respiration.

Tender, swollen, shallow

Rib fractures produce tenderness, slight edema over the fracture site, and pain that worsens with deep breathing and movement. This painful breathing causes the patient to display shallow, splinted respirations that may lead to hypoventilation.

Pain, dyspnea, cyanosis — Oh, my!

Sternal fractures, which are usually transverse and located in the middle or upper sternum, produce persistent chest pain, even at rest. If a fractured rib tears the pleura and punctures a lung, it causes pneumothorax, which usually produces severe dyspnea, cyanosis, agitation, extreme pain and, when air escapes into chest tissue, subcutaneous emphysema.

Flail foreboding

Signs and symptoms commonly seen with flail chest include:
- dyspnea
- chest wall pain
- labored and shallow respirations
- crepitus from fragments
- asymmetrical chest movements
- chest X-ray positive for fractures.

What tests tell you

A physical examination and diagnostic tests determine the extent
of injury.
• *Chest X-rays* may be used to confirm rib and sternal fractures,
pneumothorax, flail chest, pulmonary contusions, lacerated or
ruptured aorta, tension pneumothorax, diaphragmatic rupture,
lung compression, or atelectasis with hemothorax.
• *ECG* may show abnormalities with cardiac damage, including
multiple premature ventricular contractions, unexplained tachy-
cardias, atrial fibrillation, bundle-branch block (usually right), and
ST-segment changes.
• *Serial aspartate aminotransferase, alanine aminotransferase,
lactate dehydrogenase, creatine kinase (CK)*, and *CK-MB* levels
are elevated.
• *Retrograde aortography* and *transesophageal echocardiography* reveal aortic laceration or rupture.
• *Contrast studies* and *liver and spleen scans* help detect diaphragmatic rupture.
• *Echocardiography, computed tomography (CT) scans*, and
cardiac and lung scans show the extent of the injury.

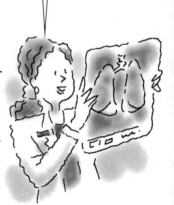

Echocardiography,
CT scans, and
cardiac and lung
scans show the
extent of the injury.

How it's treated

Blunt chest injuries call for immediate physical assessment, control of bleeding, maintenance of a patent airway, adequate ventilation, and fluid and electrolyte balance. Treatment for flail chest focuses on symptomatic and supportive care and prevention of hemothorax and pneumothorax. If hemothorax occurs, chest tube
insertion will be required. Pain medication will likely be prescribed.

What to do

Caring for a patient with a blunt chest injury requires these measures:
• Check all pulses and level of consciousness. Evaluate color and
temperature of skin, depth of respiration, use of accessory muscles, and length of inhalation compared with exhalation.
• Check pulse oximetry values for adequate oxygenation.
• Observe tracheal position. Look for jugular vein distention and
paradoxical chest motion. Listen to heart and breath sounds carefully; palpate for subcutaneous emphysema (crepitation) and a
lack of structural integrity in the ribs.

- Obtain a history of the injury. Unless severe dyspnea is present, ask the patient to locate the pain, and ask if he's having trouble breathing. Obtain an order for laboratory studies (ABG analysis, cardiac enzyme levels, complete blood count [CBC], and typing and crossmatching).
- For simple rib fractures, give a mild analgesic, encourage bed rest, and apply heat. To prevent atelectasis, instruct the patient on incentive spirometry and deep breathing, coughing, and splinting. Don't strap or tape his chest.

Pneumo needs

- For more severe fractures, intercostal nerve blocks may be needed. Obtain X-rays before and after the nerve blocks to rule out pneumothorax.
- If the patient has excessive bleeding or hemopneumothorax, intubation may be necessary. Chest tubes may be inserted to treat hemothorax and to assess the need for thoracotomy. To prevent atelectasis, turn the patient frequently and encourage coughing and deep breathing.
- If the patient has pneumothorax, he may need a chest tube placed anteriorly to the midaxillary line at the fifth intercostal space, to aspirate as much air as possible from the pleural cavity and to reexpand the lungs. Chest tubes should be attached to water-seal drainage and suction.

Fowler for flail

- If the patient has flail chest, place him in semi-Fowler's position. Reexpansion of the lung is the first definitive care measure. Administer oxygen at a high flow rate under positive pressure. Suction the patient frequently and as completely as possible. Carefully observe the patient for signs of tension pneumothorax.
- The patient with flail chest will also need I.V. therapy. Use lactated Ringer's solution or normal saline solution. Beware of both excessive and insufficient fluid resuscitation.

Give hemo the heave-ho

- For hemothorax, treat shock with I.V. infusions of lactated Ringer's solution or normal saline solution. Administer packed red blood cells for blood losses greater than 1,500 ml or circulating blood volume losses exceeding 30%. Autotransfusion is an option. Administer oxygen.
- The patient with hemothorax will also need insertion of chest tubes in the fifth or sixth intercostal space anterior to the midaxillary line to remove blood. Monitor and document vital signs and blood loss. Watch for falling blood pressure, rising pulse rate, and hemorrhage—all require thoracotomy to stop bleeding.

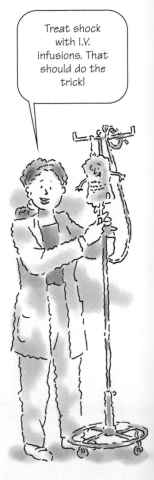

Treat shock with I.V. infusions. That should do the trick!

Colloids for contusions

• For pulmonary contusions, give limited amounts of colloids (for example, salt-poor albumin, whole blood, or plasma) to replace volume and maintain oncotic pressure. Administer an analgesic, a diuretic and, if necessary, a corticosteroid, as needed. Monitor ABG values to ensure adequate ventilation; provide oxygen therapy, mechanical ventilation, and chest tube care.

Don't forget the heart

• For suspected cardiac damage, close intensive care or telemetry may detect arrhythmias and prevent cardiogenic shock. Impose bed rest with the patient in semi-Fowler's position (unless he requires shock position). As needed, administer oxygen, an analgesic, and other supportive drugs to control heart failure or supraventricular arrhythmia.
• Watch for cardiac tamponade, which calls for pericardiocentesis. Essentially, provide the same care as for a patient who has suffered myocardial infarction.
• If the patient has myocardial rupture, septal perforation, or another cardiac laceration, immediate surgical repair is mandatory; less severe ventricular wounds require use of a digital or balloon catheter; atrial wounds require a clamp or balloon catheter.
• For the few patients with aortic rupture or laceration who reach the hospital alive, immediate surgery is mandatory, using synthetic grafts or anastomosis to repair the damage. Give large volumes of I.V. fluids (lactated Ringer's or normal saline solution) and whole blood, along with oxygen at very high flow rates; then transport the patient promptly to the operating room.

Tension and rupture

• If the patient has tension pneumothorax, insertion of a spinal or 14G to 16G needle into the second intercostal space at the midclavicular line is necessary to release pressure in the chest. After that, a chest tube will be inserted to normalize pressure and reexpand the lung. Administer oxygen under positive pressure, along with I.V. fluids.
• For a diaphragmatic rupture, insert a nasogastric tube to temporarily decompress the stomach, and prepare the patient for surgical repair.

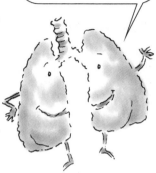

In addition to pulmonary contusions, don't forget possible cardiac damage. Monitor the patient closely to prevent cardiogenic shock...

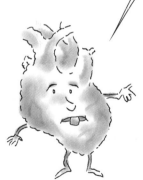

...Gee, you don't have to be so blunt about it!

Inhalation injury

Inhalation injuries result from trauma to the pulmonary system after inhalation of toxic substances or the inhalation of gases that are nontoxic but interfere with cellular respiration. Inhaled exposure forms include fog, mist, fumes, dust, gas, vapor, or smoke. Inhalation injuries commonly accompany burns.

What causes it

There are a variety of causes of inhalation injuries, including thermal inhalation, chemical inhalation, and carbon monoxide poisoning.

Thermal inhalation

Pulmonary complications remain the leading cause of death following thermal inhalation trauma. This type of trauma is commonly caused by the inhalation of hot air or steam. Mortality exceeds 50% when inhalation injury accompanies burns of the skin. This type of injury should be suspected with reports of flames in a confined area, even if burns on the surface aren't visible.

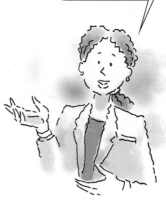

Suspect thermal inhalation injury if the patient was around flames in a confined area — even if burns on the surface aren't visible.

Chemical inhalation

A variety of gases may be generated during the burning of materials. The acids and alkalis released from burning can produce chemical burns when inhaled. The inhaled substances can reach the respiratory tract as insoluble gases and lead to permanent damage.

Synthetic materials also produce gases that can be toxic. Plastic material has the ability to produce toxic vapors when heated or burned. The inhalation of chemicals in a powder or liquid form without burning also are capable of causing pulmonary damage. Such substances as ammonia, chlorine, sulfur dioxide, and hydrogen chloride are considered pulmonary irritants.

Carbon monoxide poisoning

Carbon monoxide is a colorless, odorless, tasteless gas produced as a result of combustion and oxidation. Poisoning from carbon monoxide can occur from inhalation of small amounts of this gas over a long period of time or the inhalation of large amounts in a short period of time. Carbon monoxide is considered a chemical asphyxiant. Accidental poisoning can occur from exposure to heaters, smoke from a fire, or use of a gas lamp, gas stove, or charcoal grill in a small, poorly ventilated area.

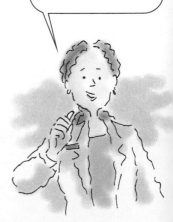

Smoke from a fire in a poorly ventilated area can cause carbon monoxide poisoning.

How it happens

The pathophysiology of each type of inhalation injury is as unique as the condition itself.

Thermal inhalation

The entire respiratory tract is at risk for damage from thermal inhalation injury; however, injury rarely progresses to the lungs. The area of greatest damage is the upper airway, where inhaled hot air or steam is confined and cooled. Reflexive closure of the vocal cords and laryngeal spasm usually prevent full inhalation of the hot air or steam, limiting injury to the lower respiratory tract. Steam inhalation is more harmful than hot air inhalation because water holds heat longer than dry air.

Chemical inhalation

Irritating gases (chlorine, hydrogen chloride, nitrogen dioxide, phosgene, and sulfur dioxide) combine with water in the lungs to form corrosive acids. These acids cause denaturization of proteins, cellular damage, and edema of the pulmonary tissues. Smoke inhalation injuries generally fall into this category. Chemical burns to the airway are similar to burns on the skin, except that they're painless because the tracheobronchial tree is insensitive to pain. The inhalation of small quantities of noxious chemicals can also damage the alveoli and bronchi.

Carbon monoxide poisoning

Several gases, such as carbon monoxide and hydrogen cyanide, aren't directly toxic to the respiratory system. Even so, these gases interfere with cellular respiration. Carbon monoxide has a greater attraction to Hb than oxygen. When carbon monoxide enters the blood, it binds with Hb to form carboxyhemoglobin. Carboxyhemoglobin reduces the oxygen-carrying capacity of Hb, which results in decreased oxygenation to the cells and tissues.

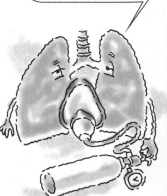

Gasp! Provide oxygen to a patient with carbon monoxide poisoning — immediately!

What to look for

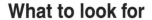

Physical findings with an inhalation injury vary depending on the gas or substance inhaled and the duration of the exposure.

Thermal inhalation

Ulcerations, erythema, and edema of the mouth and epiglottis are the initial symptoms of thermal inhalation. Edema may rapidly progress to upper airway obstruction. Stridor, wheezing, crackles, increased secretions, hoarseness, and shortness of breath may also be noted. If direct thermal injury to the upper airway occurred, burns of the face and lips, burned nasal hairs, and laryngeal edema will be present.

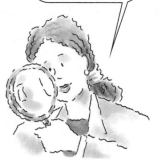

Even a patient who doesn't appear to have respiratory difficulties may suddenly develop respiratory distress.

Chemical inhalation

The most common effects of smoke or chemical inhalation include atelectasis, pulmonary edema, and tissue anoxia. Respiratory distress usually occurs early in the course of smoke inhalation, secondary to hypoxia. Even a patient who doesn't appear to have respiratory difficulties may suddenly develop respiratory distress. Intubation and mechanical ventilation equipment should be available for immediate use.

Carbon monoxide poisoning

Carboxyhemoglobin reduces the oxygen carrying capacity of Hb. This deficiency commonly causes a bright-red flush on the face and cherry-red lips. The symptoms of carbon monoxide poisoning vary with the concentration of carboxyhemoglobin. (See *Oxygen saturation in carbon monoxide poisoning.*)

Mild poisoning generally indicates a carbon monoxide level between 11% and 20%. Symptoms at this concentration commonly include headache, decreased cerebral function, decreased visual acuity, and slight shortness of breath. Moderate poisoning indicates a carbon monoxide level between 21% and 40%. Symptoms include headache, tinnitus, nausea, drowsiness, dizziness, altered mental status, confusion, stupor, irritability, hypotension, tachycardia, ECG changes, and changes in skin color.

Severe poisoning is defined as a level of carbon monoxide between 41% and 60%; symptoms include coma, seizures, and generalized instability. In the final stage (fatal poisoning), the carbon monoxide level reaches 61% to 80% and death results.

Other complications

Pulmonary complications can arise from tight eschar formation on the chest from circumferential chest burns. The eschar can restrict chest movement or impair ventilation from compression on the anatomic structures of the throat and neck. Visual assessment of the chest will reveal ease of respirations, depth of chest movement, rate of respirations, and respiratory effort.

What tests tell you

Initial laboratory studies commonly include electrolytes, liver function studies, blood urea nitrogen and creatinine, and a CBC. Obtaining these studies will provide baseline data for analysis. In addition:
- *ABG analysis* will provide valuable information on the acid-base status, ventilation, and oxygenation status of the patient.
- *Carboxyhemoglobin level* will be measured in patients with suspected carbon monoxide poisoning.
- *Cardiac monitoring* will observe for ischemic changes.
- *ECG* may show depressed ST segment, which is a common finding in the moderate stage of carbon monoxide poisoning.
- *Chest X-ray* immediately after the trauma may be normal. However, perivascular and peribronchial edema may be present as well as pulmonary edema. Diffuse pulmonary edema or patchy pneumonitis may be evident within the first 24 hours and suggest a fatal outcome.

How it's treated

These guidelines outline treatment of a patient after a toxic inhalation injury.
- Initially assess the patient's airway, breathing, and circulation.
- Obtain a history of the exposure and attempt to identify the toxic agent.
- Immediately provide oxygen to the patient. Intubation and mechanical ventilation may be required if the patient demonstrates severe respiratory distress or an altered state of mentation.
- Upper airway edema requires emergency endotracheal intubation.
- Bronchodilators, antibiotics, and I.V. fluids may be prescribed.
- The preferred treatment for carbon monoxide poisoning is administering 100% humidified oxygen continuously until carboxyhemoglobin levels fall to the nontoxic range of 10%.
- Chest physical therapy may assist in the removal of necrotic tissue.
- The use of hyperbaric oxygen for carbon monoxide poisoning remains controversial, although it's known to lower carboxyhemoglobin levels more rapidly than humidified oxygen.
- Fluid resuscitation is an important component of managing inhalation injury, but careful monitoring of fluid status is essential due to the risk of pulmonary edema.

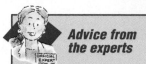

Advice from the experts

Oxygen saturation in carbon monoxide poisoning

When assessing for carbon monoxide poisoning, be aware that pulse oximetry devices measure oxygenated and deoxygenated hemoglobin but don't measure dysfunctional hemoglobin such as carboxyhemoglobin. Therefore, the oxygen saturation levels in the presence of carbon monoxide poisoning will be within normal ranges as the carboxyhemoglobin levels aren't measured.

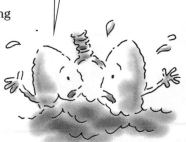

Careful monitoring of fluid status is crucial. Hold on!

What to do

Caring for a patient with an inhalation injury requires these measures:
• Carefully remove the patient's clothing to prevent additional contamination; the toxic substance may be on the fabric.
• Establish I.V. access for administration of medication, blood products, and fluid.
• Obtain laboratory samples to evaluate ventilation, oxygenation, and baseline values.
• Obtain chest X-ray, ECG, and pulmonary function studies.
• Implement cardiac monitoring to assess for ischemic changes or arrhythmias.
• Monitor for signs of pulmonary edema that may accompany fluid resuscitation.
• In the event of bronchospasms, provide oxygen, bronchodilators via a nebulizer and, possibly, aminophylline.
• Monitor fluid balance and intake and output closely.
• Administer antibiotics as prescribed.
• Assess lung sounds frequently and notify the doctor immediately of changes in lungs sounds or oxygenation.
• Provide a supportive and informative environment for the patient, patient's family, and significant others. (See *Inhalation injury in children.*)
• Monitor laboratory studies for changes that may indicate multisystem complications.

Penetrating chest injury

Depending on its size, a penetrating chest injury may cause varying degrees of damage to bones, soft tissue, blood vessels, and nerves. Mortality and morbidity from a chest wound depend on the size and severity of the wound.

Gunshot wounds are usually more serious than stab wounds because they cause more severe lacerations and rapid blood loss and a ricocheting bullet commonly damages large areas and multiple organs. Patients require prompt, aggressive treatment to increase odds of survival.

What causes it

Stab wounds from a knife or ice pick are the most common penetrating chest wounds. Gunshot wounds are a close second. Objects such as a pitchfork or any other pointed object can injure the

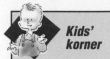

Kids' korner

Inhalation injury in children

It's essential that your care of a child with inhalation injury address the emotional and psychological needs of the child and his family. Initially, care will focus on oxygenating and stabilizing the child and managing the physical components of his injury.

However, your care must eventually encompass the psychological needs of the frightened child and the emotional needs of his parents. Parents may feel guilt if the injury could have been prevented or even if it couldn't. Be sure to provide information to the parents about their child's condition, prognosis, treatment plan, and discharge needs.

In addition to ongoing communication, psychological intervention may be needed to discuss feelings of guilt, emotional stress, or fears of the parent and child.

thorax. Wartime explosions or firearms fired at close range are the usual source of large, gaping wounds.

How it happens

Penetrating chest injuries are considered open injuries because the thoracic cavity is exposed to the pressure from the atmospheric air. Penetrating chest injuries may cause lung lacerations (bleeding and substantial air leakage through the chest tube), arterial lacerations (loss of more than 100 ml of blood per hour through the chest tube), and exsanguination. Pneumothorax (air in the pleural space causing loss of negative intrathoracic pressure and lung collapse), tension pneumothorax (intrapleural air accumulation causing potentially fatal mediastinal shift), and hemothorax can also result.

Other effects include arrhythmias, cardiac tamponade, mediastinitis, subcutaneous emphysema, esophageal perforation, and bronchopleural fistula. Tracheobronchial, abdominal, or diaphragmatic injuries can also occur.

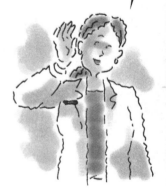

A penetrating chest injury can cause a sucking sound as the diaphragm contracts and air enters the chest cavity through the opening in the chest wall.

What to look for

In addition to the obvious chest wounds, penetrating chest injuries can also cause several other symptoms.
• A sucking sound occurs as the diaphragm contracts and air enters the chest cavity through the opening in the chest wall.
• Level of consciousness varies, depending on the extent of the injury. If the patient is awake and alert, he may be in severe pain, which will make him splint his respirations, thereby reducing his vital capacity.
• Tachycardia stems from anxiety and blood loss.
• A weak, thready pulse results from massive blood loss and hypovolemic shock.

What tests tell you

An obvious chest wound and a sucking sound during breathing confirm the diagnosis. Consider any lower thoracic chest injury a thoracicoabdominal injury until proved otherwise. Further tests to provide baseline data include:
• *pulse oximetry* and *ABG analysis* to assess respiratory status
• *chest X-rays* before and after chest tube placement to evaluate the injury and tube placement (in an emergency, don't wait for chest X-ray results before inserting the chest tube)
• *CBC*, including hemoglobin (Hb) level, hematocrit (HCT), and differential (low Hb level and HCT reflect severe blood loss; in early blood loss, these values may be normal)

• *palpation* and *auscultation* of the chest and abdomen to evaluate damage to adjacent organs and structures.

How it's treated

Penetrating chest injuries require immediate support of respiratory and circulatory systems, prompt surgical repair, and measures to prevent complications. Monitoring signs of cardiovascular compromise and hemodynamic stability is essential to the care of the patient. Supplemental oxygen will likely be required as well as intubation and mechanical ventilation.

Hemorrhage, shock, hypotension

Penetrating trauma may be associated with hemorrhage and may lead to shock or hypotension. I.V. therapy and blood product administration may be required to hemodynamically support the patient and replace fluid or blood losses. Surgery may also be required for these patients depending on the extent of the bleeding and organ and tissue damage. (See *Penetrating objects*.)

What to do

Caring for a patient with a penetrating chest injury requires these measures:
• Immediately assess airway, breathing, and circulation. Establish a patent airway, support ventilation, and monitor pulses frequently.
• Place an occlusive dressing over the sucking wound. Monitor the patient for signs of tension pneumothorax (tracheal shift, respiratory distress, tachycardia, tachypnea, diminished or absent breath sounds on the affected side). If tension pneumothorax develops, temporarily remove the occlusive dressing to create a simple pneumothorax.
• Control blood loss (also remember to look *under* the patient to estimate loss), type and crossmatch blood, and replace blood and fluids as necessary.
• Prepare the patient for chest X-rays and placement of chest tubes (using water-seal drainage) to reestablish intrathoracic pressure and drain blood in hemothorax. A second X-ray will evaluate the position of tubes and their functions.
• Emergency surgery may be needed to repair the damage caused by the injury.
• Throughout treatment, monitor central venous pressure and blood pressure to detect hypovolemia, and assess vital signs. Provide an analgesic, if needed. Tetanus and antibiotic prophylaxis may be necessary.

Advice from the experts

Penetrating objects

If an object is penetrating the chest wall or any other part of the body, it's advisable not to remove it. The object provides a sealing effect to the organs or tissues surrounding the penetrating wound. The removal of the object could result in hemorrhage.

• Reassure the patient, especially if he has been the victim of a violent crime. Report the incident to the police in accordance with local laws. Help contact the patient's family, and offer them reassurance.

Pneumothorax

Pneumothorax is an accumulation of air in the pleural cavity that leads to partial or complete lung collapse. The amount of air trapped in the intrapleural space determines the degree of lung collapse. In some cases, venous return to the heart is impeded, causing a life-threatening condition called *tension pneumothorax*.

Pneumothorax can be classified as either traumatic or spontaneous. *Traumatic pneumothorax* may be further classified as open or closed. (Note that an open [penetrating] wound may cause closed pneumothorax.) *Spontaneous pneumothorax*, which is also considered closed, is most common in older patients with chronic obstructive pulmonary disease but can occur in young, healthy patients as well. (See *Nursing care in pneumothorax*, pages 272 and 273.)

> Don't get confused. An open, or penetrating, wound may cause closed pneumothorax.

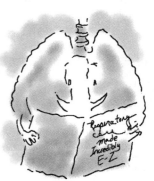

What causes it

The causes of pneumothorax vary according to classification.

Traumatic pneumothorax

Causes of open traumatic pneumothorax include:
• penetrating chest injury (stab or gunshot wound)
• insertion of a central venous catheter
• chest surgery
• transbronchial biopsy
• thoracentesis or closed pleural biopsy.
    Causes of closed traumatic pneumothorax include:
• blunt chest trauma
• air leakage from ruptured blebs
• rupture resulting from barotrauma caused by high intrathoracic pressures during mechanical ventilation
• tubercular or cancerous lesions that erode into the pleural space
• interstitial lung disease such as eosinophilic granuloma.

Spontaneous pneumothorax

Spontaneous pneumothorax is usually caused by the rupture of a subpleural bleb (a small cystic space) at the surface of a lung.

Nursing care in pneumothorax

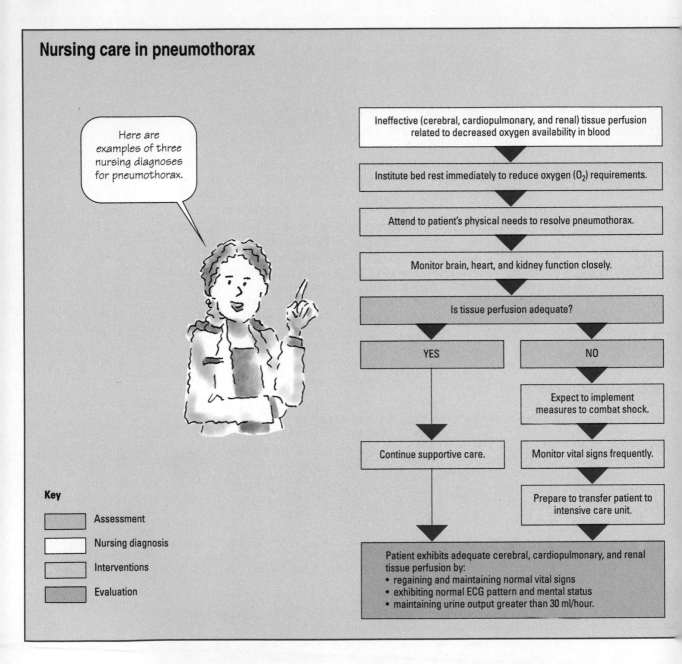

Here are examples of three nursing diagnoses for pneumothorax.

Ineffective (cerebral, cardiopulmonary, and renal) tissue perfusion related to decreased oxygen availability in blood

Institute bed rest immediately to reduce oxygen (O_2) requirements.

Attend to patient's physical needs to resolve pneumothorax.

Monitor brain, heart, and kidney function closely.

Is tissue perfusion adequate?

YES

NO

Expect to implement measures to combat shock.

Continue supportive care.

Monitor vital signs frequently.

Prepare to transfer patient to intensive care unit.

Patient exhibits adequate cerebral, cardiopulmonary, and renal tissue perfusion by:
• regaining and maintaining normal vital signs
• exhibiting normal ECG pattern and mental status
• maintaining urine output greater than 30 ml/hour.

Key

Assessment

Nursing diagnosis

Interventions

Evaluation

Tension pneumothorax

Causes of tension pneumothorax include:
• penetrating chest wound treated with an airtight dressing
• fractured ribs
• mechanical ventilation

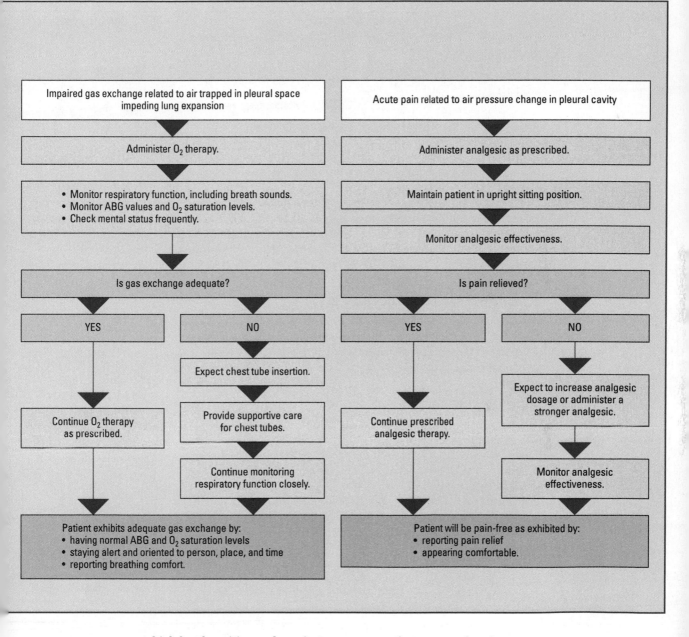

Impaired gas exchange related to air trapped in pleural space impeding lung expansion

Administer O$_2$ therapy.

- Monitor respiratory function, including breath sounds.
- Monitor ABG values and O$_2$ saturation levels.
- Check mental status frequently.

Is gas exchange adequate?

YES — NO

Expect chest tube insertion.

Continue O$_2$ therapy as prescribed.

Provide supportive care for chest tubes.

Continue monitoring respiratory function closely.

Patient exhibits adequate gas exchange by:
- having normal ABG and O$_2$ saturation levels
- staying alert and oriented to person, place, and time
- reporting breathing comfort.

Acute pain related to air pressure change in pleural cavity

Administer analgesic as prescribed.

Maintain patient in upright sitting position.

Monitor analgesic effectiveness.

Is pain relieved?

YES — NO

Expect to increase analgesic dosage or administer a stronger analgesic.

Continue prescribed analgesic therapy.

Monitor analgesic effectiveness.

Patient will be pain-free as exhibited by:
- reporting pain relief
- appearing comfortable.

- high-level positive end–expiratory pressure that causes alveolar blebs to rupture
- chest tube occlusion or malfunction. (See *Tension pneumothorax and chest tubes*, page 274.)

How it happens

The pathophysiology of pneumothorax also varies according to classification.

Traumatic pneumothorax

Open traumatic pneumothorax occurs when atmospheric air flows directly into the pleural cavity (under negative pressure). As the air pressure in the pleural cavity becomes positive, the lung on the affected side collapses, causing decreased total lung capacity. As a result, the patient develops a ventilation-perfusion imbalance that leads to hypoxia.

Closed traumatic pneumothorax occurs when an opening is created between the intrapleural space and the parenchyma of the lung. Air enters the pleural space from within the lung, causing increased pleural pressure and preventing lung expansion during inspiration.

Spontaneous pneumothorax

In spontaneous pneumothorax, the rupture of a subpleural bleb causes air leakage into the pleural spaces, which causes the lung to collapse. Hypoxia results from decreased total lung capacity, vital capacity, and lung compliance.

Tension pneumothorax

Tension pneumothorax results when air in the pleural space is under higher pressure than air in the adjacent lung. Here's what happens:
• Air enters the pleural space from the site of pleural rupture, which acts as a one-way valve. Thus, air enters the pleural space on inspiration but can't escape as the rupture site closes on expiration.
• More air enters with each inspiration and air pressure begins to exceed barometric pressure.
• The air pushes against the recoiled lung, causing compression atelectasis, and pushes against the mediastinum, compressing and displacing the heart and great vessels.
• The mediastinum eventually shifts away from the affected side, affecting venous return, and putting ever-greater pressure on the heart, great vessels, trachea, and contralateral lung.

Without immediate treatment, this emergency can rapidly become fatal. (See *Understanding tension pneumothorax.*)

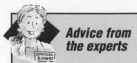

Advice from the experts

Tension pneumothorax and chest tubes

Watch for signs of tension pneumothorax in patients with chest tubes. Symptoms include:
• declining blood pressure
• profuse diaphoresis
• agitation
• cyanosis
• tachycardia
• increased respiratory rates.

Without prompt detection and treatment, this condition is commonly fatal because air becomes trapped within the pleural space when the chest tube becomes dislodged or obstructed. This trapped air leads to increased positive pressure within the patient's chest cavity, compressing the affected lung and the mediastinum and shifting them toward the opposite lung. The result is impaired venous return and cardiac output, leading to cardiac arrest.

Now I get it!

Understanding tension pneumothorax

In tension pneumothorax, air accumulates intrapleurally and can't escape. As intrapleural pressure increases, the lung on the affected side collapses.

On inspiration, the mediastinum shifts toward the unaffected lung, impairing ventilation.

On expiration, the mediastinal shift distorts the vena cava and reduces venous return.

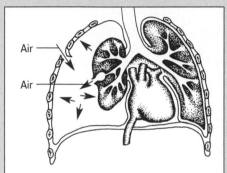

Air

Air

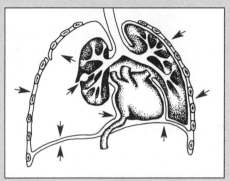

What to look for

Assessment findings depend on the severity of pneumothorax. Spontaneous pneumothorax that releases a small amount of air into the pleural space may cause no signs and symptoms. Generally, tension pneumothorax causes the most severe respiratory signs and symptoms.

Every breath hurts

Your patient's history reveals sudden, sharp, pleuritic chest pain. The patient may report that chest movement, breathing, and coughing exacerbate the pain. He may report shortness of breath.

Further findings

Inspection reveals asymmetric chest wall movement with overexpansion and rigidity on the affected side. The skin may be cool, clammy, and cyanotic. Palpation of the chest wall may reveal crackling beneath the skin (subcutaneous emphysema) and decreased vocal fremitus.

In addition, percussion may reveal hyperresonance on the affected side, auscultation may disclose decreased or absent breath

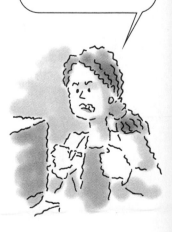

Grrr! When pressure is high, I sometimes get tense. When air pressure is high, tension of the pneumothorax kind can result.

sounds on the affected side, and vital signs may follow the pattern of respiratory distress seen with respiratory failure.

Did we mention the tension?

Tension pneumothorax also causes:
- hypotension and tachycardia due to decreased cardiac output
- tracheal deviation to the opposite side (a late sign)
- distended jugular veins due to high intrapleural pressure, mediastinal shift, and increased cardiovascular pressure.

What tests tell you

- *Chest X-rays* reveal air in the pleural space and a mediastinal shift that confirm pneumothorax.
- *ABG analysis* reveals hypoxemia, usually with elevated partial pressure of arterial carbon dioxide and normal bicarbonate ion levels in the early stages.
- *ECG* may reveal decreased QRS amplitude, precordial T-wave inversion, frontal QRS axis shifting to the right, and small precordial R voltage.

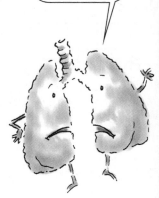

Please, Doc, cut my tension with a knife!

How it's treated

Treatment of pneumothorax depends on the cause and severity.

With trauma

Open or traumatic pneumothorax may necessitate surgical repair of affected tissues, followed by chest tube placement with an underwater seal.

With less lung collapse

Spontaneous pneumothorax with less than 30% lung collapse, no signs of increased pleural pressure, and no dyspnea or indications of physiologic compromise may be corrected with:
- bed rest to preserve energy
- monitoring of vital signs to detect physiologic compromise
- oxygen administration to improve hypoxia
- aspiration of air from the intrapleural space with a large-bore needle attached to a syringe to restore negative pressure within the pleural space.

With more lung collapse

Greater than 30% lung collapse may necessitate other measures, such as:

• placing a chest tube in the second or third intercostal space in the midclavicular line to reexpand the lung by restoring negative intrapleural pressure
• connecting the chest tube to an underwater seal or low-pressure suction to reexpand the lung.

With tension

Treatment of the patient with tension pneumothorax typically involves:
• immediate large-bore needle insertion into the pleural space through the second intercostal space to reexpand the lung, followed by insertion of a chest tube if large amounts of air escape through the needle after insertion
• analgesics to promote comfort and encourage deep breathing and coughing.

What to do

Caring for patient with a pneumothorax requires these measures:
• Assess the patient's respiratory status, including auscultation of bilateral breath sounds, at least every 2 hours. Monitor oxygen saturation levels closely for changes and obtain ABG analysis as ordered.
• Monitor hemodynamic parameters frequently as appropriate and indicated. Anticipate the need for cardiac monitoring because hypoxemia can predispose the patient to arrhythmias.
• Watch for complications, signaled by pallor, gasping respirations, and sudden chest pain. Carefully monitor vital signs at least every hour for indications of shock, increasing respiratory distress, or mediastinal shift. If your patient's respiratory status deteriorates, anticipate the need for endotracheal intubation and mechanical ventilation and assist as necessary.
• Assist with the chest tube insertion and connect to suction as ordered. Monitor the patient for possible complications associated with chest tube insertion.
• Check chest tube devices frequently for drainage and proper functioning.
• Reposition the patient to promote comfort and drainage.

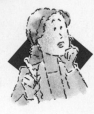

Quick quiz

1. When intentionally or accidentally removing a chest tube, it's essential to:

A. immediately apply an airtight, sterile petroleum dressing over the site.

B. increase the rate of I.V. fluid administration due to the risk of hemorrhage.

C. administer oxygen at 4 L/minute via nasal cannula and notify respiratory therapy.

D. reinsert the chest tube into the open space and notify the doctor.

Answer: A. Immediately after the removal of a chest tube, apply an airtight, sterile petroleum dressing over the site to create a seal.

2. Chemical burns to the airway from inhalation injury are usually painless because:

A. the chemical alters the patient's sense of perception.

B. the patient immediately becomes unconscious after the injury.

C. the tracheobronchial tree is insensitive to pain.

D. the burn damages the nerves and the patient can't sense the pain.

Answer: C. Chemical burns to the airway are similar to burns on the skin, except that they're painless because the tracheobronchial tree is insensitive to pain.

3. The preferred treatment for carbon monoxide poisoning is:

A. administration of 100% humidified oxygen.

B. sedation.

C. hyperbaric oxygen therapy.

D. corticosteroid therapy.

Answer: A. The preferred treatment for carbon monoxide poisoning is administering 100% humidified oxygen continuously until carboxyhemoglobin levels fall to the nontoxic range of 10%.

Scoring

☆☆☆ If you answered all three items correctly, superb. You have a penetrating knowledge of traumatic injuries!

☆☆ If you answered two items correctly, excellent. Your understanding of this chapter is anything but blunt!

☆ If you answered fewer than two items correctly, relax. Review the chapter, breathe deeply, and try again!

Neoplastic disorders

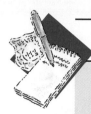

Just the facts

In this chapter, you'll learn:

♦ characteristics of laryngeal and lung cancer and their potential causes

♦ how to diagnose laryngeal and lung cancers

♦ treatment for laryngeal and lung cancers

♦ staging and prognosis for laryngeal and lung cancers.

Understanding neoplastic disorders

Neoplastic growths may be benign or malignant, depending on their likelihood to invade structures and spread through the body. Neoplastic respiratory disorders include laryngeal and lung cancer.

Laryngeal cancer

The most common form of laryngeal cancer is squamous cell carcinoma (95%); rare forms include adenocarcinoma and sarcoma. Such cancer may be intrinsic or extrinsic. An *intrinsic* tumor is on the true vocal cord and tends not to spread because underlying connective tissues lack lymph nodes. An *extrinsic* tumor is on another part of the larynx and tends to spread early. Laryngeal cancer is nine times more common in males than in females; and most commonly affects people ages 50 to 65.

> Laryngeal cancer usually strikes men ages 50 to 65.

What causes it

The cause of laryngeal cancer is unknown. Major predisposing factors include smoking and alcoholism; minor factors include chronic inhalation of noxious fumes and familial tendency.

How it happens

Initially in laryngeal cancer, the mucosa is exposed to an irritating substance and develops into a tougher mucosa by increasing its thickness or by developing a keratin layer. Cellular changes also lead to the growth of abnormal epithelial cells that eventually become malignant. These areas of epithelial cells commonly appear as white or red patches.

Metastasis to the head and neck depends on the primary site of the tumor and usually spreads to the mucosa, muscle, and bone. Systemic metastasis through the blood and lymph system is possible. If metastasis occurs, it happens most commonly in the lung or liver.

Laryngeal cancer is classified according to its location:
- supraglottis — false vocal cords
- glottis — true vocal cords
- subglottis — downward extension from the vocal cords (rare).

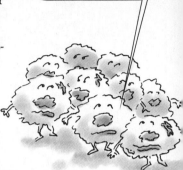

Cellular changes in laryngeal cancer lead to the growth of abnormal epithelial cells that eventually become malignant.

What to look for

With intrinsic laryngeal cancer, the dominant and earliest indication is hoarseness that persists longer than 3 weeks; with extrinsic cancer, it's a lump in the throat or pain or burning in the throat when drinking citrus juice or hot liquid. Later signs and symptoms of metastasis include dysphagia, dyspnea, cough, enlarged cervical lymph nodes, and pain that radiates to the ear.

What tests tell you

Hoarseness lasting longer than 2 weeks requires laryngoscopy to visualize the larynx. (See *Staging laryngeal cancer.*) A firm diagnosis requires xeroradiography, biopsy, laryngeal tomography, computed tomography (CT) scan or laryngography to define the borders of the lesion, and a chest X-ray to detect metastasis.

How it's treated

Early lesions are treated with surgery or radiation; advanced lesions, with surgery, radiation, and chemotherapy. Chemotherapeutic agents may include methotrexate, cisplatin, bleomycin, fluorouracil, and vincristine.

The treatment goal is to eliminate the cancer and preserve speech. If speech preservation isn't possible, speech rehabilitation may include esophageal speech or prosthetic devices. Surgical techniques to construct a new voice box are still experimental. (See *Alternative speech methods,* page 282.)

Surgical procedures vary with tumor size and can include cordectomy, partial or total laryngectomy, supraglottic laryngecto-

Staging laryngeal cancer

The TNM (tumor, node, metastasis) classification system developed by the American Joint Committee on Cancer describes laryngeal cancer stages and guides treatment. The T stages cover supraglottic, glottic, and subglottic tumors.

Primary tumor
TX—primary tumor unassessible
T0—no evidence of primary tumor
Tis—carcinoma in situ

Supraglottic tumor stages
T1—tumor confined to one subsite in supraglottis; vocal cords retain motion
T2—tumor extending to other sites in supraglottis or to glottis and vocal cords retain motion
T3—tumor confined to larynx but vocal cords lose motion; tumor extending to the postcricoid area or pre-epiglottic space
T4a—tumor extending through thyroid cartilage, to tissues beyond the larynx (such as the oropharynx or soft tissues of the neck), or esophagus
T4b—tumor invades prevertebral space, encases a carotid artery, or invades mediastinal structures

Glottic tumor stages
T1—tumor confined to vocal cords, which retain normal motion
T1a—limited to one vocal cord
T1b—involves both vocal cords
T2—tumor extending to supraglottis, subglottis, or both; vocal cords lose motion
T3—tumor confined to larynx but vocal cords lose motion

T4a—tumor extending through thyroid cartilage to tissues beyond the larynx
T4b—tumor invades prevertebral space, surrounds a carotid artery, or invades mediastinal structures

Subglottic tumor stages
T1—tumor confined to subglottis
T2—tumor extending to vocal cords; vocal cords may lose motion
T3—tumor confined to larynx with vocal cord fixation
T4a—tumor extending through cricoid or thyroid cartilage, to tissues beyond the larynx, or both
T4b—tumor invades prevertebral space, encases a carotid artery, or invades chest structure

Regional lymph nodes
NX—regional lymph nodes can't be assessed
N0—no evidence of regional lymph node metastasis
N1—metastasis in a single ipsilateral lymph node, 3 cm or less in greatest diameter
N2—metastasis in one or more ipsilateral lymph node, larger than 3 cm but less than 6 cm in greatest diameter

N2a—metastasis to single ipsilateral node, larger than 3 cm but less than 6 cm in greatest diameter
N2b—metastasis to multiple ipsilateral nodes, larger than 3 cm but less than 6 cm in greatest diameter
N2c—metastasis to bilateral or contralateral nodes, none larger than 6 cm
N3—metastasis in a node larger than 6 cm in greatest diameter

Distant metastasis
MX—distant metastasis unassessible
M0—no evidence of distant metastasis
M1—distant metastasis

Staging categories
Laryngeal cancer progresses from mild to severe as follows:
STAGE 0—Tis, N0, M0
STAGE I—T1, N0, M0
STAGE II—T2, N0, M0
STAGE III—T1, N1, M0; T2, N1, M0; T3, N0, M0; T3, N1, M0
STAGE IVA—T1, N2, M0; T2, N2, M0; T3, N2, M0; T4a, N0, M0; T4a, N1, M0; T4a, N2, M0
STAGE IVB— T4b, any N, M0; any T, N3, M0
STAGE IVC—any T, any N, M1

my, or total laryngectomy with laryngoplasty. (See *Managing laryngeal surgery complications*, page 283.) Radiation therapy alone or combined with surgery can cause such complications as airway obstruction, pain, and loss of the sense of taste.

What to do

Psychological support and good preoperative and postoperative care can minimize complications and speed recovery. In addition,

Alternative speech methods

During convalescence, your patient may work with a speech pathologist, who can teach him new ways to speak using various communication techniques, including esophageal speech, artificial larynges, and surgically implanted prostheses.

Esophageal speech

By drawing air in through the mouth, trapping it in the upper esophagus, and releasing it slowly while forming words, the patient can again communicate by voice. With training and practice, a highly motivated patient can master esophageal speech in about 1 month. Recognize that speech will sound choppy at first but words will flow more smoothly and understandably with increasing skill.

Because esophageal speech requires strength, an elderly patient or one with asthma or emphysema may find it too physically demanding to learn. In addition, because it requires frequent sessions with a speech pathologist, a chronically ill patient may find learning esophageal speech overwhelming.

Artificial larynges

The throat vibrator and the Cooper-Rand device are basic artificial larynges. Both types vibrate to produce speech that's easy to understand, although it sounds monotonous and mechanical.

Tell the patient to operate a throat vibrator by holding it in place against his neck. A pulsating disk in the device vibrates the throat tissue as the patient forms words with his mouth. The throat vibrator may be difficult to use immediately after surgery, when the patient's neck wounds are still sore.

The Cooper-Rand device vibrates sounds piped into the patient's mouth through a thin tube, which the patient positions in the corner of his mouth. Because it's easy to use, this device may be preferred soon after surgery.

Surgically implanted prostheses

Most surgical implants generate speech by vibrating when the patient manually closes the tracheostomy, forcing air upward. One such device is the Blom-Singer voice prosthesis. Only hours after it's inserted through an incision in the stoma, the patient can speak in a normal voice. The surgeon may implant the device when radiation therapy ends or within a few days (or even years) after laryngectomy.

To speak, the patient covers his stoma while exhaling. Exhaled air travels through the trachea, passes through an airflow port on the bottom of the prosthesis, and exits through a slit at the esophageal end of the prosthesis. This creates the vibrations needed to produce sound.

Not all patients are eligible for tracheoesophageal puncture, the procedure needed to insert the prosthesis. Considerations include the extent of the laryngectomy, pharyngoesophageal muscle status, stoma size and location, and the patient's mental and emotional status, visual and auditory acuity, hand-eye coordination, bimanual dexterity, and self-care skills.

---

caring for a patient with laryngeal cancer or a laryngectomy requires these measures:

Partial or total preop

• Instruct the patient to maintain good oral hygiene. If appropriate, instruct a male patient to shave off his beard.
• Encourage the patient to express his concerns before surgery. Help him choose a temporary nonspeaking method of communication such as writing.
• If appropriate, arrange for someone who has undergone laryngectomy to visit the patient. Explain postoperative procedures (suctioning, nasogastric [NG] tube

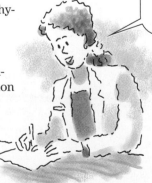

Encourage patients to use writing as a method of communication when they can't speak.

Managing laryngeal surgery complications

After your patient returns from surgery, you'll need to monitor his recovery, watching carefully for such complications as fistula formation, a ruptured carotid artery, and stenosis of the tracheostomy site.

Fistula formation

Warning signs of fistula formation include redness, swelling, and secretions on the suture line. The fistula may form between the reconstructed hypopharynx and the skin and eventually heals spontaneously, although the process may take weeks or months. Feed the patient who has a fistula through a nasogastric tube. Otherwise, food will leak through the fistula and delay healing.

Ruptured carotid artery

Bleeding, a cardinal sign of a ruptured carotid artery, may occur in a patient who received preoperative radiation therapy or in a patient with a fistula that constantly bathes the carotid artery in oral secretions. If rupture occurs, apply pressure to the site. Call for help immediately and take the patient to the operating room for carotid ligation.

Tracheostomy stenosis

Constant shortness of breath alerts you to tracheostomy stenosis, which may occur weeks to months after laryngectomy. Management includes fitting the patient with successively larger tracheostomy tubes until he can tolerate insertion of a full-sized one.

---

feeding, and care of the laryngectomy tube) and their results (the need to breath through the neck, altered speech). Also, prepare the patient for other functional losses; for example, he won't be able to smell, blow his nose, whistle, gargle, sip, or suck on a straw.

Partial postop

• Be prepared to give I.V. fluids and, typically, tube feedings for the first 2 days postoperatively; then give the patient oral fluids. Keep the tracheostomy tube (inserted during surgery) in place until edema subsides.
• Keep the patient from using his voice until he has medical permission (usually 2 to 3 days postoperatively). Then caution him to whisper until healing is complete.

Total postop

• As soon as the patient returns to his bed, place him on his side and elevate his head 30 to 45 degrees. When you move him, remember to support his neck.
• The patient will probably have a laryngectomy tube in place until his stoma heals (7 to 10 days). This tube is shorter and thicker than a tracheostomy tube but requires the same care.
• Watch for crusting and secretions around the stoma, which can cause skin breakdown. To prevent crust formation, provide adequate room humidification. Remove crusting with petroleum jelly, antimicrobial ointment, and moist gauze.
• Teach the patient stoma care.

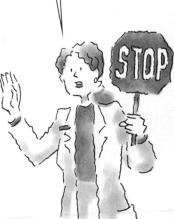

Keep the patient from using his voice until he has medical permission.

No place like home

At home after laryngectomy

Preparing a patient for discharge after laryngectomy should begin with laryngectomy education before surgery. The patient and his family should receive the following information to prepare for discharge:

• Instruct the patient about good oral hygiene practices. Suggest that the male patient shave off his beard to facilitate postoperative care in the hospital and at home.

• Instruct the patient on stoma care.

• Instruct the patient on the use of a waterproof shield to cover the stoma when bathing or showering to prevent water entry.

• Provide information on changes that will occur postoperatively, such as breathing through the neck and speech alteration. Assure the patient that there are various ways to communicate after a laryngectomy and that a speech pathologist will be available after the surgery to assist with communication method selection and skill training.

• Inform the patient that, after the laryngectomy, he won't be able to smell aromas, blow his nose, whistle, gargle, or suck on a straw.

• Encourage the patient that increasing the humidification in the home is essential (installation of a humidifier on a forced-air furnace or use of room humidifiers or vaporizers).

• Assure the patient that a home care nurse is usually involved with care after discharge and will serve as a resource for information and care.

• Provide the patient and his family with information on support groups and services. Such groups include the American Speech-Learning-Hearing Association, the International Association of Laryngectomees, the American Cancer Society, and the local chapter of the Lost Chord Club.

• Support the patient and his family through grieving. If depression is severe, refer the patient for counseling.

• Monitor the patient's vital signs. (Be especially alert for fever, which indicates infection.)

• Record fluid intake and output, and watch for dehydration.

• Provide frequent mouth care.

• Suction gently unless otherwise instructed. Don't attempt deep suctioning, which could penetrate the suture line.

• Suction through the tube and the patient's nose because he can no longer blow air through his nose; suction his mouth gently.

• After insertion of a drainage catheter (usually connected to a blood drainage system or a GI drainage system), don't stop suction until drainage is minimal. After the catheter is removed, check dressings for drainage.

• Give the patient an analgesic if necessary.

• If the patient has an NG feeding tube, check tube placement and elevate his head to prevent aspiration.

• Reassure the patient that speech rehabilitation may help him speak again. Encourage him to contact the International Association of Laryngectomees and other sources of support. (See *At home after laryngectomy.*)

Lung cancer

Even though it's largely preventable, lung cancer is the most common cause of cancer death in men and has recently become the most common cause of cancer death in women.

What causes it

Most experts agree that lung cancer is attributable to inhalation of carcinogenic pollutants by a susceptible host. Most susceptible are people who smoke or who work with or near asbestos. Pollutants in tobacco smoke cause progressive lung cell degeneration. Lung cancer is 10 times more common in smokers than in nonsmokers; 80% of lung cancer patients are or were smokers.

Cancer risk is determined by the number of cigarettes smoked daily, the depth of inhalation, how early in life smoking began, and the nicotine content of the cigarettes. Exposure to carcinogenic industrial and air pollutants (asbestos, uranium, arsenic, nickel, iron oxides, chromium, radioactive dust, and coal dust), and familial tendency also increase susceptibility.

> Lung cancer risk is determined by the number of cigarettes smoked daily, the depth of inhalation, how early in life smoking began, and the nicotine content of the cigarettes.

How it happens

Lung cancer usually develops within the wall or epithelium of the bronchial tree. The most common types are epidermoid (squamous cell) carcinoma, small-cell (oat cell) carcinoma, adenocarcinoma, and large-cell (anaplastic) carcinoma.

Although prognosis is usually poor, it varies with the extent of spread at the time of diagnosis and the growth rate of the specific cell type. Only about 14% of patients with lung cancer survive 5 years after diagnosis. Lung cancer is associated with more deaths per year than heart disease, colon cancer, and prostate cancer combined.

What to look for

Because early-stage lung cancer usually produces no symptoms, this disease is typically in an advanced state at diagnosis. These common late-stage signs and symptoms lead to diagnosis:
• *epidermoid and small-cell carcinomas* — smoker's cough, hoarseness, wheezing, dyspnea, hemoptysis, and chest pain
• *adenocarcinoma and large-cell carcinoma* — fever, weakness, weight loss, anorexia, and shoulder pain.

Not just about breathing

In addition to their obvious interference with respiratory function, lung tumors may also alter the production of hormones that regulate body function or homeostasis.

Clinical conditions that result from such changes are known as *hormonal paraneoplastic syndromes* and include:
- *gynecomastia*, which may result from large-cell carcinoma
- *hypertrophic pulmonary osteoarthropathy* (bone and joint pain from cartilage erosion due to abnormal production of growth hormone), which may result from large-cell carcinoma or adenocarcinoma
- *Cushing's* and *carcinoid syndromes*, which may result from small-cell carcinoma
- *hypercalcemia*, which may result from epidermoid tumors.

Metastatic S&S

Distant metastasis may involve any part of the body, most commonly the central nervous system, liver, and bone. Metastatic signs and symptoms vary greatly, depending the tumors' effects on intrathoracic and distant structures; they include:
- *bronchial obstruction* — hemoptysis, atelectasis, pneumonitis, and dyspnea
- *recurrent nerve invasion* — hoarseness and vocal cord paralysis
- *chest wall invasion* — piercing chest pain, increasing dyspnea, and severe shoulder pain radiating down the arm
- *local lymphatic spread* — cough, hemoptysis, stridor, and pleural effusion
- *phrenic nerve involvement* — dyspnea, shoulder pain, and unilateral paralyzed diaphragm with paradoxical motion
- *esophageal compression* — dysphagia
- *vena caval obstruction* — venous distention and edema of the face, neck, chest, or back
- *pericardial involvement* — pericardial effusion, tamponade, and arrhythmias
- *cervical thoracic sympathetic nerve involvement* — miosis, ptosis, exophthalmos, and reduced sweating.

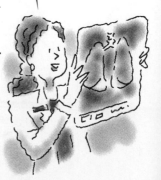

A firm diagnosis of lung cancer requires firm evidence, including chest X-ray, which can show a lesion up to 2 years before symptoms appear.

What tests tell you

Typical signs and symptoms may strongly suggest lung cancer but a firm diagnosis requires further evidence.
- *Chest X-ray* usually shows an advanced lesion but can detect a lesion up to 2 years before symptoms appear. It also indicates tumor size and location.

• *Sputum cytology* is marginally helpful in obtaining a diagnosis. It requires a specimen coughed up from the lungs and tracheo-bronchial tree, *not* postnasal secretions or saliva.
• *CT scan* of the chest may help delineate the tumor's size and its relationship to surrounding structures.
• *Bronchoscopy* can locate the tumor site. Bronchoscopic washings provide material for cytologic and histologic examination. The flexible fiber-optic bronchoscope increases the test's effectiveness.
• *Needle biopsy* of the lungs uses biplane fluoroscopic visual control or CT guidance to detect peripherally located tumors, which allows a firm diagnosis in 80% of patients.
• *Tissue biopsy* of accessible metastatic sites, including supraclavicular and mediastinal node and pleural biopsies, confirm presence of malignant neoplasm. (See *How cancer metastasizes*.)
• *Thoracentesis* allows chemical and cytologic examination of pleural fluid.

More tests

Additional studies include:
• *preoperative mediastinoscopy or mediastinotomy* to rule out involvement of mediastinal lymph nodes (which would preclude curative pulmonary resection)
• *bone scan, positron emission tomography scan, bone marrow biopsy* (recommended in small-cell carcinoma), and a *CT scan* of the brain or abdomen to detect metastasis.
• *staging,* after histologic confirmation, to determine the extent of the disease, help plan treatment, and predict prognosis.

How it's treated

Various combinations of surgery, radiation, and chemotherapy may improve the prognosis and prolong survival. Nevertheless, because treatment usually begins at an advanced stage, it's largely palliative.

Surgery

Unless the tumor is nonresectable or other conditions rule out surgery, excision is the primary treatment for stage I, stage II, or selected stage III squamous cell carcinoma, adenocarcinoma, and large-cell carcinoma. Surgery may include partial removal of a lung (wedge resection, segmental resection, lobectomy, radical lobectomy) or total removal (pneumonectomy, radical pneumonectomy).

How cancer metastasizes

Metastasis usually occurs through the bloodstream to other organs and tissues, as described here.

Cancer cells secrete enzyme and motility factors.

Basement membrane in blood vessel is disrupted.

Cancer cells escape into circulation.

Undetected cells move out of blood.

Enzymes are secreted.

Cell wall is cut.

New tissue is invaded downstream.

Chemical attraction occurs.

Malignant cells target specific site.

New site is invaded.

Cells multiply.

Metastatic tumor appears.

Preparing for external radiation therapy

• Show the patient where radiation therapy takes place and introduce him to the radiation therapist.
• Tell the patient to remove all metal objects (pins, buttons, jewelry) that may interfere with therapy. Explain that the areas to be treated will be marked with indelible ink and that *he must not scrub these areas* because it's important to radiate the same areas each time.

• Reinforce the doctor's explanation of the procedure and answer questions as honestly as you can. If you don't know the answer to a question, refer the patient to the doctor.
• Teach the patient to watch for and report adverse effects. Because radiation therapy may increase susceptibility to infection, warn him to avoid people with colds or other infections during therapy.

However, emphasize the benefits (such as outpatient treatment) instead of the adverse effects.
• Reassure the patient that treatment is painless and won't make him radioactive. Stress that he'll be under constant surveillance during radiation administration and he should call out if he needs anything.

Radiation

Preoperative radiation therapy may reduce tumor bulk to allow for surgical resection. Preradiation chemotherapy helps improve response rates.

If surgery is contraindicated, radiation therapy is ordinarily recommended for stage I and stage II lesions as well as for stage III lesions when the disease is confined to the involved hemithorax and the ipsilateral supraclavicular lymph nodes.

Generally, radiation therapy is delayed until 1 month after surgery to allow the wound to heal, and is then directed to the part of the chest most likely to develop metastasis. High-dose radiation therapy or radiation implants may also be used. (See *Preparing for external radiation therapy*.)

Chemotherapy

Another treatment is chemotherapy, including combinations of drugs, which produce a response rate of about 40% but have a minimal effect on overall survival. (See *Chemotherapy and the cell cycle*.) Promising combinations for treating small-cell carcinomas include cyclophosphamide with doxorubicin and vincristine; cyclophosphamide with doxorubicin, vincristine, and etoposide; and etoposide with cisplatin, cyclophosphamide, and doxorubicin. (See *Managing chemotherapy adverse effects*, pages 290 and 291.)

Laser therapy

Some patients may undergo laser therapy, which involves direction of laser energy through a bronchoscope to destroy local tumors.

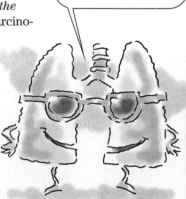

Laser therapy destroys local tumors. Glasses? Check! I'm ready!

Chemotherapy and the cell cycle

Chemotherapeutic drugs disrupt the cell cycle in one of two ways. They may be either cell-cycle specific or cell-cycle nonspecific. Cell-cycle-specific drugs, such as methotrexate, act at one or more cell-cycle phases. Cell-cycle-nonspecific drugs, such as busulfan, can act on both replicating and resting cells.

This diagram illustrates how cell-cycle-specific drugs work to disrupt the cell cycle.

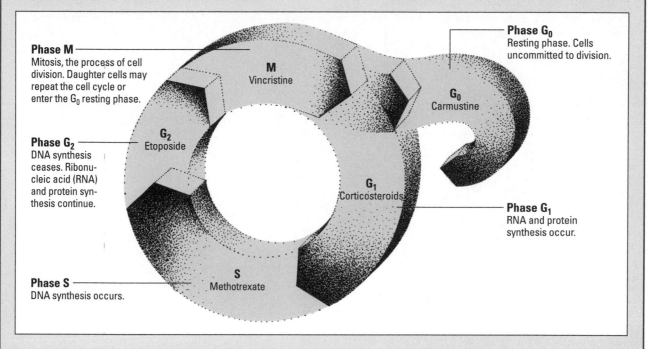

Phase M
Mitosis, the process of cell division. Daughter cells may repeat the cell cycle or enter the G_0 resting phase.

M
Vincristine

Phase G₂
DNA synthesis ceases. Ribonucleic acid (RNA) and protein synthesis continue.

G₂
Etoposide

Phase S
DNA synthesis occurs.

S
Methotrexate

G₁
Corticosteroids

G₀
Carmustine

Phase G₀
Resting phase. Cells uncommitted to division.

Phase G₁
RNA and protein synthesis occur.

What to do

Comprehensive supportive care and patient teaching can minimize complications and speed recovery from surgery, radiation, and chemotherapy.

Preop

Before surgery:
• Supplement and reinforce information about the disease and the surgical procedure.
• Explain expected postoperative procedures, such as the insertion of an indwelling urinary catheter, use of an endotracheal or chest tube (or both), dressing changes, and I.V. therapy.
• Teach the patient how to perform coughing, deep diaphragmatic breathing, and range-of-motion (ROM) exercises.

Managing chemotherapy adverse effects

This chart lists common adverse effects of chemotherapy as well as nursing actions and home care instructions.

Adverse effects	Nursing actions	Home care instructions
Bone marrow depression (leukopenia, thrombocytopenia, anemia)	• Establish baseline white blood cell (WBC) and platelet counts, hemoglobin levels, and hematocrit before therapy begins. Monitor studies during therapy. • If WBC count drops suddenly or falls below 2,000/µl, stop the drug and notify the doctor. Initiate reverse isolation if absolute granulocyte count falls below 1,000/µl. Report a platelet count below 100,000/µl. If necessary, assist with the transfusion. • Monitor temperature orally every 4 hours, and regularly inspect the skin and body orifices for signs of infection. Observe for petechiae, easy bruising, and bleeding. Check for hematuria and monitor the patient's blood pressure. Be alert for signs of anemia. • Limit S.C. and I.M. injections. If these are necessary, apply pressure for 3 to 5 minutes after injection to prevent leakage or hematoma. Report unusual bleeding after injection. • Take precautions to prevent bleeding. Use extra care with razors, nail trimmers, dental floss, toothbrushes, and other sharp or abrasive objects. • Give vitamin and iron supplements as ordered. Provide a diet high in iron.	• Instruct the patient to report fever, chills, sore throat, lethargy, unusual fatigue, or pallor immediately. • Warn him to avoid exposure to people with infections during chemotherapy and for several months after. • Explain that the patient and his family shouldn't receive immunizations during or shortly after chemotherapy because an exaggerated reaction may occur. • Tell the patient to avoid activities that could cause traumatic injury and bleeding. Advise him to report episodes of bleeding or bruising to the doctor. • Tell him to eat high-iron foods, such as liver and spinach. • Stress the importance of follow-up blood studies after completion of treatment.
Anorexia	• Assess the patient's nutritional status before and during chemotherapy. Weigh him weekly or as ordered. • Explain the need for adequate nutrition despite the loss of appetite.	• Encourage the patient's family to supply favorite foods to help him maintain adequate nutrition. • Suggest that the patient eat small, frequent meals.
Nausea and vomiting	• Before chemotherapy begins, administer antiemetics, as ordered, to reduce the severity of these reactions. • Monitor and record the frequency, character, and amount of vomitus. • Monitor serum electrolyte levels, and provide total parenteral nutrition, if necessary.	• Teach the patient and his family how to insert antiemetic suppositories. • Tell the patient to take the drug on an empty stomach, with meals, or at bedtime. GI upset indicates that the drug is working. Instruct him to report vomiting to the doctor. • Tell him to follow a high-protein diet.

Managing chemotherapy adverse effects *(continued)*

Adverse effects	Nursing actions	Home care instructions
Diarrhea and abdominal cramps	• Assess the frequency, color, consistency, and amount of diarrhea. Give antidiarrheals as ordered. • Assess the severity of cramps, and observe for signs of dehydration and acidosis, which may indicate electrolyte imbalance. • Encourage fluids and, if ordered, give I.V. fluids and potassium supplements. • Provide good skin care, especially to the perianal area.	• Teach the patient how to use antidiarrheals, and instruct him to report diarrhea to the doctor. • Encourage him to maintain adequate fluid intake and to follow a bland, low-fiber diet. • Explain that good perianal hygiene can help prevent skin breakdown and infection.
Stomatitis	• Before drug administration, observe for dry mouth, erythema, and white patches on the oral mucosa. Be alert for bleeding gums or complaints of a burning sensation when drinking acidic liquids. • Emphasize the principles of good mouth care with the patient and his family. • Provide mouth care every 4 to 6 hours with normal saline solution or half-strength hydrogen peroxide. Coat the oral mucosa with milk of magnesia. Avoid lemon-glycerin swabs because they tend to reduce saliva and change mouth pH. • To make eating more comfortable, apply a topical viscous anesthetic, such as lidocaine, before meals. Administer special mouthwashes as ordered. • Consult the dietitian to provide bland foods at medium temperatures. • Treat cracked or burning lips with petroleum jelly.	• Teach the patient good mouth care. Instruct him to rinse his mouth with 1 teaspoon of salt dissolved in 8 oz (237 ml) of warm water or hydrogen peroxide diluted to half-strength with water. • Advise him to avoid acidic, spicy, or extremely hot or cold foods. • Instruct the patient to report stomatitis to the doctor, who may order a change in medication.
Alopecia	• Reassure the patient that alopecia is usually temporary. • Inform him that he may experience discomfort before hair loss starts.	• Suggest to the patient that he have his hair cut short to make thinning hair less noticeable. • Advise the patient to wash his hair with a mild shampoo and avoid frequent brushing or combing. • Suggest wearing a hat, scarf, toupee, or wig.

Postop

After thoracic surgery:
• Maintain a patent airway, and monitor chest tubes to reestablish normal intrathoracic pressure and prevent postoperative and pulmonary complications.

- Check the patient's vital signs every 15 minutes during the first hour after surgery, every 30 minutes during the next 4 hours, and then every 2 hours. Watch for abnormal respiration and other changes.
- Suction the patient often, and encourage him to begin deep breathing and coughing as soon as possible. Check secretions often. Initially, sputum will be thick and dark with blood, but it should become thinner and grayish yellow within 1 day.
- Monitor and record closed chest drainage. Keep chest tubes patent and draining effectively.
- Watch for and report foul-smelling discharge and excessive drainage on the dressing. Usually, the dressing is removed after 24 hours, unless the wound appears infected.
- Position the patient on the surgical side to promote drainage and lung reexpansion.
- Monitor the patient's intake and output. Maintain adequate hydration.
- Watch for and treat infection, shock, hemorrhage, atelectasis, dyspnea, and mediastinal shift. (See *Chemotherapy and infection*.)
- To help prevent pulmonary embolus, apply antiembolism stockings and encourage ROM exercises.

Advice from the experts

Chemotherapy and infection

Be alert for signs of infection, particularly if the patient is also receiving radiation therapy. A low-grade fever when the granulocyte count falls below 500 µl indicates the need to take the patient's temperature often and the need to notify the doctor because an infection may be imminent.

All together now

If the patient is receiving chemotherapy and radiation:
- Explain possible adverse effects of radiation and chemotherapy. Watch for, treat, and (when possible) prevent these effects.
- Inform the patient of possible temporary hair loss, and reassure him that his hair should grow back after therapy ends. Suggest a wig, hat, or head covering.
- Check the patient's skin for petechiae, ecchymoses, chemical cellulitis, and secondary infection during treatment.
- Ask the dietary department to provide soft, nonirritating foods that are high in protein, and encourage the patient to eat high-calorie between-meal snacks.
- Give an antiemetic and an antidiarrheal as needed.
- Schedule patient care activities in a way that helps the patient conserve his energy.
- During radiation therapy, administer skin care to minimize skin breakdown. If the patient receives radiation therapy in an outpatient setting, warn him to avoid tight clothing, exposure to the sun, and harsh ointments on his chest. Teach him exercises to help prevent shoulder stiffness.

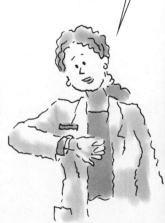

Schedule patient care activities in a way that helps the patient conserve energy.

High-risk teaching

Teach high-risk patients ways to reduce their chances of developing lung cancer.

• Refer smokers who want to quit to local branches of the American Cancer Society, Smokenders, or other smoking-cessation programs or suggest group therapy, individual counseling, or hypnosis.

• Encourage patients with recurring or chronic respiratory tract infections and those with chronic lung disease who detect changes in the character of a cough to see their doctor promptly for evaluation.

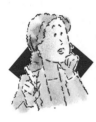

Quick quiz

1. Laryngeal cancer is classified according to:

A. the treatment required.

B. the etiology (cause).

C. its location.

D. the degree of lymph node enlargement.

Answer: C. Laryngeal cancer is classified according to its location in the supraglottis (false vocal cords), glottis (true vocal cords), or subglottis (downward extension from the vocal cords).

2. The dominant symptom of intrinsic laryngeal cancer is:

A. a lump in the throat.

B. hoarseness for longer than 3 weeks.

C. burning in the throat when drinking citrus juice or a hot liquid.

D. enlarged cervical lymph nodes.

Answer: B. With intrinsic laryngeal cancer, the dominant and earliest indication is hoarseness that persists longer than 3 weeks; with extrinsic cancer, it's a lump in the throat or pain or burning in the throat when drinking citrus juice or hot liquid. Later signs and symptoms of metastasis include dysphagia, dyspnea, cough, enlarged cervical lymph nodes, and pain radiating to the ear.

3. The treatment goal for laryngeal cancer is to:

A. facilitate swallowing.

B. teach stoma care.

C. prevent surgery.

D. eliminate the cancer and preserve speech.

Answer: D. The treatment goal for laryngeal cancer is to eliminate the cancer and preserve speech. If speech preservation isn't possible, speech rehabilitation may include esophageal speech or prosthetic devices; surgical techniques to construct a new voice box are still experimental.

4. Which of these tests can detect a lesion on the lung up to 2 years before symptoms of lung cancer appear?
    A.   Chest X-ray
    B.   CT scan of the chest
    C.   Bronchoscopy
    D.   Thoracentesis

Answer: A. Chest X-ray usually shows an advanced lesion but can detect a lesion up to 2 years before symptoms appear. It also indicates tumor size and location.

5. Preoperative radiation therapy may be used on a patient with lung cancer to:
    A.   improve response rate to chemotherapy.
    B.   destroy local tumors.
    C.   prevent infection.
    D.   reduce tumor bulk.

Answer: D. Preoperative radiation therapy may reduce tumor bulk to allow for surgical resection.

Scoring

☆☆☆   If you answered all five items correctly, zowee! Your comprehension of neoplastic respiratory disorders is without blemish.

☆☆   If you answered four items correctly, yahoo! Your knowledge of neoplasms is never-ending.

☆   If you answered fewer than four items correctly, no worries. Review the chapter and achieve benign understanding.

Respiratory emergencies

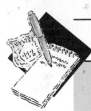

Just the facts

In this chapter, you'll learn:

♦ potential causes of respiratory emergencies

♦ how to diagnose and recognize respiratory emergencies

♦ treatments for common respiratory emergencies.

Understanding respiratory emergencies

Respiratory compromise, resulting from respiratory emergencies, is a leading cause of morbidity and mortality. Respiratory emergencies include airway obstruction, anaphylaxis, asphyxia, bronchospasm, near drowning, respiratory arrest, respiratory depression, and sudden infant death syndrome.

Airway obstruction

Maintaining a patent airway is vital to life. Coughing is the main mechanism the body uses to clear the airway. Yet, coughing may be ineffective in clearing the airway in some disease states or even under normal healthy conditions if an obstruction is present.

What causes it

A patient's upper airway can become obstructed or compromised by vomitus, food, edema, or his teeth or saliva. The most common cause is the tongue and epiglottis; obstruction is due to decreased muscle tone when a person is unconscious or unresponsive.

It's anatomic

Edema of anatomic structures in the upper airway can cause an obstruction. Edema of the tongue (caused by surgery or trauma),

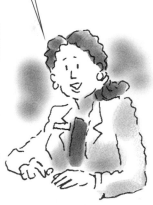

Coughing may be ineffective in clearing the airway — even in an otherwise healthy patient — if an obstruction is present.

laryngeal edema, and smoke inhalation edema are various types of edema that can lead to an obstruction. Other potential causes of an upper airway obstruction include:

- peritonsillar or pharyngeal abscesses
- tumors of the head or neck
- tenacious secretions in the airway
- cerebral disorders (stroke)
- trauma of the face, trachea, or larynx
- aspiration of a foreign object
- burns to the head, face, or neck
- croup
- epiglottiditis
- laryngospasms
- anaphylaxis.

Memory jogger

For an easy way to remember key symptoms of complete airway obstruction, just think of the 5 C's:

Choking
Cyanosis
Cessation of coughing
Consciousness level change
Cardiac arrest.

How it happens

Upper airway obstruction is an interruption in the flow of air through the nose, mouth, pharynx, or larynx. If not recognized early, it will progress to respiratory arrest. Obstruction of the upper airway is considered a life-threatening situation. Prompt detection and intervention can prevent a partial airway obstruction from progressing to a complete airway obstruction.

Partial airway obstruction commonly occurs from edema or a small foreign object that doesn't completely obstruct the airway. If the reason for the obstruction isn't detected and relieved promptly, respiratory arrest will lead to cardiac arrest and cardiopulmonary resuscitation (CPR) will be required.

What to look for

Signs of a partial airway obstruction can include diaphoresis, tachycardia, coughing, and elevated blood pressure. Experiencing no symptoms is also possible with a partial obstruction. With a complete airway obstruction these symptoms may be observed:

- choking
- gasping for air
- wheezing, whistling, or any other unusual breath sound that indicates a breathing difficulty
- cyanosis or pallor
- cessation of coughing and inability to make a sound.
- unconsciousness or change in level of consciousness (LOC)
- restlessness, agitation, panic, or increasing anxiety
- hypoxia and hypercapnia
- cardiac arrest.

What tests tell you

Physical examination may indicate decreased breath sounds. Tests aren't usually necessary to diagnose an upper airway obstruction, but may include X-rays (particularly a chest X-ray), bronchoscopy, and laryngoscopy. If symptoms of an upper airway obstruction persist, a chest X-ray, neck X-rays, laryngoscopy, or a computed tomography scan may be ordered to rule out the presence of a tumor, foreign body, or infection.

> Prompt assessment regarding the cause of an obstruction is indicated.

How it's treated

Treatment focuses on relieving the obstruction and oxygenation. (See *Opening an obstructed airway*, page 298.) Prompt assessment regarding the cause of the obstruction is indicated. When an obstruction is related to the tongue or an accumulation of tenacious secretions, the patient's head should be placed in a slightly extended position and an oral airway should be inserted. If the patient has a complete airway obstruction, is unable to cough or speak, and a foreign body obstruction is suspected, a series of abdominal thrusts should be performed to try to remove the foreign object. (See *Obstructed airway management*, pages 299 to 302.)

Emergency procedures may be required in the event of an upper airway obstruction. Such procedures as cricothyroidotomy, endotracheal (ET) intubation and tracheotomy are common and are generally preceded or followed by a direct laryngoscopy in an attempt to determine the cause of the obstruction.

Cricothyroidotomy

Cricothyroidotomy requires an excision of the cricothyroid membrane below the thyroid cartilage and the cricoid ring. A tracheostomy tube is placed through this opening to keep the newly created airway open until a tracheotomy can be performed. This procedure is used only when no other options are available to establish an airway.

Endotracheal intubation

ET intubation involves the insertion of a tube into the trachea through the nose (nasotracheal intubation) or the mouth (orotracheal intubation) by a trained healthcare professional.

Tracheotomy

Tracheotomy may be performed in an operating room or at the bedside and may be performed electively or in an emergency situ-

Opening an obstructed airway

To open an obstructed airway, use the head-tilt, chin-lift maneuver or the jaw-thrust maneuver, as described here.

Head-tilt, chin-lift maneuver

In many cases of airway obstruction, the muscles controlling the patient's tongue have relaxed, causing the tongue to obstruct the airway. If the patient doesn't appear to have a neck injury, use the head-tilt, chin-lift maneuver to open his airway. Use these four steps to carry out this maneuver:

❦ Place your hand closest to the patient's head on his forehead.

❦ Apply firm pressure—firm enough to tilt the patient's head back.

❦ Place the fingertips of your other hand under the bony portion of the patient's lower jaw, near the chin.

❦ Lift the patient's chin. Be sure to keep his mouth partially open (as shown at right). Avoid placing your fingertips on the soft tissue under the patient's chin because this may inadvertently obstruct the airway you're trying to open.

Using the jaw-thrust maneuver

If you suspect a neck injury, use the jaw-thrust maneuver to open the patient's airway. Use these four steps to carry out this maneuver:

❦ Kneel at the patient's head with your elbows on the ground.

❦ Rest your thumbs on the patient's lower jaw near the corners of his mouth, pointing your thumbs toward his feet.

❦ Place your fingertips around the lower jaw.

❦ To open the airway, lift the lower jaw with your fingertips (as shown at right).

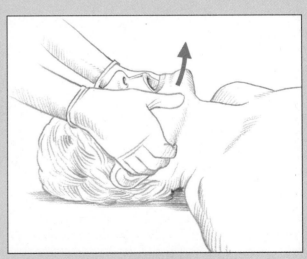

ation. It involves the incision of the skin over the trachea and the creation of a surgical wound in the trachea for placement of a tube to establish an airway (tracheostomy). This procedure may be performed if mechanical ventilation is necessary for more than

(Text continues on page 302.)

Obstructed airway management

An obstructed airway causes anoxia, which in turn leads to brain damage and death in 4 to 6 minutes. The Heimlich maneuver uses an upper-abdominal thrust to create diaphragmatic pressure in the static lung below the foreign body sufficient to expel the obstruction. The Heimlich maneuver is used in conscious adult patients. If the patient is unconscious, an abdominal thrust should be used; however, the abdominal thrust is contraindicated in pregnant women, markedly obese patients, and patients who have recently undergone abdominal surgery. For such patients, a chest thrust, which forces air out of the lungs to create an artificial cough, should be used.

The finger sweep maneuver is then used to manually remove the foreign body from the mouth. These maneuvers are contraindicated in a patient with incomplete or partial airway obstruction or when the patient can maintain adequate ventilation to dislodge the foreign body by effective coughing. However, the patient's inability to speak, cough, or breathe demands immediate action to dislodge the obstruction.

Don't give up

Keep in mind that if your patient vomits during abdominal thrusts, quickly wipe out her mouth with your fingers and resume the maneuver as necessary. Even if your efforts to clear the airway don't seem to be effective, keep trying. As oxygen deprivation increases, smooth and skeletal muscles relax, making your maneuvers more likely to succeed.

LOC check

Determine the patient's level of consciousness (LOC) by tapping her shoulder and asking, "Are you choking?" If she has a complete airway obstruction, she won't be able to answer because airflow to her vocal cords will be blocked. If she makes crowing sounds, her airway is partially obstructed, and you should encourage her to cough. This will either clear the airway or make the obstruction complete. For a complete obstruction, intervene as follows, depending on whether the patient is conscious or unconscious.

For a conscious adult

• Tell the patient that you'll try to dislodge the foreign body.
• Standing behind the patient, wrap your arms around her waist.

• Make a fist with one hand, and place the thumb side against her abdomen, slightly above the umbilicus and well below the xiphoid process. Then grasp your fist with the other hand (as shown below).

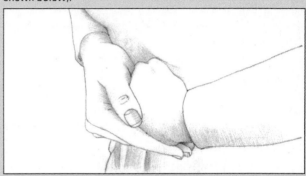

• Squeeze the patient's abdomen five times with quick inward and upward thrusts. Each thrust should be a separate and distinct movement; each should be forceful enough to create an artificial cough that will dislodge an obstruction (as shown below).

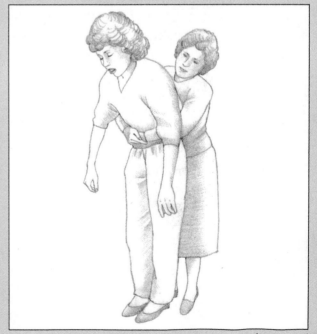

(continued)

Obstructed airway management *(continued)*

• Make sure you have a firm grasp on the patient because she may lose consciousness and need to be lowered to the floor. Look around the floor for objects that may harm her.

• If she does lose consciousness, lower her carefully to the floor. Support her head and neck to prevent injury, and place her in a supine position. Call for help or activate the emergency response system.

• Open the airway with the head-tilt and chin-lift or jaw-thrust; perform a finger sweep; and attempt to ventilate.

• If the chest doesn't rise, reposition the airway and attempt to ventilate again. If ventilation is unsuccessful, give five abdominal thrusts and follow the steps for an unconscious adult.

For an unconscious adult

• If you come upon an unconscious adult, establish unresponsiveness, ask witnesses what happened, and call for help or activate the emergency response system.

• Open the airway (head-tilt and chin-lift or jaw-thrust) and check for breathing; if the patient isn't breathing, attempt to ventilate her. If you're unable to ventilate the patient, reposition her head and try again.

• If you still can't ventilate the patient, or if a conscious patient loses consciousness during abdominal thrusts, kneel astride her thighs.

• Place the heel of one hand on top of the other. Then place your hands between her umbilicus and the tip of her xiphoid process at the midline. Push inward and upward with five quick abdominal thrusts (as shown below).

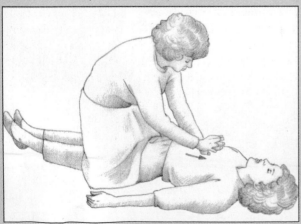

• After delivering the abdominal thrusts, open the patient's airway by grasping the tongue and lower jaw with your thumb and fingers. Lift the jaw to draw the tongue away from the back of the throat and away from any foreign body (as shown below).

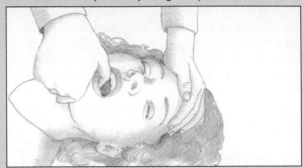

• If you can see the object, remove it by inserting your index finger deep into the throat at the base of her tongue. Using a hooking motion, remove the obstruction (as shown below). Some clinicians object to a blind finger sweep—using your finger when you can't see the obstruction—because your finger acts as a second obstruction. These clinicians believe that, in most cases, the tongue-jaw lift described above should be enough to dislodge the obstruction.

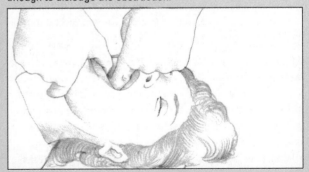

• After the object is removed, try to ventilate the patient. Then assess for spontaneous respirations, and check for a pulse. Proceed with cardiopulmonary resuscitation (CPR) if necessary.

• If the object isn't removed, try to ventilate the patient. If you can't, repeat the abdominal thrust maneuver described above in sequence until you clear the airway.

Obstructed airway management *(continued)*

For an obese or a pregnant adult

• If the patient is conscious, stand behind her and place your arms under her armpits and around her chest.

• Place the thumb side of your clenched fist against the middle of the sternum, avoiding the margins of the ribs and the xiphoid process. Grasp your fist with your other hand and perform a chest thrust with enough force to expel the foreign body (as shown below). Continue until the patient expels the obstruction or loses consciousness.

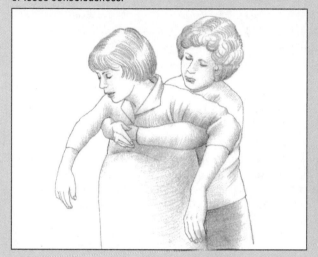

• If the patient loses consciousness, carefully lower her to the floor and place her in a supine position. Call for help or activate the emergency response system.

• Open the airway with the tongue-jaw lift; perform a finger sweep; and attempt to ventilate. If the chest doesn't rise, reposition the airway, and attempt to ventilate again. If ventilation is unsuccessful, begin chest thrusts.

• Kneel close to the patient's side, and place the heel of one hand just above the bottom of her sternum. The long axis of the heel of your hand should align with the long axis of the patient's sternum. Place the heel of your other hand on top of that, mak-

ing sure your fingers don't touch the patient's chest. Deliver each thrust forcefully enough to remove the obstruction (as shown below).

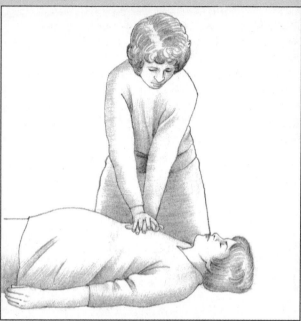

For a child

• If the child is conscious and can stand, perform abdominal thrusts using the same technique as you would with an adult, but with less force.

• If he's unconscious or lying down, kneel at his feet; if he's a large child, kneel astride his thighs. If he's lying on a treatment table, stand by his side. Deliver abdominal thrusts as you would for an adult patient, but use less force. (*Note:* Never perform a blind finger sweep on a child because you risk pushing the foreign body further back into the airway.)

(continued)

Obstructed airway management *(continued)*

For an infant

• Regardless of whether the infant is conscious, place him face down so that he's straddling your arm with his head lower than his trunk. Rest your forearm on your thigh and deliver five back blows with the heel of your hand between the infant's shoulder blades (as shown below).

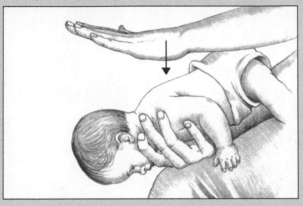

• If you haven't removed the obstruction, place your free hand on the infant's back. Supporting his neck, jaw, and chest with your other hand, turn him over onto your thigh. Keep his head lower than his trunk.

• Position your fingers. To do so, imagine a line between the infant's nipples and place the index finger of your free hand on his sternum, just below this imaginary line. Then place your middle and ring fingers next to your index finger and lift the index finger off his chest.

• Deliver five chest thrusts as you would for chest compression, but at a slower rate. Repeat the above steps until you've relieved the obstruction or the infant becomes unconscious.

• If the infant becomes unconscious, call for help, and open the airway with the tongue-jaw lift. If you see the object, remove it. (*Note:* As with a child, never perform a blind finger sweep on an infant.)

• Open the airway of the unconscious infant and attempt to ventilate; if the chest doesn't rise, reposition the airway and attempt to ventilate again.

• If ventilation is unsuccessful, give five back blows and five chest thrusts. Open the airway with the tongue-jaw lift and remove the object only if you see it.

• Continue the above sequence of attempted ventilations, back blows, and chest thrusts until the obstruction is relieved. After the object is removed, try to ventilate the infant. Assess for spontaneous ventilation; if none, give two ventilations, check for a pulse, and proceed with CPR if necessary.

1 week to prevent damage to the larynx. (See *Combating tracheotomy complications.*)

What to do

Caring for a patient with an upper airway obstruction requires these measures:

• Recognize that an upper airway obstruction is a medical emergency.

• Assess for the cause of the obstruction.

• Assess breath sounds.

• Monitor chest X-ray results and arterial blood gas (ABG) results after the obstruction is relieved.

• Observe for "seesaw" respirations.

• Monitor pulse oximetry to assess the oxygenation status of the patient.

Combating tracheotomy complications

This chart lists possible tracheotomy complications along with measures to prevent, detect, and treat them.

Complication	Prevention	Detection	Treatment
Aspiration	• Evaluate the patient's ability to swallow. • Elevate his head and inflate the cuff during feeding and for 30 minutes afterward.	• Assess for dyspnea, tachypnea, rhonchi, crackles, excessive secretions, and fever.	• Obtain chest X-ray, if ordered. • Suction excessive secretions. • Give antibiotics, if necessary.
Bleeding at tracheotomy site	• Don't pull on the tracheostomy tube; don't allow ventilator tubing to do so. • If the dressing adheres to the wound, wet it with hydrogen peroxide and remove it gently.	• Check dressings regularly; slight bleeding is normal, especially if the patient has a bleeding disorder.	• Keep the cuff inflated to prevent edema and blood aspiration. Give humidified oxygen. • Document character of bleeding. Check for prolonged clotting time. • As ordered, assist with Gelfoam application or ligation of a small bleeder.
Infection at tracheotomy site	• Always use strict sterile technique. • Thoroughly clean all tubing. • Change nebulizer or humidifier jar and all tubing daily. • Collect sputum and wound drainage specimens for culture.	• Check for purulent, foul-smelling drainage from stoma. • Be alert for other signs and symptoms of infection, including fever, malaise, increased white blood cell count, and local pain.	• As ordered, obtain culture specimens and administer antibiotics. • Inflate tracheostomy cuff to prevent aspiration. • Suction the patient frequently; avoid cross-contamination. • Change dressings when soiled.
Pneumothorax	• Assess for subcutaneous emphysema, which may indicate pneumothorax. Notify the doctor if this occurs.	• Auscultate for decreased or absent breath sounds. • Check for tachypnea, pain, and subcutaneous emphysema.	• If ordered, prepare for chest tube insertion. • Obtain chest X-ray as ordered to evaluate pneumothorax or to check placement of chest tube.
Subcutaneous emphysema	• Make sure cuffed tube is patent and properly inflated. • Avoid displacement by securing ties and using lightweight ventilator tubing and swivel valves.	• Be aware that subcutaneous emphysema is most common in mechanically ventilated patients. • Palpate neck for crepitus; listen for air leakage around cuff; and check site for unusual swelling.	• Be sure to inflate cuff properly or use a larger tube. • Suction patient, and clean tube to remove blockage. • Document extent of crepitus.
Tracheal malacia	• Avoid excessive cuff pressures. • Avoid suctioning beyond the end of the tube.	• Note dry, hacking cough and blood-streaked sputum when the tube is being manipulated.	• Minimize trauma from tube movement. • Keep tracheostomy cuff pressure below 18 mm Hg.

• Continually assess for stridor, cyanosis, and changes in LOC and notify the doctor immediately if any occur.
• Perform abdominal thrusts if a foreign object aspiration is suspected.
• Prepare for a cricothyroidotomy if the setting is outside the facility.
• Prepare for ET intubation or a tracheostomy within the hospital setting if an airway can't be established.
• Anticipate cardiac arrest if the airway obstruction isn't cleared promptly.

Anaphylaxis

Anaphylaxis is a dramatic, widespread, acute atopic reaction marked by the sudden onset of rapidly progressive urticaria and respiratory distress. A severe anaphylactic reaction may precipitate vascular collapse, leading to systemic shock and, sometimes, death.

Anaphylactic shock is a condition characterized by vasodilation of the vessels and increased capillary permeability and occurs within 1 to 2 minutes of exposure to an antigenic substance.

What causes it

The causes of anaphylactic reaction are ingestion of or other systemic exposure to a sensitizing substance or other substance.

So sensitive

Sensitizing substances include serums (usually horse serum), vaccines, allergen extracts, enzymes (such as L-asparaginase), hormones, penicillin and other antibiotics, sulfonamides, local anesthetics, salicylates, polysaccharides, diagnostic chemicals (sulfobromophthalein, sodium dehydrocholate, and radiographic contrast media), foods (legumes, nuts, berries, seafood, and egg albumin), sulfite-containing food additives, and insect venom (honeybees, wasps, hornets, yellow jackets, fire ants, mosquitoes, and certain spiders).

A common cause of anaphylaxis is penicillin, which induces anaphylaxis in 1 to 4 of every 10,000 patients treated with it. Penicillin is most likely to induce anaphylaxis after parenteral administration or prolonged therapy and in atopic patients who are allergic to other drugs or foods.

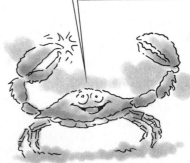

While delicious to some, seafood can cause allergic reactions in others.

How it happens

An anaphylactic reaction requires previous sensitization or exposure to the specific antigen, resulting in the production of specific immunoglobulin (Ig) E antibodies by plasma cells. This antibody production takes place in the lymph nodes and is enhanced by helper T cells. IgE antibodies then bind to membrane receptors on mast cells (found throughout connective tissue, commonly near small blood vessels) and basophils.

Haven't we met before?

On reexposure, the antigen binds to adjacent IgE antibodies or cross-linked IgE receptors, activating a series of cellular reactions that trigger degranulation — the release of powerful preformed chemical mediators (such as histamine, prostaglandins, and platelet-activating factor) from mast-cell stores. IgG or IgM enters into the reaction and activates the release of complement fractions. (See *Development of anaphylaxis*, page 306.)

Within minutes...

This acute phase of the response occurs within minutes of exposure. Because of the systemic nature of the exposure, activation of mast cells is widespread, and the massive release of these powerful mediators near blood vessels leads to vascular collapse by stimulating contraction of certain groups of smooth muscles and by increasing vascular permeability. In turn, increased vascular permeability leads to decreased peripheral resistance and plasma leakage from the circulation to extravascular tissues (which lowers blood volume, causing hypotension, hypovolemic shock, and cardiac dysfunction).

Meanwhile, back at the ranch...

In the later phase of this response (8 to 12 hours later), other mediators are synthesized and released, including chemokines, leukotrienes, and cytokines. These agents mediate the inflammatory response by recruiting eosinophils and lymphocytes. This delayed response may be less dramatic than the acute phase of anaphylaxis, but with a diffuse inflammatory response, further smooth-muscle contraction and edema can occur and progress to grave systemic symptoms.

What to look for

An anaphylactic reaction produces sudden physical distress within seconds or minutes after exposure to an allergen. A delayed or persistent reaction may occur up to 24 hours later. The severity of the reaction is inversely related to the interval between exposure

Now I get it!

Development of anaphylaxis

These illustrations show how anaphylaxis develops.

Response to antigen: Immunoglobulins (Igs) M and G recognize and bind to the antigen.

Release of chemical mediators: Activated IgE on basophils promotes the release of mediators: histamine, serotonin, and leukotrienes.

Intensified response: Mast cells release more histamine and eosinophil chemotactic factor of anaphylaxis (ECF-A), which create venule-weakening lesions.

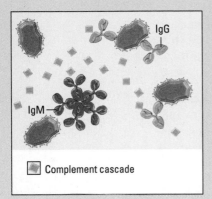

IgG

IgM

◆ Complement cascade

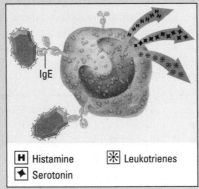

IgE

| H Histamine | ✳ Leukotrienes |
| ✦ Serotonin | |

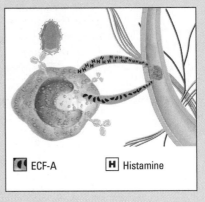

◀ ECF-A   H Histamine

Respiratory distress: In the lungs, histamine causes endothelial cell destruction and fluid leak into alveoli.

Deterioration: Meanwhile, mediators increase vascular permeability, causing fluid leak from the vessels.

Failure of compensatory mechanisms: Endothelial cell damage causes basophils and mast cells to release heparin and mediator-neutralizing substances. However, anaphylaxis is now irreversible.

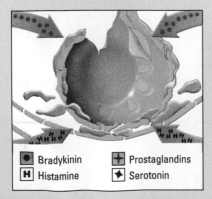

| ● Bradykinin | ✦ Prostaglandins |
| H Histamine | ✦ Serotonin |

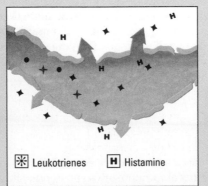

✳ Leukotrienes   H Histamine

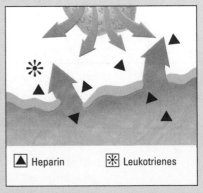

▲ Heparin   ✳ Leukotrienes

to the allergen and the onset of symptoms. Usually, the first signs and symptoms include a feeling of impending doom or fright, weakness, sweating, sneezing, shortness of breath, nasal pruritus, urticaria, and angioedema, followed rapidly by symptoms in one or more target organs.

In the system

Systemic effects of anaphylaxis include:
• *cardiovascular*—hypotension, shock and, sometimes, cardiac arrhythmias, which, if untreated, may precipitate circulatory collapse
• *respiratory*—nasal mucosal edema, profuse watery rhinorrhea, itching, nasal congestion, sudden sneezing attacks, and edema of the upper respiratory tract resulting in hypopharyngeal and laryngeal obstruction (hoarseness, stridor, and dyspnea) that's an early sign of acute respiratory failure, which can be fatal
• *GI and genitourinary*—severe stomach cramps, nausea, diarrhea, and urinary urgency and incontinence.

What tests tell you

Anaphylaxis can be diagnosed by the rapid onset of severe respiratory or cardiovascular symptoms after ingestion or injection of a drug, vaccine, diagnostic agent, food or food additive, or after an insect sting. If these symptoms occur without a known allergic stimulus, rule out other possible causes of shock (such as acute myocardial infarction, status asthmaticus, and heart failure).

How it's treated

Treatment for anaphylaxis focuses on promotion of adequate ventilation and tissue perfusion. Maintaining a patent airway, ensuring oxygenation, restoring vascular volume, and managing the effects of chemical mediators are included in the management of this condition.

What to do

Caring for a patient with anaphylaxis requires these measures:
• Anaphylaxis is always an emergency. It requires an *immediate* injection of 0.1 to 0.5 ml of epinephrine 1:1,000 aqueous solution, repeated every 5 to 20 minutes as necessary.
• If the patient is in the early stages of anaphylaxis, hasn't yet lost consciousness, and is still normotensive, give epinephrine I.M. or subcutaneously (S.C.); help it move into the circulation faster by massaging the injection site. For severe reactions when the pa-

Anaphylaxis is always an emergency.

tient has lost consciousness and is hypotensive, give epinephrine I.V.

• Maintain airway patency. Observe the patient for early signs and symptoms of laryngeal edema (stridor, hoarseness, and dyspnea), which will probably necessitate ET tube insertion or a tracheotomy and oxygen therapy.

• If the patient is experiencing cardiac arrest, begin CPR, including closed-chest heart massage, assisted ventilation, and sodium bicarbonate; further therapy depends on the patient's response.

• Watch for hypotension and shock, and maintain circulatory volume with a volume expander (plasma, a plasma expander, saline solution, or albumin) as needed. Stabilize blood pressure with the I.V. vasopressors norepinephrine and dopamine. Monitor blood pressure, central venous pressure, and urine output as a response index.

After the hubbub

• After the initial emergency, administer such medications as S.C. epinephrine, a longer-acting epinephrine, a corticosteroid, I.V. diphenhydramine for long-term management, and aminophylline I.V. over 10 to 20 minutes for bronchospasm. (*Caution:* Rapid infusion of aminophylline may cause or aggravate severe hypotension.)

• Even after the acute anaphylactic event has been controlled, patients must be counseled about the risks of delayed signs and symptoms. Recurrence of shortness of breath, chest tightness, sweating, angioedema, or other signs and symptoms must be reported immediately.

• To prevent anaphylaxis, teach the patient to avoid exposure to known allergens. (See *Preventing anaphylaxis.*)

Weeding out the usual suspects

• If the patient has a food or drug allergy, he must learn to avoid the offender in all forms. If the patient has an allergy to insect stings, he should avoid open fields and wooded areas during the insect season and should carry an anaphylaxis kit whenever he goes outdoors. Show him how to use the kit. (See *How to use an anaphylaxis kit.*) If the patient is prone to anaphylaxis, he should wear medical identification naming his allergies.

• If a patient must receive a drug to which he's allergic, prevent a severe reaction by making sure he receives careful desensitization with gradually increasing doses of the antigen or advance administration of steroids.

• A patient with history of allergies should receive a drug with a high anaphylactic potential only after cautious pretesting for sen-

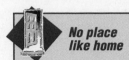

No place like home

Preventing anaphylaxis

To help prevent a future episode, instruct the patient to avoid exposure to known allergens, such as foods, drugs, and insects.

• Tell the patient not to consume the offending item in any combination or form. Caution him to read food labels before purchasing and to check with restaurant personnel about the contents of menu items before ordering.

• Advise the patient to avoid insect stings by not wearing scented colognes or deodorants and by staying away from open fields and wooded areas during the insect season.

• Recommend that the patient carry an anaphylaxis kit whenever he's outdoors; ensure that he knows how and when to use it.

• Tell the patient to always wear medical identification naming his allergies.

No place like home

How to use an anaphylaxis kit

If the doctor has prescribed an anaphylaxis kit for the patient to use in an emergency, explain that the kit contains everything he needs to treat an allergic reaction:
• prefilled syringe containing two doses of epinephrine
• alcohol swabs
• tourniquet
• antihistamine tablets.

Instruct the patient to notify the doctor at once if anaphylaxis occurs (or to ask someone else to call) and to use the anaphylaxis kit as outlined here.

Getting ready
• Take the prefilled syringe from the kit and remove the needle cap. Hold the syringe with the needle pointing up. Expel air from the syringe by pushing in the plunger until it stops.
• Next, clean about 4″ (10 cm) of the skin on your arm or thigh with an alcohol swab. (If you're right-handed, clean your left arm or thigh; if you're left-handed, your right arm or thigh.)

Injecting the epinephrine
• Rotate the plunger one-quarter turn to the right so that it's aligned with the slot.

Insert the entire needle—like a dart—into the skin.
• Push down on the plunger until it stops. It will inject 0.3 ml of the drug. Withdraw the needle. (*Note:* This dose is for patients older than age 12. The dose and administration for infants and for children ages 12 and younger must be directed by a doctor.)

Removing the insect's stinger
• Quickly remove the insect's stinger if it's visible. Use a dull object, such as a fingernail or tweezers, to pull it straight out. If the stinger can't be removed quickly, stop trying. Go on to the next step.

Applying the tourniquet
• If you were stung on an arm or a leg, apply a tourniquet between the sting site and your heart. Tighten the tourniquet by pulling the string.
• After 10 minutes, release the tourniquet by pulling on the metal ring.

Taking the antihistamine tablets
• Chew and swallow the antihistamine tablets. (Children ages 12 and younger

should follow the directions supplied by the doctor or provided in the kit.)

Following up
• Apply ice packs—if available—to the sting site. Avoid exertion, keep warm, and see a doctor or go to an emergency facility immediately.
• *Important:* If you don't notice an improvement within 10 minutes, give yourself a second injection by following the directions in the kit. If the syringe has a preset second dose, don't depress the plunger until you're ready to give the second injection. Proceed as before, following the injection instructions.

Special instructions
• Keep the kit handy for emergency treatment at all times.
• Ask the pharmacist for storage guidelines.
• Periodically check the epinephrine in the preloaded syringe. A pinkish brown solution must be replaced.
• Note the kit's expiration date and replace the kit before that date.

sitivity. Closely monitor the patient during testing, and make sure you have resuscitative equipment and epinephrine ready.
• Closely monitor a patient undergoing diagnostic tests that use radiographic contrast dyes, such as cardiac catheterization, excretory urography, and angiography.

Asphyxia

Asphyxia is a condition of insufficient oxygen intake and is one of the leading causes of fatal injuries in children. Asphyxiation in children is most commonly caused by a foreign body obstruction.

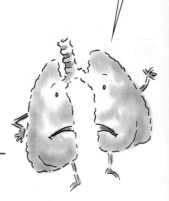

Asphyxia results from any condition or substance that inhibits respiration.

What causes it

Asphyxia results from any condition or substance that inhibits respiration, such as:
• hypoventilation due to narcotic abuse, medullary disease or hemorrhage, pneumothorax, respiratory muscle paralysis, or cardiopulmonary arrest
• intrapulmonary obstruction, as in airway obstruction, severe asthma, foreign body aspiration, pulmonary edema, pneumonia, and near drowning
• extrapulmonary obstruction, as in tracheal compression from a tumor, strangulation, trauma, or suffocation
• inhalation of toxic agents, as in carbon monoxide poisoning, smoke inhalation, and excessive oxygen inhalation.

How it happens

Asphyxia results in cardiopulmonary arrest because it's a condition of insufficient oxygen and accumulating carbon dioxide in the blood and tissues due to interference with respiration. Without prompt treatment, it's fatal.

What to look for

Depending on the duration and degree of asphyxia, common symptoms include anxiety, dyspnea, agitation, and confusion leading to coma, altered respiratory rate (apnea, bradypnea, occasional tachypnea), decreased breath sounds, central and peripheral cyanosis (cherry-red mucous membranes in late-stage carbon monoxide poisoning), seizures, and fast, slow, or absent pulse.

What tests tell you

Diagnosis is based on the patient history and laboratory results. ABG measurement, the most important test, indicates decreased partial pressure of arterial oxygen (PaO_2) — less than 60 mm Hg — and increased partial pressure of arterial carbon dioxide ($PaCO_2$) — more than 50 mm Hg. Chest X-rays may show a foreign body, pulmonary edema, or atelectasis. Toxicology tests may show drugs, chemicals, or abnormal hemoglobin. Pulmonary function tests may indicate respiratory muscle weakness.

How it's treated

Asphyxia requires immediate respiratory support — with CPR, ET intubation, and supplemental oxygen as needed. In addition, treatment requires elimination of an underlying cause, including:
• bronchoscopy for extraction of a foreign body
• narcotic antagonist (such as naloxone) for a narcotic overdose
• gastric lavage for poisoning
• withholding supplemental oxygen for carbon dioxide narcosis due to excessive oxygen therapy.

What to do

Caring for a patient with asphyxia requires these measures:
• Provide immediate circulatory and respiratory support.
• Maintain adequate oxygenation.
• Manage the underlying cause of asphyxia.
• Establish I.V. access for medication and fluid administration.
• Consider that respiratory distress is frightening, so reassure the patient during treatment.
• Give prescribed medications.
• Suction carefully, as needed, and encourage deep breathing.
• Closely monitor vital signs and laboratory test results.
• To prevent drug-induced asphyxia, warn patients about the danger of taking alcohol with other central nervous system (CNS) depressants.

Bronchospasm

The onset of bronchospasm may be sudden, commonly resulting from anesthesia induction, or onset may be progressive over several minutes.

What causes it

A variety of conditions can cause bronchospasm. The most common condition associated with bronchospasm is asthma. Other causes include:
• allergic response to a drug or anesthesia
• history of pulmonary obstructive disease or allergies

• irritation of the airway from suctioning or airway insertion during an emergency
• increased irritation from an ET tube
• vigorous physical activity.

How it happens

Bronchospasms result from the tightening of the muscles surrounding the bronchial tubes, which results in narrowing of the air passages and an interruption in the normal flow of air into and out of the lungs. If bronchospasms aren't promptly diagnosed and treated, air exchange is hindered as air is trapped in the alveolar sacs of the lungs. Bronchospasms are commonly caused by a hyperreactive response to an allergen.

Exercise-induced bronchospasms generally occur during exercise or within minutes of stopping. Hyperventilation of air that's cooler and dryer than the air in the respiratory tract results in the loss of heat or water from the lungs during episodes of physical exertion. Exercise-induced bronchospasms should be anticipated in all patients with a history of asthma.

Bronchospasms can occur during the induction of anesthesia or at any time during the anesthetic or postoperative period. The severity of bronchospasm during the induction of anesthesia may be life-threatening and inability to ventilate the patient may result. Patients at risk for bronchospasms related to anesthesia include those with a history of reactive airway disease, patients with a significant smoking history, or those with a recent history of upper respiratory tract infection.

> Exercise-induced bronchospasms generally occur during exercise or within minutes of stopping.

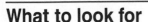

What to look for

Signs of bronchospasm can be sudden or occur over time. Such signs may include:
• slight cough with no further sound
• wheezing
• little or no movement of the chest
• inability to ventilate even with positive pressure
• change in oxygen saturation values
• change in LOC
• color change to pale or cyanotic due to lack of oxygen
• dyspnea
• respiratory distress at rest
• diminished breath sounds due to air trapping.

What tests tell you

These tests may be used to diagnose bronchospasms:
• *Pulmonary function tests* reveal decreased vital capacity and increased total lung and residual capacities during an acute asthma attack, if asthma is the suspected cause. Peak and expiratory flow rate measurements are less than 60% of baseline.
• *Pulse oximetry* commonly shows decreased oxygen saturation.
• *Chest X-ray* may show hyperinflation with areas of atelectasis and flat diaphragm due to increased intrathoracic volume.
• *ABG analysis* reveals decreasing Pao_2 and increasing $Paco_2$.
• *Electrocardiogram (ECG)* may show sinus tachycardia.

How it's treated

The patient with bronchospasms is monitored closely for respiratory failure. Oxygen, bronchodilators, epinephrine, corticosteroids, and nebulizer therapies may be ordered. The patient may be intubated and placed on mechanical ventilation if $Paco_2$ increases or respiratory arrest occurs.

Asthma chronicles

If the patient has a history of asthma, consider these interventions:
• identifying and avoiding precipitating factors, such as environmental allergens or irritants, to prevent future attacks
• desensitization to specific antigens if the stimuli can't be removed entirely; this decreases the severity of asthma attacks with future exposure
• bronchodilators (such as epinephrine and albuterol) to decrease bronchoconstriction, reduce bronchial airway edema, and increase pulmonary ventilation
• anticholinergics to increase the effects of bronchodilators
• corticosteroids (such as methylprednisolone) to decrease bronchoconstriction, reduce bronchial airway edema, and increase pulmonary ventilation
• S.C. epinephrine to counteract the effects of asthma attack mediators

'Tis the season

• mast-cell stabilizers (cromolyn [Intal] and nedocromil [Tilade]) in patients with atopic asthma who have seasonal disease that, when given prophylactically, block the acute obstructive effects of antigen exposure by inhibiting the degranulation of mast cells,

thereby preventing the release of chemical mediators responsible for anaphylaxis
• humidified oxygen to correct dyspnea, cyanosis, and hypoxemia and to maintain an oxygen saturation greater than 90%
• mechanical ventilation, which is necessary if the patient doesn't respond to initial ventilatory support and drugs or develops respiratory failure
• relaxation exercises to increase circulation and aid recovery from an asthma attack.

What to do

Caring for a patient with bronchospasms requires these measures:
• Conduct careful and frequent assessment of the patient's respiratory status, especially if the patient isn't intubated. Check the respiratory rate, auscultate breath sounds, and monitor oxygen saturation.

What a wheeze

• Be alert for a patient who was wheezing but suddenly stops and continues to show signs of respiratory distress. In this case, the absence of wheezing may be due to severe bronchial constriction that narrows the airways severely during inhalation and exhalation. As a result, so little air passes through the narrowed airways that no sound is made. This lack of sound is a sign of imminent respiratory collapse; the patient needs intubation and mechanical ventilation. Reassure the patient and stay with him. Help him to relax as much as possible.
• Assess the patient's mental status for confusion, agitation, or lethargy.
• Assess the patient's heart rate and rhythm. Be alert for cardiac arrhythmias related to bronchodilator therapy or hypoxemia.
• Obtain ordered tests and report results promptly.
• Administer medications as ordered (particularly bronchodilators).
• I.V. fluids are commonly ordered to replace insensible fluid loss from hyperventilation.

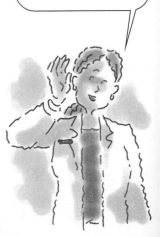

Be alert for a patient who was wheezing but suddenly stops and continues to show signs of respiratory distress. This lack of sound may be a sign of imminent respiratory collapse.

Near drowning

Near drowning refers to surviving—temporarily, at least—the physiologic effects of hypoxemia and acidosis that result from submersion in fluid. Although no statistics are available for deaths from near-drowning, in the United States, drowning claims about 8,000 lives annually.

What causes it

Near drowning results from an inability to swim or, in swimmers, from panic, a boating accident, a heart attack or a blow to the head while in the water, drinking heavily before swimming, or a suicide attempt.

Only nearly

Near drowning occurs in three forms:
• *dry* — the victim doesn't aspirate fluid but suffers respiratory obstruction or asphyxia (10% to 15% of patients)
• *wet* — the victim aspirates fluid and suffers from asphyxia or secondary changes due to fluid aspiration (about 85% of patients)
• *secondary* — the victim suffers a recurrence of respiratory distress (usually aspiration pneumonia or pulmonary edema) within minutes or 1 to 2 days after a near-drowning incident.

How it happens

Regardless of the tonicity of the fluid aspirated, hypoxemia is the most serious consequence of near drowning, followed by metabolic acidosis. Other consequences depend on the kind of water aspirated. After fresh-water aspiration, the fresh water moves quickly across the alveolar-capillary membrane and goes into the microcirculation. Lung surfactant is destroyed, producing alveolar instability. This instability, known as *atelectasis*, and $\dot{V}/\dot{Q}$ mismatch lead to pulmonary edema and hypoxemia.

Too much salt

After saltwater aspiration, the hypertonicity of seawater exerts an osmotic force, which pulls fluid from pulmonary capillaries into the alveoli. The resulting intrapulmonary shunt causes hypoxemia. In addition, if the pulmonary capillary membrane is injured, it can induce pulmonary edema. In wet or secondary near drowning, pulmonary edema and hypoxemia occur secondary to aspiration. (See *Physiologic changes in near drowning*, page 316.)

Physiologic changes in near drowning

This flowchart shows the primary cellular alterations that occur during near drowning. Separate pathways are shown for saltwater and freshwater incidents. Hypothermia presents a separate pathway that may preserve neurologic function by decreasing the metabolic rate. All pathways lead to diffuse pulmonary edema.

```
                              Submersion
                                  │
          ┌───────────────────────┴───────────────────────┐
          ▼                                                ▼
Water temperature greater than 68° F (20° C)      Water temperature less than 68° F
          │                                                │
    ┌─────┴─────┐                                          ▼
    ▼           ▼                                  Rapid cooling of body
Saltwater   Freshwater                                     │
aspiration  aspiration                                     ▼
    │           │                            Catecholamine release caused by
    ▼           ▼                            struggle before loss of consciousness
Fluid drawn   Water moves across                          │
into alveoli; alveolar-capillary                          ▼
washes out    membrane                             Vasoconstriction
surfactant        │                                       │
    │             ▼                                        ▼
    ▼         Surfactant is destroyed       Decreased cerebral and cardiac oxygen
Protein-rich      │                         consumption from cooled body and
exudate floods    ▼                         shunting of blood to brain and heart
alveoli       Alveolar instability                        │
    │         and atelectasis                             ▼
    ▼             │                            Body in near-dormant state
Reduced           │                                       │
compliance        │                                       ▼
    │             │                         Rewarming leading to systemic
    ▼             ▼                         vasodilation and hypotension; fluid
Widespread atelectasis causes               challenges to increase blood pressure
ventilation perfusion mismatch
    │
    ▼
Intrapulmonary shunting
    │
    ▼
Pulmonary edema  ◄───────────────────────────────────────┘
```

What to look for

Near-drowning victims can display a host of clinical problems, including:

- apnea or shallow or gasping respirations
- substernal chest pain
- asystole, tachycardia, bradycardia
- restlessness, irritability, lethargy
- fever
- confusion, unconsciousness
- vomiting
- abdominal distention
- cough that produces a pink, frothy fluid.

What tests tell you

Diagnosis requires a history of near drowning, including the type of water aspirated, along with characteristic features and auscultation of crackles and rhonchi. In addition:
• *ABG analysis* shows decreased oxygen content, low bicarbonate levels, and low pH.
• *Electrolyte levels* may be elevated or decreased, depending on the type of water aspirated.
• *White blood cell count* may show leukocytosis.
• *ECG* shows arrhythmias and waveform changes.

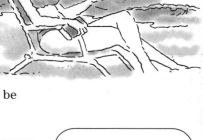

Diagnosis of near drowning sometimes depends on the type of water aspirated.

How it's treated

Emergency treatment begins with CPR and administration of 100% oxygen. If hypothermia is an issue, measures must be taken to warm the patient. In addition, hemodynamic monitoring should be instituted and ongoing support and monitoring of circulation and oxygenation must be maintained.

What to do

Caring for a near-drowning patient requires these measures:
• Stabilize the patient's neck in case he has a cervical injury.
• When the patient arrives at the hospital, assess for a patent airway. Establish one if necessary. Continue CPR, intubate the patient, and provide respiratory assistance, such as mechanical ventilation with positive end-expiratory pressure, if needed.
• Assess ABG and pulse oximetry values.
• If the patient's abdomen is distended, insert a nasogastric tube. (The patient will be intubated first if he's unconscious.)
• Start I.V. lines and insert an indwelling urinary catheter.
• Give medications as ordered. Drug treatment for near-drowning victims is controversial; it may include sodium bicarbonate for acidosis, corticosteroids and osmotic diuretics for cerebral edema, antibiotics to prevent infections, and bronchodilators to ease bronchospasms.
• Remember that all near-drowning victims should be admitted for an observation period of 24 to 48 hours because of the possibility of developing delayed drowning symptoms.
• Observe for pulmonary complications and signs of delayed drowning (confusion, substernal pain, adventitious breath sounds).
• Suction often.

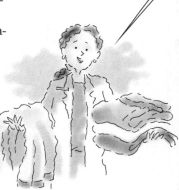

If hypothermia is an issue, measures must be taken to warm the patient.

- Monitor vital signs, intake and output, and peripheral pulses.
- Pulmonary artery catheters may be useful in assessing cardio-pulmonary status.
- Check for skin perfusion and watch for signs of infection.
- To facilitate breathing, raise the head of the bed slightly.
- To prevent near drowning, advise swimmers to avoid drinking alcohol before swimming, observe water safety rules, and take a water safety course sponsored by the Red Cross or YMCA.

Respiratory arrest

Respiratory compromise can have an abrupt or insidious onset. Respiratory arrest is the third in a series of three stages of respiratory compromise:

- *Respiratory distress* may be mild or severe and results in changes in respiratory rate, respiratory mechanism, or both.
- *Respiratory failure* indicates that the respiratory system can no longer meet the oxygen requirements of the body and, if not corrected, will progress to respiratory arrest.
- *Respiratory arrest* is the cessation of respiration (including episodes of prolonged apnea).

What causes it

Effective pulmonary gas exchange involves a variety of functions, including a clear airway, normal lungs and chest wall, and adequate pulmonary circulation. A compromise of any of these anatomic structures or functions can affect respiration.

Conditions that may induce this compromise include:

- stroke
- complete airway obstruction
- cardiac arrest
- shock
- heart disease
- cardiac arrhythmias
- seizures
- poisoning or inhalation of toxic substances
- injury to the lungs or chest
- near-drowning or suffocation
- emphysema or asthma
- allergic reactions
- hyperventilation
- drugs
- prematurity
- head or brain stem injury.

How it happens

Primary respiratory arrest results from airway obstruction, decreased respiratory drive, or respiratory muscle weakness. While airway obstruction can be partial or complete, the most common cause in an unconscious victim is upper airway obstruction due to tongue displacement into the oropharynx secondary to a loss of muscle tone.

Other potential causes of airway obstruction include:
- accumulation of blood, mucus, or vomitus
- foreign-body aspiration
- spasms or edema of the larynx
- edema of the pharynx
- inflammation of the upper airway
- neoplasm
- trauma.

How low can you go?

Lower airway obstruction is less common and may be related to the aspiration of gastric contents, severe bronchospasms, or conditions that fill the alveoli of the lungs with fluid, as in pulmonary hemorrhage.

Close second

Secondary respiratory arrest results from insufficient circulation. *Complete respiratory arrest* is the absence of spontaneous ventilatory movement with cyanosis and may develop quickly in a conscious victim due to a foreign body obstruction. If the respiratory arrest is prolonged, cardiac arrest will follow due to impairment of cardiac oxygenation and function related to hypoxemia.

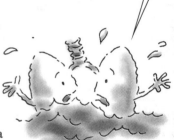

Lower airway obstruction is less common and may be related to conditions that fill my alveoli with fluid. Yipes!

What to look for

Impending respiratory arrest is characterized by a depressed sensorium, gasping for air, and an irregular respiratory pattern. Tachycardia, diaphoresis, and hypertension due to agitation or carbon dioxide retention are early signs of respiratory arrest or impending respiratory arrest. Other symptoms include:
- absence of spontaneous breathing
- no rise or fall of the chest
- inability to feel the movement of air from the mouth or nose
- color change (typically, cyanosis) due to lack of oxygen.

What tests tell you

Tests generally aren't necessary to diagnose cessation of respirations. Auscultating the chest demonstrates the presence or absence of breath sounds. Placing a hand on the chest allows assessment of chest movement with respirations or lack of movement in respiratory arrest. Observing the chest wall for movement will also provide basic information the presence or absence of breathing. If tests are ordered, they may include:

- *chest X-ray* to identify a suspected obstruction
- *ABG analysis* that may reveal hypoxemia or hypercapnia
- *bronchoscopy* and *laryngoscopy* to identify a suspected obstruction.

How it's treated

Respiratory arrest is a medical emergency. Treatment focuses on correcting the cause of the arrest, establishing an airway, and providing oxygenation. If respiratory arrest is related to an obstructed airway, intervention will focus on relieving the obstruction through a series of subdiaphragmatic, abdominal thrusts in a child or adult or five back blows followed by five chest thrusts in an infant. If the airway is patent and cardiac arrest occurs, CPR must be implemented.

What to do

Caring for a patient with respiratory arrest requires these measures:

- Assess for respirations and circulation.
- Assess for airway patency.
- Initiate basic life support in the absence of circulation and respirations and in the presence of a patent airway.
- If the airway is obstructed, attempt to clear the obstruction using subdiaphragmatic, abdominal thrusts or back blows, and chest thrusts in an infant. A pregnant woman usually requires chest thrusts.
- If a cervical spine injury is suspected after a fall, use the modified jaw thrust technique to open the airway.
- Assess breath sounds.
- Monitor chest X-ray and ABG results after the obstruction is relieved.

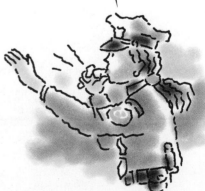

Stop right there! We need to determine the cause of this arrest!

Up and down and up and down

- Observe for "seesaw" respirations.
- Use pulse oximetry to assess the oxygenation status of the patient.
- Continually assess for stridor, cyanosis, and changes in LOC and notify the doctor immediately if any of these signs occur.
- Prepare for ET intubation or a tracheostomy within the hospital setting if an airway can't be established.
- Anticipate cardiac arrest if the obstruction isn't cleared promptly.
- Administer oxygen.
- Initiate or continue cardiac monitoring.
- Place an I.V. line for fluid and medication administration, if an I.V. isn't already present.
- Administer medications as ordered.

Respiratory depression

Respiratory depression implies inadequate ventilation. If this condition isn't corrected, it will lead to acidemia.

What causes it

Respiratory depression may be caused by an impairment at various levels of the respiratory system, including the CNS, upper and lower airways, and alveolar spaces or chest wall, as well as impairment of normal mechanisms of ventilation or the blood and circulatory system. Causes of these conditions include:

- cerebral trauma from birth injuries
- intracranial tumors
- vascular lesions
- CNS infections (meningitis, encephalitis, or sepsis)
- drug overdose (see *Poisoning in children*)
- severe asphyxia
- aspiration
- strangulation
- pulmonary edema
- pneumothorax
- flail chest
- carbon monoxide or cyanide poisoning
- severe anemia
- tetanus
- anesthesia.

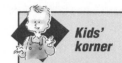

Kids' korner

Poisoning in children

Because of their curiosity and ignorance, children are the most common group of poison victims. In fact, accidental poisoning—usually from the ingestion of salicylates (aspirin) and acetaminophen (Tylenol), cleaning agents, insecticides, paints, cosmetics, and plants—is the fourth leading cause of death in children.

Assessment of the patient with a toxic ingestion must include a simultaneous history; assessment of airway, breathing, and circulation; and initiation of life support as indicated.

The patient's history from the parent or caregivers should reveal the source of poison and the form of exposure (ingestion, inhalation, injection, or skin contact). Assessment findings vary with the poison.

How it happens

Respiratory depression is a serious complication and commonly occurs in patients sedated with anesthesia or medications such as opioids. (See *Central apnea.*) In respiratory depression, the respiratory rate may decrease gradually or abruptly cease. Any change from respiratory function reflected in prior assessments and data must be considered as potential respiratory depression. If the condition goes uncorrected, progressive carbon dioxide retention and hypoxemia can result in systemic acidemia.

What to look for

Respiratory depression requires urgent assessment and intervention. These signs may indicate respiratory depression:
• respiratory rates below 10 (with normal adult respiratory rates of 12 to 18 breaths per minute)
• shortness of breath
• tachycardia
• dyspnea
• change in the depth of respirations
• restlessness or agitation
• unresponsiveness
• depressed LOC
• air hunger
• pale or cyanotic skin color
• hypoventilation, with an overdose of sedatives or opiates (see *Common antidotes*)
• signs of an overdose, which may include diaphoresis, dilated or constricted pupils, coma, tremors, seizure activity, or neurologic posturing.

What tests tell you

Suspicion of respiratory depression necessitates ABG analysis to confirm the presence of hypoxemia and hypercapnia (hypercarbia) because clinical assessment of the change in ventilatory status is unreliable when considered alone. Additional diagnostic tests may help diagnose respiratory depression.
• *Pulse oximetry* will show decreased oxygen saturation values.
• *Chest X-ray* may reveal pulmonary pathology.
• *ABG analysis* may reveal low PaO_2 and high $PaCO_2$ levels.

Central apnea

Central apnea results from the depressant effect of anesthesia on the respiratory centers in the brain (cerebral medulla). The onset of central apnea is common during the induction of I.V. anesthesia.

Anesthesia induction agents usually include a hypnotic agent, such as thiopental and propofol, and an opioid such as fentanyl. Neuromuscular blocking agents may also be administered to paralyze the patient for tracheal intubation.

A diagnosis of central apnea is based on the absence of respiratory effort in the patient.

Treatment is consistent with managing respiratory distress in general. However, reversal of the anesthetic administered is generally avoided because it would reverse the anesthetic state that the anesthesiologist or nurse anesthetist is attempting to achieve.

Common antidotes

This chart lists drugs or toxins commonly involved in respiratory depression and their antidotes.

Drug or toxin	Antidote
Acetaminophen	Acetylcysteine (Mucomyst, Acetadote)
Anticholinergics, tricyclic antidepressants	Physostigmine (Antilirium)
Benzodiazepines	Flumazenil (Romazicon)
Calcium channel blockers	Calcium chloride
Cyanide	Amyl nitrate, sodium nitrate, and sodium thiosulfate; methylene blue
Digoxin, cardiac glycosides	Digoxin immune fab (Digibind)
Ethylene glycol or methanol	Fomepizole (Antizol)
Heparin	Protamine sulfate
Insulin	Glucagon
Iron	Deferoxamine (Desferal)
Lead	Edetate calcium disodium (Calcium Disodium Versenate)
Opioids	Naloxone (Narcan), nalmefene (Revex), naltrexone (Depade, ReVia)
Organophosphates, anticholinesterases	Atropine, pralidoxime (Protopam)

- *Blood glucose monitoring* helps rule out hypoglycemia as the cause of the patient's altered LOC.
- *ECG* reveals ischemia and arrhythmias.
- *Toxicology studies* (including drug screens) of drug levels in the mouth, vomitus, urine, stool, or blood or on the victim's hands or clothing assist in confirming respiratory depression related to a drug overdose.
- *Pulmonary function tests* will show a low tidal volume below 10 ml/kg.

How it's treated

Initial treatment for respiratory depression includes support for the patient's airway, breathing, and circulation and administration of an antidote if an overdose is diagnosed. Ventilation with a bag and mask, tracheal intubation, or reversal of the agent causing the respiratory depression is commonly required.

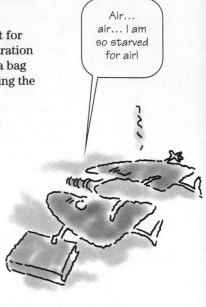

Air... air... I am so starved for air!

What to do

Caring for a patient with respiratory depression requires these measures:
• Immediately assess the patient's airway, breathing, and circulation. Institute emergency resuscitative measures as necessary.
• Monitor neurologic, cardiac, and respiratory status closely, at least every 15 minutes or more frequently depending on the patient's condition.
• Assess LOC for such changes as increasing confusion, restlessness, or decreased responsiveness.
• Auscultate lung sounds for crackles, rhonchi, or stridor.
• Observe for signs of airway obstruction, including labored breathing, severe hoarseness, and dyspnea.
• Administer supplemental humidified oxygen as ordered.
• Monitor oxygen saturation via continuous pulse oximetry and serial ABG analysis for evidence of hypoxemia and anticipate the need for ET intubation and mechanical ventilation should the patient's respiratory status deteriorate.
• Administer I.V. fluid therapy as ordered.
• Obtain laboratory specimens to assess for drug, electrolyte, and glucose levels.
• Anticipate administering normal saline solution and vasopressors if the patient is hypotensive and dextrose 5% in water if the patient is hypoglycemic.
• Place the patient in semi-Fowler's position to maximize chest expansion. Keep the patient as quiet and comfortable as possible to minimize oxygen demands.
• Administer bronchodilators as ordered.

Listen and look

• Perform oropharyngeal or tracheal suctioning as indicated by the patient's inability to clear the airway or evidence of abnormal breath sounds.
• Monitor vital signs continuously for changes.

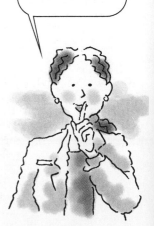

Keep the patient as quiet and comfortable as possible to minimize oxygen demands.

• Assist with pulmonary artery catheter insertion if indicated to evaluate hemodynamic status. Monitor hemodynamic parameters, including central venous pressure, pulmonary artery wedge pressure, cardiac output (and cardiac index), frequently.

• Institute continuous cardiac monitoring to evaluate for possible arrhythmias. If the patient develops heart block, prepare for cardiac pacing. Administer antiarrhythmics as ordered.

• Assess intake and output every hour; insert an indwelling urinary catheter as indicated to ensure accurate urine measurement.

• Administer antidote as ordered and available. When administering flumazenil and naloxone, watch for signs of withdrawal. Flumazenil may precipitate seizures especially in patients who have ingested cyclic antidepressants or have been on long-term sedation with benzodiazepines.

• Monitor the patient experiencing respiratory depression from an overdose for the return of overdose symptoms because the drug may last longer than the dose of antidote.

• Monitor laboratory test results.

Sudden infant death syndrome

Sudden infant death syndrome (SIDS), a medical mystery of early infancy, is the leading cause of death among apparently healthy infants ages 1 month to 1 year. Most deaths occur between age 1 and 4 months. The syndrome, also called *crib death*, occurs at the rate of 2 in every 1,000 live births. Each year in the United States, about 7,000 infants die of SIDS. Although the syndrome was known in ancient times, its cause remains obscure.

Positive decline

Incidence of SIDS declines rapidly between ages 4 and 12 months. About 60% of victims are male infants who die in their sleep, without warning, sound, or struggle. The incidence is slightly higher in preterm infants, Inuit infants, disadvantaged Black infants, infants of mothers under age 20, and infants of multiple births.

Increased incidence

The incidence of SIDS is 2 to 3 times more likely in Black children than in White children. Native American children are 5 times more susceptible than White children. Incidence is 10 times higher in SIDS siblings than in children without SIDS siblings. The occurrence of SIDS is slightly higher in infants whose mothers smoke than in children of mothers who don't smoke. It's up to 10 times more com-

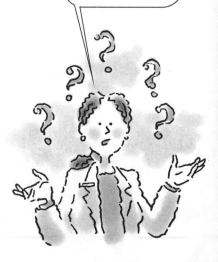

Unfortunately, the cause of SIDS still eludes us.

mon in infants whose mothers are drug addicts than in children of non-drug-addicted mothers.

That time of year?

Infants most commonly succumb to SIDS in the fall and winter. Many have a history of respiratory tract infections, suggesting viral infection as a cause. Studies show conflicting data about abnormal hepatic or pancreatic function. Although the link between apneic episodes and SIDS remains unclear, about 60% of infants with near-miss respiratory events have second episodes of apnea to which some succumb.

What causes it

There are numerous theories regarding the etiology of SIDS; yet, the cause remains unknown. At one time, SIDS was attributed to abuse or to accidental suffocation during sleep. On postmortem examination, some SIDS-diagnosed infants show changes indicating chronic hypoxia, hypoxemia, and large-airway obstruction, leading researchers to suspect more than one cause.

How it happens

Two leading hypotheses regarding the cause of SIDS are hypoxemia and apnea. The hypoxemia theory suggests that SIDS occurs because of damage to the respiratory control center in the brain from chronic hypoxemia. The apnea theory holds that SIDS victims experience prolonged periods of sleep apnea and eventually die during an episode.

Another proposed cause involves *Clostridium botulinum* toxin, which has been linked to a few SIDS deaths. A disproved theory is an association between SIDS and diphtheria, tetanus, and pertussis vaccines. Bottle-feeding and advanced parental age don't cause the syndrome, although breast-fed infants are at decreased risk for SIDS. Because the syndrome is always fatal, it has no complications.

Hypoxemia and apnea are two leading theories about the pathophysiology of SIDS.

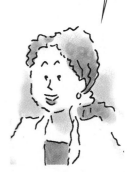

What to look for

The patient history supplied by the parents may reveal that they found the infant wedged in a crib corner or with blankets wrapped around his head. Despite such findings, autopsy results rule out suffocation as the cause of death. The history may also note frothy, blood-tinged sputum found around the infant's mouth or on the crib sheets. However, autopsy findings show a patent airway, ruling out aspiration of vomitus as the cause of death. In addition, parents typically report that the infant didn't cry and showed no signs of disturbed sleep.

Reports of the infant found in a peculiar position or tangled in his blankets suggest movement before death, possibly from terminal spasm. Occasionally, the history may reveal a respiratory tract infection.

Start from the beginning

Documentation of events before discovery of the infant's death should be part of the history. The bruising, possible fractured ribs, and appearance of blood in the infant's mouth, nose, or ears from internal bleeding is commonly confused with abuse. Although abuse shouldn't be dismissed as a possibility, never assume that abuse caused the infant's death without obtaining further information. Also avoid assessment questions that may suggest parental responsibility for the death.

Other signs

Depending on how long the infant has been dead, inspection may reveal an infant with mottled complexion and extremely cyanotic lips and fingertips. You may also see pooled blood in the legs and feet. These markings may be mistaken for bruises. The infant's diaper may be wet and full of stool.

What tests tell you

Diagnosis of SIDS requires an autopsy to rule out other causes of death. Characteristic histologic findings on autopsy include small or normal adrenal glands and petechiae over the visceral surfaces of the pleura, within the thymus (which is enlarged), and in the epicardium. Autopsy also reveals well-preserved lymphoid structures; signs of chronic hypoxemia such as increased pulmonary artery smooth muscle; edematous, congestive lungs fully expanded; liquid (not clotted) blood in the heart; and stomach curd inside the trachea.

How it's treated

Because most infants can't be resuscitated, treatment focuses on emotional support for the family. Any infant found apneic and successfully resuscitated, as well as any infant who has a sibling with apnea, may be at risk for SIDS. In such instances, a home apnea monitor may be recommended until the at-risk infant passes the age of vulnerability.

What to do

Caring for a family dealing with death of their child from SIDS requires these measures:
• Make sure both parents are present when the child's death is confirmed. The parents may lash out at emergency department personnel, the baby-sitter, or anyone else involved in the child's care — even at each other. Stay calm and let them express their feelings. Reassure them that they aren't to blame.
• Let the parents see the infant in a private room. Allow them to express their grief. Stay in the room with them, if appropriate. Offer to call clergy, friends, or relatives. Return the infant's belongings to the parents.
• If your facility's policy is to assign a home health nurse to the family, she should provide the continuing reassurance and assistance the parents need. Assist her in gathering the information necessary to implement appropriate follow-up care.

Go to the info

• After the parents and other family members recover from the initial shock, explain the need for an autopsy to confirm the diagnosis. In some states, this is legally mandatory. At this time, provide the family with basic facts about SIDS, and encourage them to consent to the autopsy. Be sure they receive the autopsy report promptly.

• Refer the parents and family to community and health care facility support services. Participants in such a program should contact the parents, ensure that they receive the autopsy report promptly, introduce them to a professional counselor, and maintain supportive telephone contact. Refer the parents to a local SIDS parents' group if one is available. Advise parents to contact the SIDS hot line (1-800-221-SIDS).

• If the parents decide to have another child, provide appropriate information to help them cope with pregnancy and the first year of the new infant's life. (See *Back to sleep*.)

• Teach family members how to operate home apnea and cardiac monitors, if appropriate. If parents of healthy infants inquire about monitors for home use, explain that monitoring is recommended only for siblings of SIDS victims because of its high cost and sometimes disruptive effects on family dynamics.

• Teach family members and caregivers how to perform one-person CPR or refer them to classes conducted by the American Red Cross if appropriate.

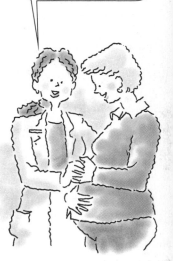

If the parents decide to have another child, provide appropriate information to help them cope with pregnancy and the first year of the infant's life.

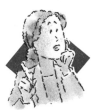

Quick quiz

1. An upper airway obstruction is an interruption in the flow of air through the:

    A.   lungs.
    B.   alveoli.
    C.   pharynx.
    D.   main stem bronchus.

Answer: C. Upper airway obstruction is an interruption in the flow of air through the nose, mouth, pharynx, or larynx.

2. Which statement best describes the symptoms of a partial airway obstruction?

    A.   Gasping for air and cyanosis
    B.   Diaphoresis, tachycardia, and elevated blood pressure
    C.   Cessation of coughing or speaking
    D.   Cardiac arrest

Answer: B. Partial airway obstruction commonly occurs from edema or a small foreign object that doesn't completely obstruct the airway. Signs of a partial airway obstruction include diaphoresis, tachycardia, coughing, and elevated blood pressure. Experiencing no symptoms is also possible with a partial obstruction.

3. The initial drug of choice for treating anaphylaxis is:
   A.   diphenhydramine.
   B.   dopamine.
   C.   albuterol.
   D.   epinephrine.

Answer: D. Anaphylaxis is always an emergency. It requires an *immediate* injection of 0.1 to 0.5 ml of epinephrine 1:1,000 aqueous solution, repeated every 5 to 20 minutes as necessary. If the patient is in the early stages of anaphylaxis, hasn't yet lost consciousness, and is still normotensive, give epinephrine I.M. or S.C., and help it move into the circulation faster by massaging the injection site. For severe reactions, when the patient has lost consciousness and is hypotensive, give epinephrine I.V.

4. In a near drowning victim, these ABG results would be expected:
   A.   elevated bicarbonate level, elevated pH, and decreased oxygen content.
   B.   low bicarbonate level, low pH, and decreased oxygen content.
   C.   elevated bicarbonate level, elevated pH, and elevated oxygen content.
   D.   decreased bicarbonate level, decreased pH, and decreased oxygen content.

Answer: B. ABG analysis shows decreased oxygen content, low bicarbonate levels, and low pH.

5. The "Back to Sleep" educational initiative started in 1992 has decreased the incidence of SIDS in the United States by more than:
   A.   15%.
   B.   25%.
   C.   40%.
   D.   50%.

Answer: C. Since the implementation of the "Back to Sleep" initiative in 1992, the incidence of SIDS has decreased by more than 40% in the United States. In 1992, SIDS was the leading cause of death in the United States for infants less than age 1 year and now it's the third leading cause of death following congenital anomalies and prematurity.

6. Extrapulmonary obstructions in asphyxia can be caused by:
   A.   strangulation.
   B.   severe asthma.
   C.   foreign body aspiration.
   D.   near drowning.

Answer: A. An extrapulmonary obstruction results from tracheal compression from a tumor, strangulation, trauma, or suffocation. An intrapulmonary obstruction is caused by an airway obstruction, severe asthma, foreign body aspiration, pulmonary edema, pneumonia, and near drowning.

7. The antidote commonly prescribed for an opioid overdose is:
   A.   naloxone.
   B.   flumazenil.
   C.   atropine.
   D.   ethanol.

Answer: A. Naloxone, nalmefene, and naltrexone are the commonly used antidotes for the opioid class of drugs.

8. The most common condition associated with bronchospasm is:
   A.   pneumonia.
   B.   near drowning.
   C.   idiopathic pulmonary fibrosis.
   D.   asthma.

Answer: D. A variety of conditions can cause bronchospasm. The most common condition associated with bronchospasm is asthma.

Scoring

☆☆☆ If you answered all eight items correctly, fantastic! You're clearly breathing easy about respiratory emergencies.

☆☆ If you answered five to seven items correctly, superb! You must have extra pulmonary perception.

☆ If you answered fewer than five items correctly, don't hyperventilate. Review the chapter, breathe easy, and try again.

Appendices and index

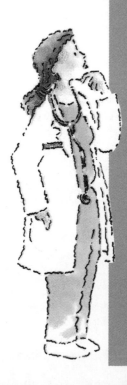

Glossary

acinus: the chief respiratory unit for gas exchange

acute respiratory distress syndrome (ARDS): form of pulmonary edema that leads to acute respiratory failure resulting from increased permeability of the alveolo-capillary membrane

adventitious breath sounds: abnormal sounds regardless of their location when auscultated

Allen's test: test to assess a patient's collateral arterial blood supply performed before obtaining an arterial blood gas sample

allergen: substance that induces an allergy or a hypersensitivity reaction

anaphylaxis: severe allergic reaction to a foreign substance

anoxia: absence of oxygen in the tissues

antitussive: pharmacologic agent that suppresses or inhibits coughing

apnea: absence of breathing

arterial blood gas (ABG) analysis: measurement of the arterial pH, partial pressures of oxygen and carbon dioxide, and other levels used to evaluate acid-base balance, and gas exchange

asthma: chronic disorder in which airways are hyperresponsive

atelectasis: collapse of a section of alveoli or an entire lung due to obstruction, lack of surfactant, or compression of the chest wall

barrel chest: abnormal chest shape in which the chest appears round and bulging with a greater than normal front to back diameter

Biot's respirations: rapid, deep breathing with abrupt pauses between each breath; equal depth to each breath

bradypnea: decreased rate but regular breathing

bronchial breath sounds: breath sounds heard next to the trachea, sounding loud, high-pitched, and discontinuous

bronchiectasis: an irreversible condition marked by chronic abnormal dilation of bronchi and destruction of bronchial walls

bronchitis: acute inflammatory condition affecting the mucous membranes of the bronchial tree

bronchodilator: pharmacologic agent that relaxes the smooth muscles of the bronchioles to improve airflow

bronchoscopy: direct inspection of the trachea and bronchi through a flexible fiber-optic or rigid bronchoscope

bronchovesicular breath sounds: breath sounds heard next to the sternum between the scapula; continuous, medium pitched sounds heard during inhalation and exhalation

capnogram: carbon dioxide waveform produced in end tidal carbon dioxide monitoring

chest physiotherapy (PT): postural drainage techniques, chest percussion and vibration, and coughing and deep-breathing exercises used to mobilize and eliminate secretions, reexpand lung tissue, and promote efficient use of respiratory muscles

Cheyne-Stokes respirations: breaths that gradually become faster and deeper than normal, then slower; alternates with periods of apnea

chronic obstructive pulmonary disease (COPD): long-term pulmonary disorder characterized by air flow resistance

clubbing: angle of the fingernail entering the skin at an angle greater than or equal to 180 degrees; indication of long-term hypoxia

continuous positive airway pressure (CPAP): mode of ventilation that maintains positive pressure in the airways throughout the patient's respiratory cycle

crackles: intermittent nonmusical brief sounds caused by collapsed or fluid-filled alveoli popping open; don't clear with coughing

cyanosis: bluish discoloration of the skin and mucous membranes that results from an excessive amount of deoxygenated hemoglobin in the blood or a structural defect in the hemoglobin molecule

diffusion: gas movement through a semipermeable membrane from an area of greater concentration to one of lesser concentration

dyspnea: difficulty or a feeling of uncomfortable breathing

emphysema: form of chronic obstructive pulmonary disease involving abnormal, permanent enlargement of the acini accompanied by destruction of the alveolar walls

empyema: collection of pus within the pleural space

endotracheal intubation: oral or nasal insertion of a flexible tube through the larynx into the trachea to control the airway and mechanically ventilate the patient

expectorants: pharmacologic agents that thin mucus to aid in clearing it more easily out of the airways

forced vital capacity: amount of air that can be exhaled after maximum inspiration

functional residual capacity: amount of air remaining in lungs after normal expiration

hemothorax: collapse of part or all of the lung due to blood collecting in the pleural space

hyperpnea: deep breathing at a normal rate

hypoxemia: oxygen deficit in arterial blood (lower than 80 mm Hg)

hypoxia: reduction of oxygen in body tissues to below normal levels

immunocompetence: ability of cells to distinguish antigens from substances that belong to the body and to launch an immune response

incentive spirometry: use of a breathing device to help promote lung expansion after prolonged bedrest or surgery; the device requires that the patient take a deep breath and hold it for several seconds

inspiratory capacity: amount of air that can be inhaled after normal expiration

Kussmaul's respirations: rapid, deep breathing without pauses; usually sounding labored with deep breaths resembling sighs

leukocyte: white blood cell that protects the body against microorganisms causing disease

lobectomy: surgical removal of one of the five lung lobes

lymphocyte: leukocyte produced by lymphoid tissue that participates in immunity

macrophage: highly phagocytic cells that are stimulated by inflammation

mediastinum: space between the lungs that contains the heart and pericardium, thoracic aorta, pulmonary artery and veins, venae cavae and azygos veins, thymus, lymph nodes and vessels, trachea, esophagus and thoracic duct, and the vagus, cardiac, and phrenic nerves

metabolic acidosis: condition resulting from excess acid retention or excess bicarbonate loss; the lungs increase the rate and depth of ventilation to eliminate excess carbon dioxide, thus reducing carbonic acid levels

metabolic alkalosis: condition resulting from excess bicarbonate retention; the rate and depth of ventilation decrease so that carbon dioxide can be retained; this increases carbonic acid levels

metered dose inhaler (MDI): device used to trigger the release of measured doses of aerosol drug from a canister; also called a *puffer*

minute volume: amount of air breathed per minute

mixed venous oxygen saturation: measurement indicative of the oxygen saturation of venous blood

nares: nostrils

nebulizer: device that uses compressed gas to convert liquid drugs into a fine aerosol for inhalation

nonrebreather mask: type of oxygen delivery system that involves a one-way inspiratory valve that opens on inhalation and directs oxygen from a reservoir bag into the mask; patient breathes air only from the bag

oropharyngeal airway: curved rubber or plastic device inserted into the mouth to the posterior pharynx to establish or maintain a patent airway

oropharynx: posterior wall of the mouth

orthopnea: shortness of breath when lying down

oxygen saturation: ratio of actual hemoglobin oxygen content to potential maximum oxygen content carrying capacity of the hemoglobin

partial pressure of arterial carbon dioxide (Paco$_2$): measurement reflecting the adequacy of ventilation of the lungs

partial pressure of arterial oxygen (Pao$_2$): measurement reflecting the body's ability to pick up oxygen from the lungs

pectus carinatum: pigeon chest appearing with a sternum protruding beyond the front of the abdomen

pH: measurement of the percentage of hydrogen ions in a solution; normal pH is 7.35 to 7.45 for arterial blood

pleura: membrane that totally encloses the lung

pleural effusion: collection of fluid in the pleural space

pleural friction rub: low-pitched, grating, rubbing sound heard on inhalation and exhalation

pneumonia: acute infection of the lung parenchyma that commonly impairs gas exchange

pneumothorax: collapse of part or all of the lung due to air in the pleural space

pulmonary edema: abnormal fluid accumulation in the lungs; a life-threatening condition

pulmonary embolism: sudden obstruction of a pulmonary blood vessel by foreign substances or a blood clot

pulmonary hypertension: chronically elevated pulmonary artery pressure higher than 30 mm Hg and a mean pulmonary artery pressure higher than 18 mm Hg

pulmonary perfusion: blood flow from the right side of the heart, through the pulmonary circulation, and into the left side of the heart

pulse oximetry: relatively simple, noninvasive procedure used to monitor arterial oxygen saturation

residual volume: amount of air remaining in the lungs after forced expiration

respiratory acidosis: acid-base disturbance caused by failure of the lungs to eliminate sufficient carbon dioxide; $Paco_2$ above 45 mm Hg and pH below 7.35

respiratory alkalosis: acid-base imbalance that occurs when the lungs eliminate more carbon dioxide than normal; partial pressure of arterial carbon dioxide below 35 mm Hg and pH above 7.45

respiratory failure: condition that occurs when the lungs can't sufficiently maintain arterial oxygenation or eliminate carbon dioxide

rhonchi: low-pitched snoring and rattling sounds occurring primarily on exhalation; change or disappear with coughing

spacer: holding chamber device that attaches to the mouthpiece of an inhaler; useful in making sure that a patient gets the entire dose of drug each time

sputum: material expectorated from a patient's lungs and bronchi during deep coughing

status asthmaticus: emergency, life-threatening situation resulting from an acute asthma attack that goes untreated or in which the person doesn't respond to drug therapy after 24 hours

stridor: low, high-pitched crowing sound audible without a stethoscope; caused by an upper airway obstruction

synchronized intermittent mandatory ventilation (SIMV): mechanical ventilation in which the ventilator delivers a set number of specific-volume breaths; the patient may breathe spontaneously between the SIMV breaths at volumes that differ from those on the machine

systemic decongestants: pharmacologic agents that stimulate the sympathetic nervous system to reduce swelling of the respiratory tract's vascular network

tachypnea: shallow breathing with increased respiratory rate

tactile fremitus: palpable vibrations caused by the transmission of air through the bronchopulmonary system

tension pneumothorax: air trapped within the pleural space

thoracentesis: pleural fluid aspiration to obtain a sample of pleural fluid for analysis, relieve lung compression and, occasionally, obtain a lung tissue biopsy specimen

thoracotomy: surgical removal of all or part of a lung

tidal volume: amount of air inhaled or exhaled during normal breathing

topical decongestants: pharmacologic agents that act directly on the alpha receptors of the vascular smooth muscle in the nose, causing the arterioles to constrict

tracheal breath sounds: breath sounds heard over the trachea, sounding harsh and discontinuous

tracheal suction: removal of secretions from the trachea or bronchi by means of a catheter inserted through the mouth or nose, a tracheal stoma, a tracheostomy tube, or an endotracheal tube

tracheotomy: surgical opening into the trachea to provide an airway

type I alveolar cells: most abundant type of epithelial cells in the alveoli; thin, flat, squamous cells across which gas exchange occurs

type II alveolar cells: epithelial cells in the alveoli that secrete surfactant, a substance that coats the alveolus and promotes gas exchange by lowering surface tension

V̇/Q̇ ratio: ratio of ventilation (amount of air in the alveoli) to perfusion (amount of blood in the pulmonary capillaries); expresses the effectiveness of gas exchange

ventilation: gas distribution into and out of the pulmonary airways

Venturi mask: type of oxygen delivery system allowing mixture of a specific volume of air and oxygen to deliver a highly accurate oxygen concentration

vesicular sounds: breath sounds heard over most of both lungs, sounding soft and low pitched; prolonged during inhalation and shortened during exhalation

vital capacity: amount of air that can be exhaled after normal inspiration

wedge resection: surgical removal of a small portion of the lung without regard to its segments

wheezes: high-pitched sounds first heard on exhalation; occur when airflow is blocked

Quick-reference guide to laboratory tests

Arterial blood gases
pH: 7.35 to 7.45 (SI, 7.35 to 7.45)
Pao$_2$: 80 to 100 mm Hg (SI, 10. 6 to 13.3 kPa)
Paco$_2$: 35 to 45 mm Hg (SI, 4.7 to 5.3 kPa)
O$_2$CT: 15% to 23% (SI, 0.15 to 0.23)
Sao$_2$: 94% to 100% (SI, 0.94 to 1.00)
HCO$_3^-$: 22 to 25 mEq/L (SI, 22 to 25 mmol/L)

Hematocrit
Males
  – 42% to 52% (SI, 0.42 to 0.52)
Females
  – 36% to 48% (SI, 0.36 to 0.48)
Children
  – *10 years:* 36% to 40% (SI, 0.36 to 0.40
Infants
  – *3 months:* 30% to 36% (SI, 0.30 to 0.36)
  – *1 year:* 29% to 41% (SI, 0.29 to 0.41)
Neonates
  – *At birth:* 55% to 68% (SI, 0.55 to 0.68)
  – *1 week:* 47% to 65% (SI, 0.47 to 0.65)
  – *1 month:* 37% to 49% (SI, 0.37 to 0.49)

Hemoglobin (Hb) electrophoresis
Hb A: 95% (SI, 0.95)
Hb A$_2$: 1.5% to 3% (SI, 0.015 to 0.03)
Hb F: < 2% (SI, <0.02)

Red blood cell count
Males: 4.5 to 5.5. million/μl (SI, 4.5 to 5.5 $\times$ 10^{12}/L)
Females: 4 to 5 million/μl (SI, 4 to 5 $\times$ 10^{12}/L)
Neonates: 4.4 to 5.8 million/μl (SI, 4.4 to 5.8 $\times$ 10^{12}/L)
2 months: 3 to 3.8 million/μl (SI, 3 to 3.8 $\times$ 10^{12}/L)
Children: 4.6 to 4.8 million/μl (SI, 4.6 to 4.8 $\times$ 10^{12}/L)

White blood cell count
4,000 to 10,000/μl (SI, 4 to 10 $\times$ 10^9/L)

White blood cell differential, blood
Adults
  – *Neutrophils:* 54% to 75% (SI, 0.54 to 0.75)
  – *Lymphocytes:* 25% to 40% (SI, 0.25 to 0.40)
  – *Monocytes* 2% to 8% (SI, 0.02 to 0.08)
  – *Eosinophils:* 1% to 4% (SI, 0.01 to 0.04)
  – *Basophils:* 0 to 1% (SI, 0 to 0.01)

References and Internet resources

Barnes, K. *Paediatrics: A Clinical Guide for Nurse Practitioners.* Philadelphia: Butterworth Heinemann, 2003.

Baum, G.L. (ed). *Baum's Textbook of Pulmonary Diseases*, 7th ed. Philadelphia: Lippincott Williams & Wilkins, 2004.

Behrman, R.E., et al. *Nelson Textbook of Pediatrics*, 17th ed. Philadelphia: W.B. Saunders, 2004.

Betz, C.L. and Sowden, L. *Mosby's Pediatric Nursing Reference*, 5th ed. St. Louis: Mosby–Year Book Inc., 2004.

Bickley, L.S., and Szilagyi, P.G. *Bates' Guide to Physical Examination and History Taking*, 8th ed. Philadelphia: Lippincott Williams & Wilkins, 2003.

Burns, S. M. "Working with Respiratory Waveforms: How to use Bedside Graphics," *AACN Clinical Issues* 14(2):133-44, quiz 264, May 2003.

Cavanaugh, B.M. *Nurses' Manual of Laboratory and Diagnostic Tests*, 4th ed. Philadelphia: F.A. Davis Co., 2003.

Centers for Disease Control and Prevention "Guideline for Environmental Infection Control in Health-Care Facilities, 2003." Available: *www.cdc.gov/ncidod/hip/enviro/guide. htm.*

Critical Care Nursing Made Incredibly Easy. Springhouse, Pa.: Lippincott Williams & Wilkins, 2004.

Emergency Nurses Association. *Core Curriculum for Pediatric Emergency Nursing.* Sudbury, Mass.: Jones & Bartlett Pubs., 2003.

Dreyfuss, D. and Saumon, G. "Evidence-based Medicine or Fuzzy Logic: What is Best for ARDS Management?" *Intensive Care Medicine* 28(3):230-34, March 2002.

Feigin, R.D., et al. (ed). *Textbook of Pediatric Infectious diseases*, 5th ed. Philadelphia: W.B. Saunders, 2004.

Fischbach, F.T., et al. *A Manual of Laboratory and Diagnostic Tests*, 7th ed. Philadelphia: Lippincott Williams & Wilkins, 2004.

Gattinoni, L., et.al. "Effect of Prone Positioning on the Survival of Patients with Acute Respiratory Failure," *The New England Journal of Medicine* 345(8):568-73, August 2001.

Haynes, J.M. "Assessing the Need for Bronchodilator Therapy: Don't Believe Everything You Hear," *Respiratory Care* 48(6):621, June 2003.

Hijazi, Z.M., et al. *Essential Pediatric Cardiology.* New York: McGraw-Hill Book Co., 2004.

Hockenberry M., et al. *Wong's Nursing Care of Infants and Children*, 7th ed. St. Louis: Mosby–Year Book, Inc., 2003.

Iregui, M., et.al. "Use of a Handheld Computer by Respiratory Care Practitioners to Improve the Efficiency of Weaning Patients from Mechanical Ventilation," *Critical Care Medicine* 30(9):2038-43, September 2002. Available: *www.medscape.com/viewarticle/ 442647.*

Kercsmar, C.M. "Current Trends in Management of Pediatric Asthma," *Respiratory Care* 48(3):194-205; discussion 205-8, March 2003.

Medical-Surgical Nursing Made Incredibly Easy. Springhouse, Pa.: Lippincott Williams & Wilkins, 2004.

Nursing 2004 Drug Handbook, 24th ed. Springhouse, Pa.: Lippincott Williams & Wilkins, 2004.

Porth, C.M., and Kunert, M.P. *Pathophysiology Concepts of Altered Health States*, 6th ed. Philadelphia: Lippincott Williams & Wilkins, 2002.

Professional Guide to Diseases, 7th ed. Springhouse, Pa.: Springhouse Corp., 2001.

Rotta, A.T., and Wiryawan, B. "Respiratory Emergencies in Children," *Respiratory Care* 48(3):248-58; discussion 258-60, March 2003.

Schieken, L.S. "Asthma Pathophysiology and the Scientific Rationale for Combination Therapy," *Allergy and Asthma Proceedings* 23(4):247-51, July-August 2002.

Smeltzer, S.C., and Bare, B.G. *Brunner and Suddarth's Textbook of Medical Surgical Nursing*, 10th ed. Philadelphia: Lippincott Williams & Wilkins, 2004.

Wilkins, R.L., et al. *Egan's Fundamentals of Respiratory Care*, 8th ed. St. Louis: Mosby–Year Book, Inc., 2003.

Index

t refers to a table; i refers to an illustration; **boldface** refers to a full-color illustration.

t refers to a table; i refers to an illustration; **boldface** refers to a full-color illustration.

t refers to a table; i refers to an illustration; **boldface** refers to a full-color illustration.

t refers to a table; i refers to an illustration; **boldface** refers to a full-color illustration.

t refers to a table; i refers to an illustration; **boldface** refers to a full-color illustration.

—